AUTISM AND JOINT ATTENTION

Autism and Joint Attention

Development, Neuroscience, and Clinical Fundamentals

PETER C. MUNDY

THE GUILFORD PRESS
New York   London

© 2016 The Guilford Press
A Division of Guilford Publications, Inc.
370 Seventh Avenue, Suite 1200, New York, NY 10001
www.guilford.com

Printed in the United States of America

This book is printed on acid-free paper.

Last digit is print number: 9   8   7   6   5   4   3   2   1

The author has checked with sources believed to be reliable in his efforts to
provide information that is complete and generally in accord with the standards
of practice that are accepted at the time of publication. However, in view of the
possibility of human error or changes in behavioral, mental health, or medical
sciences, neither the author, nor the editors and publisher, nor any other party
who has been involved in the preparation or publication of this work warrants
that the information contained herein is in every respect accurate or complete,
and they are not responsible for any errors or omissions or the results obtained
from the use of such information. Readers are encouraged to confirm the
information contained in this book with other sources.

Library of Congress Cataloging-in-Publication Data is available from the
publisher.

ISBN 978-1-4625-2509-6

About the Author

Peter C. Mundy, PhD, is Professor and Lisa Capps Endowed Chair of Neurodevelopmental Disorders and Education in the School of Education and the Department of Psychiatry and Behavioral Sciences at the University of California, Davis (UC Davis). He is also Director of Educational Research at the UC Davis MIND Institute. A developmental and clinical psychologist, Dr. Mundy has been working on defining the nature of autism and developmental disabilities for over 30 years. An author of the Early Social Communication Scales, which was selected by Autism Speaks as a recommended measure for clinical trials, he is an associate editor of *Autism Research* and serves as an editorial board member or consulting editor for numerous other journals.

Preface

One of the challenges faced in today's science of autism spectrum disorders (ASD) is that the amount of information to master and the number of different perspectives to consider increase with the number of scientists engaged in examining autism. This is both a boon and a bane for the field. There are now many more scientists from a wider array of disciplines working to understand autism than ever before. This is illustrated by the growth in the number of scientific articles published on ASD. In the four-plus decades between the discovery of ASD in the early 1940s and December 1989, approximately 4,577 peer-reviewed scientific papers and 495 books were published on ASD. In the last two-plus decades, approximately 39,822 peer-reviewed articles and 5,875 books were published (ProQuest.com/PsycINFO search, September 19, 2015). This recent flood of information has substantially enriched our understanding of the genetic and neurodevelopmental factors that may be involved in ASD, and has improved our methods of early identification, diagnosis, and treatment. However, the wealth of new observations comes at a cost: It is increasingly difficult for researchers to recognize or share a common picture of autism across what is now a vastly multidisciplinary science. Each scientific discipline, and each level of analysis within a discipline, emphasizes concepts, methods, and even language that may or may not be familiar to other groups of scientists. The tendency to adopt discipline-specific concepts and a language speeds progress *within* a discipline, but may impede progress and consensus *across* disciplines.

There is nothing unique about the science of autism in this regard. Science is ultimately a form of human collaboration and communication. From many disparate voices and points of view, valid, commonly held concepts ultimately emerge. In the early years of a science, though, the process can be a bit cacophonous. Such is the case in the science of autism today. The advancing diversity of the research on autism has increased the challenge of reaching a consensus on what, if any, developmental processes are *central* or *essential* to ASD. Some may regard this assertion as a bit hyperbolic. Perhaps, but people are complex. When neurodevelopmental disorders interact with human nature, complexity is multiplied, so a precise description of the essential nature of a disorder is going to be difficult and time-consuming to establish. In this regard, one of two possibilities may best describe the present state of affairs in research on autism. One is that we have yet to develop sufficiently robust theory or research approaches to guide us to the right places to look for the answers to the question of what processes or dimensions are essential to autism. The alternative, though, is that we *have* already begun to look in the right places, but that amidst the daily deluge of new data we have yet to fully appreciate and effectively communicate what we have observed. In my view, this second possibility very much describes our current understanding of the role of the development of joint attention in the human nature of autism.

Joint attention refers to the fluid, exquisitely well-honed human ability to adopt a common point of reference with other people. The name for this dimension of behavior comes from the observation that prelinguistic infants learn to share information and experiences with other people by coordinating their visual, auditory, or tactile attention on objects or events with these people. Hence joint attention first involves coordinating attention with other people to the external world. However, a dynamic dance between social-cognitive neurodevelopment and practice with joint attention to external objects in early infancy leads to the emergence of the capacity to socially coordinate attention to internal mental objects in later infancy. This internalized cognitive capacity for joint attention, and adopting a common point of reference, is fundamental to learning language, developing collaborative and cooperative behavior, and advances in social-cognitive development. Moreover, joint attention is also fundamental to our sense of social relatedness and intersubjectivity when it is accompanied by the perception of sharing meaning and experience with another person.

Given this description of joint attention, it may not come as a surprise that differences in joint attention are among the most important characteristics of autism spectrum development yet identified. Indeed, in my mind, no other symptom dimension has more evidence for its centrality to

ASD. Joint attention measures are consistently observed to be important in the early identification and the later diagnosis of preschool children. Because joint attention is pivotal to human learning, language, and social relatedness, targeted preschool interventions lead to improvements in children with ASD. Early joint attention difficulties also appear to be part of a continuous line of developmental disturbance expressed as social-cognitive or theory-of-mind problems in children and adults with ASD.

Since 1979, an uninterrupted line of 500 studies has attested to the importance of joint attention in autism syndrome development (ProQuest.com/PsycINFO search, September 19, 2015). Nevertheless, there is a decided lack of agreement among scientists about the meaning and importance of joint attention phenomena in the study of ASD (e.g., Charman, 2003; Leekam, 2005). Leekam eloquently described the lack of consensus this way:

> Ask any clinician to describe the earliest and most significant impairments in autism, and the chances are that they will put joint attention at the top of the list. Ask them to explain why children with autism have this impairment, and they will be less likely to give you a straightforward answer. The truth is that, despite advances in our knowledge of autism over the last twenty to thirty years, we still have contradictory interpretations for one of the most robust and predictive behavioral indicators of autism. (2005, p. 205)

Each of the "contradictory interpretations" of joint attention phenomena in ASD holds more than a grain of truth. However, many researchers assign a rather static role for joint attention in autism spectrum development, and thus the field has not yet fully appreciated the significance of what joint attention research brings to the current and future science of ASD. Understanding joint attention will not completely explain autism, but it is very likely that no explanation of autism will be complete without a definitive understanding of joint attention's role in its etiology. This volume has been developed to address the need for greater clarity in recognizing the role of joint attention in the human nature of autism spectrum development.

Framework of the Book

The book has been developed for students of the science of ASD, including researchers, parents, teachers, and professionals, as well as people who directly experience autism syndrome development. Because the readers of this volume may vary in their goals, interests, and expertise, the text also varies its presentation of old and new information on the science of autism, as well as the technical level of presentation. Though all the chapters are connected, each chapter has been written as an individual essay that may be read on its own or in combination with other chapters. All the chapters have been written with the goal of presenting evidence from developmental, clinical, neurocognitive, and genetic/molecular research for the hypothesis that joint attention is a fundamental dimension of the phenotype and endophenotype of ASD.

The chapters are organized into three general topics. An introduction to joint attention and its role in the diagnosis of autism is provided in Chapters 1, 2, and 3. These chapters comprise the least technical sections of the book and are intended to provide an introduction that is informative for a wide range of readers. The role of joint attention in social development and social learning, and in the difficulties in these areas that define ASD, is described in Chapters 4, 5, and 6. These chapters involve a more technical discussion of social cognition, developmental science, and intervention science. Nevertheless, Chapter 6 is intended for a wide range of readers interested in better understanding treatment and education for children affected by ASD. Finally, the neuroscience and genetics of joint attention in autism are covered in Chapters 7 and 8. These chapters involve what may be the most technical discussions of the book. They are primarily intended to translate the developmental science of joint attention to applications for readers interested in the biological sciences of autism.

Chapter 1 begins with a review of the historical shifts that have occurred in the conceptualization and diagnosis of ASD. This chapter is not so much about joint attention as it is about the difficulty and complexity involved in trying to define any major facet of human nature, including the nature of autism. Chapter 1 discusses the problems with the initial conceptualization of the prototype of autism as a pervasively unresponsive child. It also discusses the observation that the presentation of autism varies significantly across people; this variability or heterogeneity has made it difficult to categorically define the nature of autism, and thus has complicated both the basic and clinical science of autism. This chapter's contention, though, is that we should expect any category of human nature (including the category of ASD) to have fuzzy boundaries, and that this expectation is important to a more veridical understanding of this syndrome. Heterogeneity is not specific to autism; it is a phenomenon associated with all clinical and nonclinical categories applied to people.

Chapter 2 begins the discussion of the book's central topic by describing how the study of joint attention in ASD has informed and begun to change the conceptualization and diagnosis of ASD. In conjunction with the philosophy of the National Institute of Mental Health

Research Domain Criteria, this chapter discusses the benefits of shifting away from research on ASD as a *category of disorder* to examining ASD as *part of human nature*. From this perspective, ASD is defined in terms of a specific outcome of the interaction of individual differences in the development of critical dimensions of human development. This chapter begins the argument that joint attention is best conceived as one of the distinct dimensions of human development involved in ASD, and not one that can be understood or explained by other important and perhaps better-recognized dimensions.

Chapter 3 reviews the impact that joint attention research has had on advancing diagnosis, screening, and risk measurement for ASD. It describes how joint attention measures, nomenclature, and developmental research have been included in the "gold-standard" diagnostic measures for autism that have been developed since 1990. Sections of this chapter are also devoted to how joint attention measures informed and improved early screening instruments for ASD. Finally, insights derived from joint attention studies of infant siblings of children with autism are reviewed, to provide a better understanding of when in infancy differences in joint attention may indicate risk for autism syndrome development.

Chapter 4 advances the discussion of learning and joint attention, especially in connection with the relations between early joint attention development and childhood/adult social-cognitive development. One of the competing hypotheses about why children with autism have difficulty with joint attention is that it reflects their social-cognitive or theory-of-mind deficits. In discussing this idea, this chapter describes in detail a model of the *learning-to* and *learning-from* phases of joint attention development. This model serves as a means of better understanding how in development children learn to manage the self-referenced (interoceptive and proprioceptive) and external (exteroceptive) information-processing demands of joint attention. It also discusses how learning to manage this type of multichannel information processing may be difficult for children with autism. According to this model, this difficulty leads to later problems with the development of social cognition, language, and social learning.

Chapter 5 discusses three other competing hypotheses. Two of these involve the related ideas that joint attention development and its role in autism may be well explained as part of more primary social orienting or face processing. This chapter provides more details to support the assertion that joint attention is a form of information processing that is fundamental to human learning, and that it cannot be explained satisfactorily in terms of either orienting or face processing. The chapter also reviews data suggesting that joint attention develops early in the first 6 months of life and may be no less primary in development than social orienting or face processing. The chapter goes on to present the idea that a motivation disturbance in ASD may involve early difficulty with joint attention. A new perspective is discussed here that suggests that this disturbance involves a reduced arousal or reward response to the perception of attention to self, rather than the reduced reward value of attending to other people. The third competing hypothesis discussed in this chapter is that difficulty with joint attention is a circumscribed phenomenon of infancy that has limited validity in basic and clinical research with older individuals with ASD. In response to this hypothesis, the chapter discusses how joint attention plays a lifelong role in learning, intersubjectivity, and cooperative engagement with others. Consequently, it will be important to develop new, sensitive measures of joint attention for both children and adults, to provide a clearer understanding of the role of joint attention in ASD throughout the lifespan.

Chapter 6 concludes the discussion of the role of joint attention in learning with a review of experimental treatment research on this topic. This review highlights advances in effective targeted interventions for joint attention development in autism. The development of targeted intervention treatments for joint attention was one of the first types of treatment research funded in 1997 by the National Institutes of Health Collaborative Programs of Excellence in Autism. A lot has been learned since then, the highlights of which are described at some length in this chapter.

Chapter 7 begins with an overview of how far developmental cognitive neuroscience has come in identifying the discrete neural networks involved in joint attention. Numerous neuroimaging and electroencephalographic studies on this topic are described. These range from two studies of the neural substrates of joint attention in 5- and 6-month-old infants, to multiple studies of the cortical correlates of differences in joint attention between children and adults with and without ASD. This chapter explores why there is considerable overlap in the neural network activated by joint attention tasks and those activated by social-cognitive tasks. It also explores the implications of data currently suggesting that the differences in default network and frontoparietal control network activation may be primary to the differences in joint attention that characterize ASD.

Finally, Chapter 8 moves to the frontier of research on the genetic and related molecular mechanisms that may affect joint attention development in human nature, including the human nature of autism. Research on genetic studies of joint attention in ASD, as well as comparative studies of joint attention in primates, are discussed. In addition, the incipient literature on the genetics of social cognition is described. The review of the literature in this chapter leads to potentially important new hypotheses and observations. One is that data across studies converge on the idea that dopamine-transported genes may interact with oxytocin as well as vasopressin receptor genes in ways that influence joint attention. Moreover, these interactions may reflect repurposing of the actions of these genes in ways that may be different from their repertoire of action in other primates and mammals. These ideas lead to a crucial conclusion of the book: More consideration of the neurodevelopmental and metabolic factors involved in joint attention may be as important to the future study of autism's etiology as joint attention research has been to advances in the clinical assessment and treatment of ASD in the recent past.

Acknowledgments

The development of my theory and research described in this book was supported and made possible by many people and institutions. Above all, the love, camaraderie, and clinical acumen of my wife, Kim Fuller, as well as the light of day provided by our daughter, Erin Mundy McCook, have been the necessary ingredients in all of this.

Extramural grants over the last 30 years from the National Institutes of Health and other federal research funding agencies have made it possible to pursue much of the research and theory described in this volume. Beginning in 1982, these grants have included Nos. RO1NS-2543, RO117662, RO1NS26121, RO1HD38052, RO1MH071273, and R21MH085904, as well as Grant No. SP08984 from the Substance Abuse and Mental Health Services Administration and Grant No. UR3/CCU421965 from the Centers for Disease Control and Prevention. Funding for the research and ideas provided in the book has also been provided by the Dan and Claire Marino Foundation. Finally, the support of Mark Friedman and Marjorie Solomon for the Lisa Capp Endowment to the UC Davis Department of Psychiatry and the MIND Institute, and current support from Institute of Education Sciences Grant No. R324A110174, have been indispensable in the development of this book.

The data and ideas herein are shared products of many people and several collaborations. These began at the University of Miami during my graduate work with Keith Scott on developmental disabilities, and with Jeff Seibert and Ann Hogan on the theory and measurement of joint attention. This was followed by the great opportunity to work with Marian

Sigman and Connie Kasari on a program of studies on autism and joint attention at UCLA for 10 years. A return to the University of Miami as a faculty member allowed me to work with Kim Oller, Heather Henderson, Daniel Messinger, Stephen Sheinkopf, Amy Vaughan Van Hecke, Michael Alessandri, and others in countless ways that informed central tenets of this book. Furthermore, many of the ideas in this volume were stimulated by many lively discussions with Peter and Jessica Hobson over the past 20 years. I'd also like to thank Nathan Fox for providing a foundation for my understanding of neuroscience in general, and the neuroscience of joint attention in particular.

Now at UC Davis, my opportunities to work on ideas with Ann Mastergeorge, Marjorie Solomon, Emily Solari, Nancy McIntyre, Lindsay Swain, Tasha Oswald, Stephanie Novotny, Bill Jarrold, Kwanguk Kim, Matt Zajic, and many others—including the entire faculty of the MIND Institute during the Friday morning research seminars—have both motivated and refined many of the thoughts that follow. Finally, I'd like to thank the editors at The Guilford Press for their patience, support, and frequent rescues of the text from my error-prone ways.

Contents

Chapter 1

A Brief History
of the Concept of Autism

Autism involves a common impairment of
affective relatedness to others.
—LEO KANNER

We are drowning in information, but starved
for knowledge.
—JOHN NAISBITT

Autism and the Myth of the Unresponsive Child

Pick up a journal article or book on autism, and you are likely to read a
sentence somewhat like this: "Autism is a biologically based condition that
is characterized by impaired social interaction, impaired social communication, and the presence of repetitive behaviors and thoughts." Others
might argue that an impairment of social imagination warrants inclusion,
perhaps in place of repetitive behaviors and thoughts (Wing, Gould, &
Gillberg, 2011). Nevertheless, there is a general consensus that autism is
of biological origin and that autism syndrome development is characterized by differences in social interaction, social communication, and cognition. Even though this triad of descriptors adheres closely to a seminal
description of autism published in 1943, it took the next 50 years to reach
agreement on even this very general conceptualization of what autism is
and is not.

At Johns Hopkins University and the University of Vienna, Leo Kanner (1943) and Hans Asperger (1944), respectively and independently, discovered evidence of the distinct syndrome of what is now called *autism spectrum disorder* (ASD). Kanner, for his part, displayed impressive clinical acumen when he was able to discern three common characteristics of a subgroup of children within a larger clinical sample of children. Kanner observed that some children appeared to have (1) a common impairment of affective relatedness to others, which (2) resulted in a disorder that primarily involved impairments of the capacity for typical social interactions, and (3) was of such a unique and robust presentation that it was likely to be caused by biologically based processes. The recognition of the biological, affective, and social-behavioral syndrome triumvirate of autism was a remarkable achievement, and is as valid today as it was in 1943.

Unfortunately, Kanner's initial perspective did not fit well with the *zeitgeist*, or dominant school of thought at the time. In 1943, the psychodynamic model dominated thinking about atypical human development. This model emphasized the primacy of early experience and interaction to a much greater extent than biological factors in explaining all aspects of human mental development. Advocates of this school of thought brought sufficient pressure to bear that Kanner recanted his hypothesis of a biological etiology, and adopted an early-experience explanation of ASD (Kanner, 1949). Such is the power of the zeitgeist in a science, then and now.

In the ensuing 30 years, the science of autism drifted from one perspective to another. The psychodynamic perspective described autism as a disorder brought on by an aloof parenting style, which caused children to grow up to be severely emotionally disengaged from all people; a famous advocate of this view was Bruno Bettelheim (1959). This notion was personified in the metaphor of the so-called "refrigerator parent," whose interactive style caused autism. It also led to development of the prototype of the "robotic" child with autism, who exhibited a pattern of pervasively aloof, unresponsive, and emotionally flat behavior (Bettelheim, 1959).

By the early 1960s and 1970s, compelling, albeit indirect, evidence for the biological nature of ASD had been presented to counter the psychodynamic model. This evidence included observations that autism was linked to gender, with more male than female children affected. It was also based on observations of consistent estimates of the prevalence of autism across cultures; observations of familial risk for the disorder; and, perhaps most importantly, observations that parents of children with ASD did not systematically differ from other parents in their interactive style with their children (e.g., McAdoo & DeMyer, 1978; Rimland, 1964). However, even after the "refrigerator parent" model of autism was rejected, the prototype of people with ASD as emotionless, aloof, and unresponsive remained for a long time to come.

Little evidence to permit a critical appraisal of the aloof-phenotype hypothesis was available until the 1980s. There was practically no information on the social development of children with autism, because few methods for precise research on social development were available. In contrast, *relatively* more robust methods for appraising sensory, perceptual, or language development were at hand. So it is not surprising that research and theory in the 1960s and 1970s emphasized the possible role that impairments in language, perception, and sensory processing might play in the etiology of autism (Hermelin & O'Connor, 1970; Ornitz & Ritvo, 1968; Rutter, 1968, 1978). At this time, the nascent science of the biological and neurodevelopmental etiology of ASD began to emerge (Cohen, Caparulo, & Shaywitz, 1978; Damasio & Maurer, 1978).

The blossoming of evidence-based studies of ASD in the 1960s and 1970s provided much-needed guidance. However, there were disadvantages as well as advantages: Real progress was made in the science of ASD, but the available paradigms were not necessarily the most relevant to defining the nature of ASD. This problem is not uncommon in a science and is often illustrated with the following parable (based on Kaplan, 1964):

> A policeman sees a man searching for something under a streetlight and asks the man what he has lost. The man says he lost his keys. So the policeman joins his search under the streetlight. After a few minutes, the policeman asks if the man if he is sure he lost them here. The man shakes his head and says that he lost the keys in the park across the street. The confounded policeman asks, "Then why are you searching for them over here?" The man replies, "This is where the light is!"

The point of this vignette is that in science we often look for answers by using the best available research tools, because they provide the best light through which to study nature. However, there may be little coherent theory guiding the use of these tools. Without that, there is no guarantee that these tools will direct the collective spotlights of science to the best places to look in the investigation of natural phenomena. In the history of autism, one untoward consequence of the early emphasis on language, perception, and sensory process paradigms in research was to turn the spotlight of attention away from the fundamental social features of autism spectrum development. Indeed, social-emotional behaviors were relegated to the status of epiphenomena in many early models of ASD (Mundy & Sigman, 1989a). Thus, even though Kanner had emphasized the social nature of autism, the view of this aspect of the syndrome was severely occluded. For example, in 1978 Pat Howlin provided a "state of the art" review of our knowledge of social development in autism. Her review required only 7 pages and included only 39 citations. Moreover, only a handful of those papers actually reported empirical research on the social behavior of ASD (Mundy & Sigman, 1989a).

So it was that we knew very little about its social symptoms when ASD was first described (as *infantile autism*) in the American Psychiatric Association's (1980) *Diagnostic and Statistical Manual of Mental Disorders*, third edition (DSM-III). Prior to DSM-III, autism had been described as an early-onset variant of psychotic disorders. Worldwide, it was rudimentarily described under the labels *schizophrenic reaction, childhood type*, or *schizophrenia, childhood type* (American Psychiatric Association, 1952, 1968; World Health Organization, 1977).

The *nosology*, or set of symptom criteria, used to describe infantile autism in DSM-III in 1980 included only six items: (A) onset before 30 months of age; (B) a pervasive lack of responsiveness to other people; (C) gross deficits in language development; (D) if speech is present, peculiar speech patterns (such as immediate or delayed echolalia, metaphorical language, or pronominal reversal); (E) bizarre responses to various aspects of the environment (e.g., resistance to change, peculiar interest in or attachments to animate or inanimate objects); and (F) absence of delusions, hallucinations, loosening of associations, and incoherence as in schizophrenia. Only one item in this set of symptoms was specific to the *social* nature of autism. This rather broad and indefinite descriptor of a "pervasive lack of responsiveness to other people" reflected and reified the prototype of the aloof child with autism spectrum development.

Moreover, since this description of the social nature of autism was not based on empirical data, its accuracy and validity were unknown at the time of DSM-III's publication. Certainly, at this time we simply had no idea *how* to precisely examine and describe the social symptom domain of ASD. An irony here was that Kanner (1943) had argued that atypical social development was *most central* to the nature of autism, but in the ensuing four decades, science paid little attention to this central feature.

Fortunately, the inclusion of infantile autism in DSM-III led to a more vital interest in autism among clinical and developmental scientists, with a resultant explosion of research on the social nature of autism spectrum development. Only a few years after Howlin's 1978 publication, she realized the need to publish a second review on social development in children with ASD. Rather than the 7 pages and 39 citations of her 1978 paper, this new review required 24 pages and 116 citations to cover the science adequately (Howlin, 1986).

The Demise of the Unresponsive Prototype

The welcome increase in information on the social nature of ASD occurred because of translational research. The science of human development took great strides forward from the 1960s through 1980s, especially with the emergence of the subspecialty of infant developmental science. As this occurred, research groups in the United States, the United Kingdom, and throughout the world began to recognize that theory and methods used in the study of human infancy could be powerfully applied to characterize the early development of children with ASD (e.g., Baron-Cohen, Leslie, & Frith, 1985; Dawson & McKissick, 1984; Hobson, Ouston, & Lee, 1988; Rogers & Pennington, 1991; Sigman & Ungerer, 1984). This new wave of research applied theory and research on such topics as infant imitation, sensorimotor development, social learning, preverbal communication, and attachment, as well as social-cognitive development, to the study of young children with ASD. One immediate and vital impact of this surge of translational research was the recognition that describing the social behavior of ASD singularly in terms of a "pervasive lack of responsiveness to others" was at best too limited, and at worst a prototype that had misguided the field for years.

Many studies were published that were not consistent with the "pervasive lack of responsiveness" characterization of children with autism (Mundy & Sigman, 1989a). Some studies indicated that the social behaviors of many children with autism increased over age *and* in response to peers or adults who actively engaged them in social interactions (e.g., Clark & Rutter, 1981; Lord, 1984; Rutter, 1986; Strain, Kerr, & Ragland, 1979). Other observations suggested that *modeling* techniques, which demanded that children with autism attend to, respond, and learn from the actions of others, were viable intervention approaches for some children (Charlop, Schreibman, & Tryon, 1983; Egel, Richman, & Koegel, 1981). Innovative investigations also began to reveal that some children with autism were very aware when others imitated their actions, and that they increased their social behaviors in response to imitation (Dawson & Adams, 1984; Tiegerman & Primavera, 1984). The latter observation was to become a mainstay of later developments in early intervention methods (see Chapter 6).

Perhaps the most surprising set of observations was that many young children with autism displayed clear evidence of attachment behaviors during separation and reunion with their parents or caregivers (Sigman & Ungerer, 1984; Sigman & Mundy, 1989). This was a major violation of the concept of a *pervasive* lack of responsiveness in affected children. The research paradigms used in these studies measured attachments in terms of evidence of a child's systematic responsiveness to a specific caregiver, especially caregiver separations and reunions. They indicated that there were few differences in the attachment behaviors displayed by 3- to 6-year-olds with autism, compared to 3- to 6-year-olds with other developmental disorders such as Down syndrome. The conclusion was that children with ASD were as attached to their parents as any other comparable groups of children were. Research from 16 additional studies subsequently supported this seminal observation (Rutgers, Bakermans-Kranenburg, van IJzendoorn, & Berckelaer-Onnes, 2004).

Thus, shortly after the publication of DSM-III, a body of evidence became available that was not consistent with the idea that all children with autism displayed a pervasive lack of responsive to all people. It's also useful to note that this evidence was also not consistent with the notion that all children with autism paid little attention to people, and especially not consistent with the prominent hypothesis of the time that an aversion to attending to people was a clear, chronic, and defining characteristic of autism (Richer, 1978; Tinbergen & Tinbergen, 1983).

Even prior to DSM-III, important observations had been published that were inconsistent with the "pervasive lack of responsiveness" characterization of autism. Lorna Wing and Judith Gould (1979) published the fundamental observation that there were at least three different patterns of social behaviors evident in groups of children with autism. Some children with autism did appear to be socially *aloof,* much as the description of a "pervasive lack of responsiveness" suggested. Often these aloof children were also affected by what are now called intellectual and developmental disabilities (IDD). In contrast, other children with mild to no IDD were not so clearly pervasively underresponsive. Instead, some were *passive,* but socially responsive in structured situations. A third group of children were proactive in initiating interactions, but their interactive style could best be described as *active but odd.* These children were the least similar to the unresponsive prototype of autism. They often sought out social interactions, but were frequently maladaptive in initiating or maintaining interactions with other people (Wing & Gould, 1979). Subsequently, these behavioral differences were replicated in several studies (e.g., Volkmar, Cohen, Bregman, Hooks, & Stevenson, 1989; Fein et al., 1999). The recognition that the social-behavioral phenotype of people with autism varies significantly across individuals is now considered fundamental to science. Indeed, it was the work of Wing and Gould (1979) that first directly suggested the concept of a *spectrum* of autism to the field.

In summary, by the early 1990s, developmental and observational research indicated that key elements of the DSM-III nosology of ASD were incorrect. Children with ASD, as a group, did not display a pervasive lack of responsiveness to others. The focus on a nonresponsive pattern of social behavior as a defining characteristic of autism was at best inaccurate, and at worst misleading. It promoted an invalid diagnostic prototype of the syndrome that excluded many affected children who made eye contact with some frequency, or displayed caregiver attachment, or exhibited any of several other social behaviors. The persistence of this inaccurate prototype probably contributed significantly to a historic underestimation of the prevalence of ASD prior to the late 1990s (Wing & Potter, 2002).

The Dimensional Approach to the Social Nature of Autism

Significant steps toward a more valid and precise description of autism in our diagnostic systems have followed the increase in empirical studies of the behavioral development of affected children (e.g., American Psychiatric Association, 1987, 1994, 2000, 2013; Lord, Rutter, & Le Couteur, 1994). However, even with this progress, we have not yet achieved a definitive, comprehensive description. The task of developing such a description is challenging because the nature of autism is complex. We are hard pressed to make advances in developmental science, neuroscience, genetics, and several other disciplines fast enough to have all the tools and ideas we need to address its complexities. This leaves a number of questions and issues open for debate.

Among the most perplexing yet unresolved issues are the nature and meaning of the individual differences, or *symptom heterogeneity*, recognized by Wing and Gould (1979). It remains very difficult to articulate one set of symptoms that appears to be equally applicable to all people affected by autism, at all phases of development. Yet the acknowledgment of symptom heterogeneity challenges the very idea that autism reflects a single, definable clinical category of developmental disorder. Some have made a cogent case for abandoning the idea that autism is a single category of neurodevelopmental disorder (e.g., Coleman & Gillberg, 2012). Instead, it could be described in plural form, as *the autisms*. According to advocates of this view, the autisms represent a group of conditions with multiple etiologies, and consequently no *universal* signs or symptoms are expected to be present in a high percentage of cases (Coleman & Gillberg, 2012, p. 6). This viewpoint accords well with current difficulties in identifying genetic, neurodevelopmental, or psychological causes or explanations that can clearly account for the varied social, communication, and repetitive behavior symptoms of ASD (Happé, Ronald, & Plomin, 2006).

Of course, autism is a significant part of human nature, and human nature is inherently variable. Perhaps, then, we should be cautious before adopting the autisms perspective, with all its connotations. Indeed, a related but less sweeping approach to saying that there are many separate types of autism is to abandon the search for a single cause and/or core dimension that entirely explains autism. Instead, we may need to understand the etiology of autism in terms of a complex interaction of varying degrees of atypical development within individuals across multiple biobehavioral dimensions (Cuthbert & Insel, 2013; Happé et al., 2006).

According to this perspective, we may be loath to explain one dimension of ASD in terms of another, for fear of losing information that is vital to developing an accurate picture of the human nature of autism. Consequently, an essential goal of research is to identify all the distinctive biobehavioral dimensions that play a significant role in autism, and to understand their dynamic interaction throughout the course of autism spectrum development. This will be no small task, but it is a necessary one. To contribute to what will need to be a multidisciplinary effort, this book describes evidence from the science of developmental psychopathology that joint attention is a distinctive and very significant dimension in the lifespan of development of the category of ASD (Mundy & Sigman, 1989a, 1989b).

Joint attention refers to our human ability to coordinate our attention with that of other people (see Figure 1.1). Joint attention allows us to fluidly adopt a common point of reference or point of view with others. Much of human learning in structured or unstructured instructional opportunities is fundamentally dependent on our well-honed ability to attend to a common point of reference with others. The development of joint attention to objects, events, and eventually ideas is an essential process in our human capacity for reference, language development, and instructional learning. However, joint attention is not just part of language and learning, it's also part of human social engagement. Joint attention is significantly related to a sense of relatedness to others in the development of children with autism or typical development (e.g., Mundy, Sigman, & Kasari, 1994). Social relatedness is built around shared experiences with others, and the opportunity to repeatedly process information about a common referent, such as an event, with other people during episodes of joint attention is essential to sharing experiences. Without joint attention, or if joint attention were too effortful or unrewarding, the quality and quantity of our human capacity for shared experiences would be vastly different.

Observations of the relative speed and quality of joint attention development in preschool children have helped us define the category of autism for the past three decades. It is no more than one distinctive

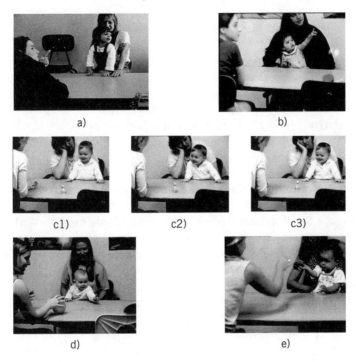

a)   b)

c1)   c2)   c3)

d)   e)

FIGURE 1.1. Illustrations of different types of infant social attention coordination behaviors: (a) *responding to joint attention* (RJA), involving following another person's gaze and pointing gesture; (b) *initiating joint attention* (IJA), involving a conventional gesture of pointing to share attention regarding a poster in the room; (c1, c2, c3) IJA involving alternating eye contact to share attention with respect to a toy; (d) *initiating behavior request* (IBR), involving pointing to elicit aid in obtaining an out-of-reach object; and (e) *responding to behavior request* (RBR), involving following an adult's open-palm "give it to me" gesture. From Mundy et al. (2007). Copyright 2007 by John Wiley & Sons, Inc. Reprinted by permission.

dimension of the diagnostic category, but no less either. The study of joint attention does not lead to a full understanding of the category of autism. Nevertheless, a full understanding of autism may not be possible without understanding joint attention. I use the word *category* advisedly, because it is a term that is often misunderstood when applied to individual differences in the development of people or their mental lives. Therefore, before I delve much further into the significance of the joint attention dimension for autism, which is the goal of the next chapter, it is important to discuss what a category of neurodevelopmental disorder is and is not.

The Fuzzy Nature of Human Nature

One difficulty in our current attempts to define or test the categorical nature of autism is that we don't yet have fully realized developmental models of autism. We have very few large-scale longitudinal data on the individual development of people affected by autism. Therefore, we understand relatively little about changes that may occur across age, either in symptoms or in behaviorally, cognitively, neurologically, or genetically defined dimensions. In other words, we have yet to chart either the *developmental phenotype* or a *developmental endophenotype* of ASD. It's curious that we have engaged in the study of a neurodevelopmental disorder without investing greater effort in research that uses longitudinal methods to describe the developmental phenotype and endophenotype. Without precise knowledge of either, we often find the scientific conversation muddled, such as when we use the phrase "the phenotype of autism" as though a single set of characteristics is (or should be) applicable to all people with ASD at all ages. Fortunately, this concern is coming of age and emphasis on the importance of longitudinal research is increasing.

Another issue that may often confuse us is the degree to which symptom heterogeneity in ASD is different from heterogeneity in other conditions. However, ASD may not be unique in presenting with a confounding level of symptom variability. Such variability is characteristic even of conditions that stem from understood and relatively circumscribed genetic or chromosomal causes (Wachs, 2000). Children affected by fragile X syndrome display a very wide range of developmental symptom expression (Bregman, Dykens, Watson, Ort, & Leckman, 1987), as do individuals with trisomy 21 or Down syndrome (Wachs, 2000). Even in single-gene-dominant disorders such as tuberous sclerosis or Alpert syndrome, where the expectation for homogeneous presentation is greatest, we observe significant variations in cognitive outcome among affected individuals (Abuleo, 1991).

Individual differences in symptom presentation present an even greater challenge for diagnosis and treatment in disorders without known genetic etiologies or polygenic etiologies. This applies to children and adults affected by developmental problems including, but not limited to, attention-deficit/hyperactivity disorder (ADHD), Tourette syndrome, and schizophrenia (e.g. Castellanos, Sonuga-Barke, Milham, & Tannock, 2006; Freeman et al., 2000; Pinto et al., 2008; Siever & Davis, 2004).

A recent description of the variable nature of schizophrenia symptom expression emphasizes that heterogeneity is common to many (if not all) significant categorical differences in human neurocognitive and behavioral development:

> The kinds of symptoms that are utilized to make a diagnosis of schizo-
> phrenia differ between affected people and may change from one year
> to the next within the same person as the disease progresses. Different
> subtypes of schizophrenia are defined according to the most signifi-
> cant and predominant characteristics present in each person at each
> point in time. The result is that one person may be diagnosed with dif-
> ferent subtypes over the course of his illness. (Bengston, 2013)

Bengston's description of schizophrenia provides a useful perspective
on the vicissitudes of describing the essential nature of neurodevelopmental disorders such as ASD, which by their very nature may change in
appearance across age. Symptom heterogeneity was explicitly recognized
as a characteristic of schizophrenia in the research and clinical communities with the adoption of the term *schizophrenia spectrum disorders* several decades ago (e.g., Doane, West, Goldstein, Rodnick, & Jones, 1981).
Knowingly or not, the autism research community has followed suit by
adopting a similar designation in the most recent version of DSM. Instead
of the term *pervasive developmental disabilities* used in DSM-IV (American
Psychiatric Association, 1994), the categorical label is now *autism spectrum
disorder* (ASD) in DSM-5 (American Psychiatric Association, 2013).

It is not the case, then, that heterogeneity of symptoms is a unique
and confounding feature of the category of ASD. Rather, heterogeneity is
part of all categories of human neurodevelopmental differences. This has
long been recognized in the longstanding debate about the pros and cons
of categorical or dimensional approaches to any and all mental conditions (Meehl, 1995). Pickles and Angold (2003) have suggested that much
of this debate is misconceived. They argue that we most often approach
the identification or diagnosis of psychological and developmental disturbance in children or adults with measures of multiple dimensions. However, when it comes time to make a decision, such as determining whether
the disturbance is at a level that warrants treatment, we use criterion
scores on each dimensional measure alone, or summed across dimensions, to make a choice regarding whether an individual displays characteristics associated with a dichotomously conceived categorical disorder
(e.g., not-autism vs. autism).

Almost always, this type of categorical decision is probabilistic. We
compare the criterion scores of an individual to reference scores derived
from large samples of children or adults. We then estimate the likelihood
that the individual scores outside the typical range of scores on one or
more dimensions. If the individual does this, we may conclude that the
person's scores fall within the range of scores characteristic of one categorical condition or another. We also know that the chance of error for
this estimation is usually on the order of 1–5%. Although this explicit

recognition of the probabilistic nature of our categorical decisions fades into the background when we decide whether not a child "meets criteria" for ASD, it always remains a decision about *how probable* it is that the child's behavior meets these criteria. This is also often true when we use similar methods for estimating the probability that individuals meet criteria for IDD, ADHD, anxiety disorders, and so forth

To suggest that it is appropriate to rely on probability to make a categorical decision may seem like an oxymoron, or so-called "soft science." This would seem to violate the syllogism that if autism is a specific category of developmental disorders, then there is an absolute set of necessary and sufficient symptoms that clearly defines the category and distinguishes it from all other categories of disorders. However, this logic may be in error. Science has long recognized that many natural categories are ill defined. There is no simple set of criteria features that determines the membership of all exemplars of a category. Category membership is often not based on characteristics measurable on dichotomous scales (present–absent), but rather on characteristics that can only be assessed on continuous scales, where measurement is relative. For example, most of us would agree that we naturally perceive a category of tall people, but how would we define the category? We could validly define it as all people taller than ourselves, or of an average height, or above the 98th percentile for height. In each case category, membership is not absolute. Rather, it is based on a judgment about comparative measurements of height across people. So categories of neurodevelopmental and mental conditions are based on comparative measurements across people.

Of course, correctly defining a category of neurodevelopment such as ASD is more complex because of the need to measure more than one behavioral or biological dimension. Although we are trying to increase the precision of the multidimensional measurement, any multidimensional system is problematic. Different combination of measurements across dimensions may lead to the same degree of certainty or probability of a valid match between the characteristics of an individual and category membership (Martin & Caramazza, 1980). Moreover, in a *developmental* disorder, the set of dimensions measured as well as their criterion scores may be expected to change as a child's age or levels of achievement change. For example, the chance that a primary symptom of ASD, "difficulties in sharing imaginative play or in making friends" (American Psychiatric Association, 2013, p. 50), will be useful in the identification of ASD before age 3 is relatively low, but its value in the categorical diagnosis is likely to increase through subsequent years. With more research with more people, what we recognize as the criteria for a categorical decision may change. For example, what was once classified as normal blood pressure (a systolic pressure of 120–139 mm Hg and a diastolic pressure of 80–89 mm Hg) in 1997 is now categorized as prehypertension (*www. health.harvard.edu/heart-health/blood-pressure-normal-maybe-now-it-isnt*).

In truth, the nature of categories can be considered from two points of view, described as *classical set theory* and *fuzzy set theory* (i.e., *fuzzy logic*). These alternative perspectives have been succinctly characterized by Kaushal, Mohan, and Sandhu (2010) in this way:

> In classical set theory, an item is either a part of a set or not. There is no in-between; there are no partial members. For example, a cat is a member of a set of mammals, and a frog is not. Such sets are called crisp sets. Fuzzy set theory recognizes that very few crisp sets actually exist. Fuzzy logic allows partial set membership; it allows gradual transitions between fully a member of the set and fully not a member of the set. Being partially a member of a given set, a given element is also partially not a member of that set. Traditional logic recognizes only full or null membership in a set and requires that a given assertion be either true or false. Fuzzy logic, however, allows partial truth and partial falseness. (pp. 313–314)

Fuzzy logic, and its mathematical and statistical applications, have been used effectively to improve many areas of science. It has applications when what seems like a dichotomous or linear process turns out to be more complex and conditional than expected. For example, it has had effective applications in research on decision making in artificial intelligence; in research on grammatical and semantic processing in linguistics; and even in the study of fuzzy protein complexes, which evince structural ambiguity or require multiplicity for biological function (Tompa & Fuxreiter, 2008).

It may well be that recognition of the mathematics of fuzzy logic will have useful applications in efforts to develop a more rigorous approach to the nosology of autism. This may be the case because human development and human developmental disorders reflect stochastic systems. A *stochastic system* is one that undergoes continual change or instability, and for which any subsequent state (or prediction of subsequent state such as a diagnosis) must be determined probabilistically. Stochastic processes play fundamental roles in physics, biology, economics, and many if not most of the other sciences. Indeed, gene expression has stochastic characteristics (Fraser & Marcotte, 2004). We must embrace the stochastic nature of ASD. It may be time to abandon the search for single causes of a single autism (Happé et al., 2006). However, we should not abandon the search for single dimensions of development that, in stochastic combination with other dimensions and factors, give rise to ASD.

A similar message comes from the literature on a dynamic systems approach to human development (e.g., Gleick, 1987; Thelen, 1989; Berta-lanffy, 1968). Systems perspectives acknowledge that linear deterministic models rarely hold for natural and especially biological processes. It encourages the perspective that multiple determinant, conditional, and nonlinear development perspectives are more likely to lead to veridical "common" causal explanations for any aspect of human development (Wachs, 2000). Wachs (2000) has stated that we should embrace the complexity of dynamic systems in all applications of developmental science:

> Variable outcomes as a function of specific developmental influences may be inherent in the developmental process itself . . . Human developmental scientists should assume that there will be variability in individual developmental outcomes and begin to look for [new] conceptual and methodological approaches to help us understand why such variability is occurring. (p. 10)

Systems theories of human development recommend that variability of symptom expression and outcome should be an expectation not a surprise in the study of ASD. It should be a central topic of inquiry in the science of ASD (Spencer et al., 2006). According to this perspective, there is no flaw in the logic of defining the necessary common dimensions that define the categorical nature of autism. The flaw only comes from thinking that (1) the common dimensions of autism affect the development of all children one singular deterministic fashion; and (2) the science is about defining a single primary dimension or process, rather than a set of dimensions *and their interactions*, that gives rise to the multiply determined but ultimately common nature of autism.

It may be a little too early in our science to abandon any ideas—and certainly not the idea that autism is a definable neurodevelopmental disorder category, or that certain signs and symptoms can be expected to be present in a high percentage of cases. Rather, we can expect the combination of symptoms of the disorder to vary across individuals and ages, but with time we will uncover dimensions and processes are that are common to symptoms and the nature of the disorder. Of course, we can expect the search for those commonalities to be challenging and to be complicated by a number of factors. One of these is the interaction between dimensions that play a specific role in autism spectrum development, and dimensions that are important to significant human variation but not necessarily to ASD.

The Moderator Model of Autism

Differences among people affected by ASD may be the result of variability in the primary dimensions involved in autism (autism specific dimensions) and in how autism-specific dimensions interact with a variety of nonspecific dimensions of human nature that give rise to significant behavioral variations across all people (moderator dimensions). The interaction of moderator dimensions with autism specific dimensions may be part of the reason that defining the fuzzy category of autism in so challenging. This assertion is central to the *moderator model* or *modifier model* of autism (Burnette et al., 2011; Mundy et al., 2007).

Autism is a relatively common part of the human condition. Recent data indicate that it affects as many as 1 in 68 children (Centers for Disease Control and Prevention [CDC], 2014). However, in a very real sense, there are no "autistic children" or "autistic adults." This is because autism does not define or describe the totality of any individual, as may be implied by such commonly used but inaccurate terms as "autistic children." Rather, autism affects the development of only part of an individual, albeit a very important part. The set of factors that constitutes autism may be expected to interact with a system of genetic and environmental factors contributing to the wide ranges of rates of development, temperament/personality dimensions, and cognitive dimensions that define the variability of human nature. It seems likely that these general dimensions of human individual differences interact with the multiple, but (let us hope) relatively circumscribed, set of dimensions of autism. This interaction of *syndrome-specific* and *non-syndrome-specific determinants* probably contributes to patterns of symptom heterogeneity in ASD, to a greater or lesser degree, at different points in development. If so, symptom variability in ASD may reflect the nonlinear or complex determinant pathways of a dynamic system (Barton, 1994), and may not unequivocally indicate the presences of differences in etiological processes within this developmental disorder category.

One part of the dynamic system of autism is illustrated in Figure 1.2, which depicts two major paths to developmental variability and symptom expression in people affected by ASD. One path involves the interactions among multiple initial causal processes (ICPs in the figure), which involve multiple major genetic determinants and variable expressivity as well as penetrance of gene expression, caused by largely unknown epigenetic gene–gene and gene–environment interaction processes. The dynamic interactive processes in the primary genetic etiology of ASD are such that they alone would be expected to lead to significant variations along major axes of development, such as IQ, associated with varied symptom presentations (Geschwind, 2011). However, this does not automatically indicate a lack of common causal processes that define the disorder. It does mean, though, that ASD is very complex and that its causes are both difficult both to conceive and to perceive.

A complication that is illustrated in the moderator model in Figure 1.2 is that processes not specific to autism affect and refract the expression

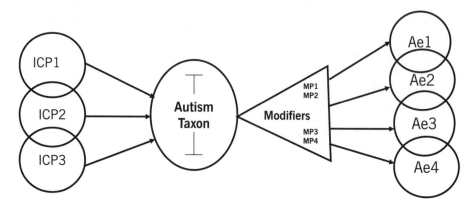

FIGURE 1.2. Phenotypic variability in autism may arise from at least two sources: syndrome-specific *initial causal processes* (ICPs) and non-syndrome-specific *modifier processes* (MPs). Varied constellations of genetic and neurodevelopmental ICPs contribute to differences in ASD expression at different ages across the course of autism in individuals. In addition, phenotypic variability in the expression of autism at any age (Ae1, Ae2, . . .) may be caused by the interactions of the ICPs of autism with non-syndrome-specific MPs, such as variation in the temperament dimensions of avoidance and approach tendencies associated with the behavioral inhibition and activation systems respectively. From Burnette et al. (2011). Copyright 2011 by Springer New York LLC. Reprinted by permission.

of ASD. Theoretically, this interaction between major core processes and nonspecific individual-difference processes significantly complicates the phenotypic expression of ASD across individuals; it also complicates attempts to define the nature of ASD. For example, recent studies have provided examples of how symptom expression in ASD may vary in interaction with dimensions of temperament that are not necessarily specific to ASD (e.g., Burnette et al., 2011; Clifford et al., 2013; Sutton et al., 2005; Schriber, Robins, & Solomon, 2014; Schwartz et al., 2009).

The study by Burnette et al. (2011) examined a frontal electro-encephalographic (EEG) index of the relative impact of bias toward behavioral activation and behavioral inhibition in sample of higher-functioning school-age children with ASD. The *behavioral inhibition system* (BIS) is a neural network that theoretically controls the experience of sensitivity to cues of punishment, loss of reward or novelty, and avoidance-associated emotions such as anxiety and fear. The *behavioral activation system* (BAS) is a neural network that controls the experience of sensitivity to reward and goal-directed approach behaviors, as well as approach-associated emotions such as pleasure and anger (Gray, 1981; Carver & White, 1994).

Burnette et al. (2011) observed no evidence of group differences in BIS or BAS that were specific to higher-functioning children with ASD. Instead, just like their typically developing peers, about 50% of these children displayed EEG patterns related to activation bias and the other half displayed patterns related to inhibition bias. This observation fit well with Wing and Gould's (1979) long-standing observation that people affected by ASD can display social inhibition tendencies associated with aloof, withdrawn patterns of behavior, *or* socially active tendencies associated with approaching but odd patterns of behavior.

Burnette et al. (2011) also observed that differences in the EEG index of BAS were associated with parent reports of milder expression of social symptoms and later age of symptom onset in these children with ASD. With respect to the latter, parents of children with the EEG marker of BIS bias reported recognizing symptoms of autism in their children at about 2 years. Alternatively, parents of children with EEG markers of BAS reported that they did not recognize symptoms until their children were about 4 years of age. EEG markers of BAS were also associated with higher levels of child self-reported outward expressions of anger and symptoms of obsessive–compulsive disorder. Thus this study provided evidence that the dimensions of behavioral activation and behavioral inhibition may moderate the expression of ASD in higher-functioning children with respect to intensity of social symptom presentation, age of symptom identification, and comorbid emotional characteristics.

Differences in active/approach and passive/avoidance tendencies have also been associated with differences in intervention responsiveness and developmental course in studies of ASD. Beglinger and Smith (2005) used a measure of the Wing and Gould (1979) typology and observed that aloof preschool children were less responsive to early intervention than socially active children were. Sherer and Schreibman (2005) also reported that children with ASD who displayed more approach and less avoidance had better responses to pivotal response training. In a third study, Garon et al. (2009) observed 34 of 138 infant siblings of children with autism who were ultimately diagnosed with ASD. Sixteen of the children in this sample displayed relatively clear symptoms by 24 months, and 18 expressed clear symptom presentation later, at 36 months of age. One distinguishing characteristics of these two subgroups was that ASD was identified later in life for children with higher ratings of behavioral approach. Garon et al. (2009, p. 73) noted the striking parallel of this finding with elements of the moderator/modifier model of autism.

The assumptions associated with the moderator model are significant for the study of ASD. They help to make us aware of the need for great precision in defining what we mean by the word *social* when we speak of "the social phenotype of ASD." Not all aspects of social behavior are part of the ASD phenotype. This is critical to understand, because revolutions in the field of ASD research that are expected in genomics and neuroscience may be absolutely reliant on the precision of phenotypic descriptions of ASD (Konopka & Geschwind, 2010). The observation that BAS and BIS may affect ASD, but are probably not central to the nature of ASD, is illustrative of this point. There is much to be learned from animal models of ASD. However, to the extent that an animal model of ASD is based on manipulations that give rise to aloof/avoidant or active but odd behaviors, caution in interpreting the validity of the model may well be advisable.

Recognizing the nature of the variable expression of ASD also brings to mind the observation that many features of autism are clearly evident in the general population. This range of expression from adaptive to less adaptive behaviors is called the *broad autism phenotype* (BAP). Some features of the BAP, such as an intense, obsessive, or seemingly limited interest in particular topic or idea, can have very adaptive expressions in the work of businesspeople, scientists, artists, and many others. This tendency for what we label as a disorder to be defined by features associated with less extreme and adaptive behavioral expressions is part of the fuzzy nature of human categories. It is also characteristic of most of our current categories of mental disorders, rather than a feature peculiar to ASD. For example, Kay Redfield Jamison (1995) famously observed that that single-mindedness of endeavor and unfailing confidence about decisions in the presence of contradictory evidence can be symptoms of bipolar I disorder. However, while extremes of this characteristic of human nature can be very unfortunate for an individual, less extreme expressions can be vital in the general population.

So facets of autism may also be viewed as the extreme expressions of a constellation of sensory, perceptual, cognitive, social-communicative, and emotional tendencies that often have less problematic or beneficial expressions in people. This *continuous dimension* viewpoint may be taken as an argument against a categorical or taxonomic view of autism. In actuality, many if not all forms of psychopathology and even physical disease processes can be viewed as variations on continuous dimensions of human cognitive and social development (Insel et al., 2010). This issue has been a recognized but unresolved complication in theories on mental disorders for decades (Meehl, 1995), including developmental disorders (Achenbach, 1966; Pickles & Angold, 2003). In the final analysis, though, we shift from a dimensional to a categorical approach whenever clinical decisions about individuals must be made with respect to their candidacy for interventions.

The practical need for this type of shift has been recognized as part of the essential duality of dimensional and categorical approaches to human developmental psychopathology (Pickles & Angold, 2003). The issue is not whether a dimensional or categorical approach is more appropriate for the science of ASD, because they are both appropriate. What is important is to recognize all of the dimensions of human nature that are distinctly involved in autism spectrum development. Considerable progress has been made in this regard over the last few decades (e.g., Lord et al., 1989, 1994). However, we still have miles to go to identify all the physiological, genetic, neurodevelopmental, cognitive, social, and emotional dimensions that characterize autism spectrum development across the lifespan. To identify these, we will need to be open to innovative ideas coming from well outside the bounds of the science of ASD alone. Just as assuredly, though, critical information regarding the identity of these dimensions will come directly from what we learn from the study of autism spectrum development in people.

Chapter 2

The Dimension of Joint Attention and ASD Diagnosis

The term *dimension of joint attention* is used in this book to integrate the present discussion with the recent systematic attempts by the National Institute of Mental Health (NIMH) to advance the science through a dimensional approach to psychopathology (Cuthbert & Insel, 2013). As part of these efforts, the Research Domain Criteria (RDoC) were developed as an alternative to the use of symptom-based categories of disorders in organizing clinical research. The RDoC approach is designed to identify the brain–behavior dimensions that are needed for precisely describing all facets of atypical mental development. Once these dimensions are identified, research can then be implemented to determine the subsets of which dimensions, and their dynamic interactions in development, are most central to understanding different types of psychopathology. The hope is that starting with dimensions and building up to categories of disorders will lead more directly to targeted treatments or "precision medicine" for neurodevelopmental disorders and psychopathology (Cuthbert & Insel, 2013, p. 3). The initial RDoC system (as of October 2012) includes 5 domains and 23 superordinate dimensions, which are also referred to as *constructs*. Table 2.1 presents an outline of the initial RDoC.

TABLE 2.1. The RDoC of the NIMH as of October 2012

Negative valence domain	Positive valence systems	Cognitive systems	Systems for social processes	Arousal/ modulatory systems
Acute threat ("fear")	Approach motivation	Attention	Affiliation and attachment	Arousal
Potential threat ("anxiety")	Initial responsiveness to reward	Perception	Social communication	Biological rhythms
Sustained threat	Sustained responsiveness to reward	Working memory	Perception and understanding of self	Sleep–wake
Loss	Reward learning	Declarative memory	Perception and understanding of others	
Frustrative nonreward	Habit	Language behavior		
		Cognitive (effortful) control		

Note. From Cuthbert and Insel (2013). Copyright 2013 by B. N. Cuthbert and T. R. Insel. This is an Open Access article distributed under the terms of the Creative Commons Attribution License (*http://creativecommons.org/licenses/by/2.0*), which permits unrestricted use, distribution, and reproduction in any medium, provided the original work is properly cited.

Joint Attention and the RDoC

To identify broad domains of brain–behavior dimensions, the RDoC system relies on two sources of information. First, the selection of domains and dimensions is based on the consensus decisions of large working groups of scientists about the nature of the basic cognitive and motivational functions that the human brain has evolved to perform. In addition, there needs to be compelling evidence for a distinct and specified set of biological processes associated with the development and functions of each dimension (Cuthbert & Insel, 2013). In no small way, the remainder of this book presents a comprehensive argument that joint attention is one of the vital cognitive and motivational functions the human brain has evolved to perform.

The initial RDoC system is designed to spur the science of mental health forward. Its initial content and organization presented challenges that required the systematization of a rapidly changing and complex network of information. It may be best viewed as a snapshot of the study of mental development and clinical conditions at a particular point in time (late 2012). Hence the content of the RDoC is not expected to be fixed, complete, or accurate in all its features. One example of how the RDoC is currently incomplete is how it classifies joint attention within the system.

Joint attention falls within the Systems for Social Processes domain of the RDoC. This domain includes four constructs, or superordinate dimensions: Attachment and Affiliation, Social Communication, Perception and Understanding of Self, and Perception and Understanding of Others (see Table 2.1). A more complete description of all the dimensions in the current RDoC, and of paradigms for their measurement, is available through an NIMH web link (*www.nimh.nih.gov/research-priorities/rdoc/rdoc-constructs. shtml*). Within this taxonomy, joint attention falls within Social Communication, but not as a distinct mental function with a specified course of neurodevelopment. Rather, it is conceived of in much more limited fashion. It is designated as a method of measurement (or paradigm) for research on Reception and Production of Facial Communication (see Table 2.2).

This allocation within the RDoC has some logic to it. Joint attention is clearly pivotal to human social communication (Adamson, 1995). Moreover, episodes of joint attention can involve both the processing of another person's gaze and head direction information, and the expression of one's own facial affect and gaze direction during episodes of joint attention (e.g., Brooks & Meltzoff, 2002; Kasari, Freeman, & Paparella, 2000; Mundy & Crowson, 1997). However, subsuming it under facial communication in the RDoC speaks to the current lack of a comprehensive understanding of joint attention in the sciences, either as a major human mental function, or as a major dimension of autism.

Joint attention may involve face processing. However, we need not study face processing at all to study joint attention. We do not measure face processing in neurocognitive studies of declarative pointing in children and adults (Brunetti et al., 2014; Henderson, Yoder, Yale, & McDuffie, 2002), and declarative pointing is a quintessential joint attention behavior. We also do not measure or consider face processing in studies of the development of joint attention in children affected by blindness (Bigelow, 2003), or in the study of joint attention mediated by sophisticated auditory perception in dolphins (Pack & Herman, 2006). Moreover, cognitive neuroscience indicates that there is little overlap between the brain systems that are most prominent in joint attention processing and those that are most prominent in face processing (e.g., Brunetti et al., 2014; Calder et al., 2007; Gordon, Eilbott, Feldman, Pelphrey, & Vander Wyk, 2013).

So although there may be a plausible connection between joint attention and face processing, it is not a deep connection. The mental processes involved in joint attention include, but in no way are defined by, those associated with face processing.

This is because the essential component of joint attention involves sharing a common point of reference (or point of view) with another person with respect to a third physical or mental object or event. In other words, the study of joint attention is the study of the human cognitive and neurocognitive capacity for social reference (Bruner, 1975; Bates, Camaioni, & Volterra, 1975; Mundy & Newell, 2007; Tomasello, Carpenter, Call, Behne, & Moll, 2005; Mundy & Newell, 2007). Indeed, it is fair to argue that nothing is more basic to social communication development than our exquisitely honed human capacity to coordinate our attention with that of another person and/or to refer the attention of another person to a common point of interest. The referential function is such a ubiquitous part of human social communication that it may be hard to perceive as a distinct dimension of human mental development. Nevertheless, it is a distinct dimension—or at least this is the story that the last four decades of research and theory on joint attention seem to tell.

Joint attention, at its most basic, involves the gradual development of integrated multichannel information processing. To engage in joint attention, we need to process information about our own point of reference (i.e., self-referenced information processing), the point of reference of another person (i.e., other-person-referenced information processing). And, critically, information about whether the information processing of self and other is spatially co-directed to reference a particular object or event in the world. We must thoroughly practice self–other processing of a common focus of attention in the first years of life, in order to develop the cognitive wherewithal to engage easily in the referential function of language (e.g., Colonnesi, Stams, Koster, & Noom, 2010) and human levels of sophisticated social communication.

Thus the study of joint attention does not seem to be well placed in its current minor role within the Systems for Social Processes domain of the RDoC. Rather, it seems to lie at the nexus of many of the subordinate dimensions of Social Communication recognized in the RDoC. This book presents evidence that joint attention is involved in the development of all subordinate domains of the Systems for Social Processes domain (see Table 2.1), except for Attachment in the Affiliation and Attachment construct. To appreciate this assertion, we need to adopt a developmental perspective on the Systems for Social Processes domain and understand the role of joint attention in human learning and social-cognitive development. Understanding this role starts with a deeper appreciation of human attention development (Mundy & Newell, 2007).

TABLE 2.2. Units of Analysis for Reception and Production of Facial Communication, as Subdimensions within the Social Communication Construct of the Systems for Social Processes Domain in the RDoC

			Reception of facial communication: Units of analysis				
Genes	Molecules	Cells	Circuits	Physiology	Behavior	Self-reports	Paradigms
OXTR	Oxytocin	Face-selective neurons: FTA, STS, amygdala	VI-FFA-STS-amygdala	SCR	Identification of emotion	Face dimensional rating scales	Emotional face expression tests
CNTNAP2	Vasopressin		VI-FFA-STS-VS	HR/BP/respiration	Eye gaze detection		Face feature manipulation (e.g., morphing)
5HTT	Serotonin		IFG-INS-amygdala/VS	Pupil dilation	Scanning patterns	Arousal ratings	Still face paradigm
COMT	GABA	Neurons with mirror properties	OFC-ACC-amygdala-striatum	Startle reflex	Behavioral observation/coding systems		Distress paradigms
FMR1	FMRP		Amygdala-brainstem	Facial EMG	Implicit mimicry		Social reward paradigms
BDFN	Testosterone		Resting state networks	ERP N170, N250; ECoG			Emotional Stroop/emotional go/no-go
Other autism risk genes	Dopamine			Frontal brain asymmetry (decreased alpha to faces)			Social Flanker, other attention paradigms
				Local cerebral blood flow changes			Dynamic social stimulus tasks
				Network dynamics, including within and between network structure (e.g., coherence, functional connectivity)			Conditioning paradigms
							Joint attention tasks

Production of facial communication: Units of analysis

Genes	Molecules	Cells	Circuits	Physiology	Behavior	Self-reports	Paradigms
CNTNAP2	Contactin AP		Eye movements: PPC-SC-SNc-SEF-FEF-CB	Facial EMG	Eye gaze aversion/contact	Berkeley Expressivity Questionnaire	Imitation of affect
FOXP2				SC, HR variability, pupil dilation			Directed facial action tasks expression: FACS and FACES coding systems; other automated facial analysis
SHANK3					Head turning		
NRX1			Facial expression: Regions including PAG, AC	Photoplethysmography (skin color measure of capillary dilation; temperature)	Reciprocal eye contact		"Thin slices" of nonverbal behavior test
OXTR					Reciprocal emotional expression		
Other autism risk genes				NIRS	Facial affect production		Relived memories paradigm
				Tear production	**Joint attention**		Human–computer action
					Behavioral observation/coding systems		Social games (e.g., cyberball)
							Provocative tasks/settings to elicit expressions

Note. Adapted from a table in the Social Processes: Workshop Proceedings of February 2012, retrieved on November 22, 2014, from *www.nimh.nih.gov/research-priorities/rdoc/rdoc-social-processes_143400.pdf* (in the public domain). Items in the "Behavior" column relevant to joint attention are given in **boldface.** *OXTR,* oxytocin receptor gene; *CNTNAP2,* human contactin-associated protein-like 2 gene; *COMT,* catechol-*O*-methytransferase gene; *5HTT,* serotonin transporter gene; *FTA,* fusiform temporal area; STS, superior temporal gyrus; *FMR1,* fragile X mental retardation (protein) gene; *BDFN,* brain-derived neurotrophic factor gene; IFG, inferior frontal gyrus; INS, insular cortex; OFC, orbital V1-FFA-STS, primary visual cortex–fusiform areas–superior temporal gyrus; VS, ventral surface; frontal cortex; ACC or AC, anterior cingulate cortex; SCR or SC, skin conductance response; HR, heart rate; BP, blood pressure; EMG, electromyography; ERP, EEG evoked response potential; N170 and N250, parameters of EEG evoked responses; ECoG, single channel electrocorticogram; PPC-SC-SNc-SEF-FEF-CB, basal ganglia and cortical regions involved in reward-oriented eye movements such as the superior colliculus (SC), substantia nigra pars compacta (SNc), supplemental eye-fields (SEF), frontal eye-fields (FEF); PAG, periaqueductal gray.

Attention and Joint Attention

One misinterpretation of joint attention is that the term *attention* is often confused with the related term *orienting*. *Orienting* refers to processes whereby we direct our sensory organs toward a stimulus. However, *attention* refers to the active process of information processing that occurs once we have oriented to a stimulus. The *spotlight model* of attention illustrates this point. At any moment in time, there is always more information available to us through our sensory and mental processes than we can embrace. To deal with this problem, attention can be thought of as a movable spotlight that we use to highlight or select information to process that is most relevant to our immediate goals. When information is illuminated by the spotlight of attention, information processing proceeds in a more efficient manner, partly because information from other stimuli outside the spotlight may be inhibited (Sperling & Weichselgartner, 1995).

We often share our own personal, moment-to-moment attention spotlight with other people. We do this more frequently, more easily, and in more ways than most if not all other animals do (see Facebook or other types of social media for examples!). Adopting a common attention spotlight with regard to a referent in the world, or in our minds, is necessary but not sufficient for us to share experience and information with one another. On a cognitive level, sharing of our attention spotlights is fundamental learning from one another via instruction. On an emotional level, sharing our attention spotlights allows us to experience a sense of intersubjectivity, which contributes to connections or affiliations among people. The capacity for sharing this metaphoric spotlight, of course, is joint attention. Research suggests that joint attention not only allows us to share information with others, but also deepens or changes the encoding of stimulus information in both infants and adults in ways that are not observed when information is individually spotlighted. This enhanced encoding in joint attention is an important element of human social cognition (Kim & Mundy, 2012; see Chapter 3).

Now let us consider individuals with autism spectrum development, who, for reasons of ability or motivation, do not easily share or coordinate their attention spotlight with that of another person. At any time in a social interaction, their attention spotlight may diverge from the consensus point of view or topic of the interaction. This is not necessarily because they are distracted by information outside the spotlight, as may be the case for someone affected by ADHD. Rather, in autism this occurs because the aptitude for establishing coordinated attention is not as strong or compelling as it is for other people. Individuals with moderate or intermittent difficulty or motivation for joint attention may frequently refer to information in their own attention spotlight, but not the common spotlight of others. This may lead to patterns of learning, communication, or behavior that seem tangential or idiosyncratic to others. More seriously, individuals with chronic or severe difficulty in socially coordinating their attention spotlight to a common point of reference may appear to be almost "blind" to what matters to others in a social interactions. Thus, in its most intense presentation, attenuation of joint attention development can contribute to severe disturbances in language and intellectual development, as well as in social development.

To better appreciate the role of joint attention disturbance across the lifespan, rather than as just a phenomenon of infant development, let's consider the type of problems a bright child with ASD may experience in an elementary school because of the inability to coordinate his or her attention spotlight easily or eagerly with that of others. An autobiographical story first published in *The New Yorker* in 2007, "Parallel Play: A Lifetime of Restless Isolation Explained," provides such a scenario. In this article (and a subsequent book), Tim Page provided the following recollection of his life as a very bright but undiagnosed second-grade student with ASD in the 1960s:

> My second-grade teacher never liked me much, and one assignment I turned in annoyed her so extravagantly that the red pencil with which she scrawled "See me!" broke through the lined paper. Our class had been asked to write about a recent field trip, and, as was so often the case in those days, I had noticed the wrong things.
>
>> Well, we went to Boston, Massachusetts through the town of Warrenville, Connecticut on Route 44A. It was very pretty and there was a church that reminded me of pictures of Russia from our book that is published by Time-Life. We arrived in Boston at 9:17. At 11 we went on a big tour of Boston on Gray Line 43, made by the Superior Bus Company like School Bus Six, which goes down Hunting Lodge Road where Maria lives and then on to Separatist Road and then to South Eagleville before it comes to our school. We saw lots of good things like the Boston Massacre site. The tour ended at 1:05. Before I knew it we were going home. We went through Warrenville again but it was too dark to see much. A few days later it was Easter. We got a cuckoo clock.
>
> It is an unconventional but hardly unobservant report. In truth, I didn't care one bit about Boston on that spring day in 1963. Instead, I wanted to learn about Warrenville, a village a few miles northeast of the town of Mansfield, Connecticut, where we were then living. I had memorized the map of Mansfield, and knew all the school-bus routes by heart—a litany I would sing out to anybody I could corner. But Warrenville was in the town of Ashford, for which I had no guide, and I remember the blissful sense of resolution I felt when I certified

that Route 44A crossed Route 89 in the town center, for I had long hypothesized that they might meet there. Of such joys and pains was my childhood composed.

I received a grade of "Unsatisfactory" in Social Development from the Mansfield Public Schools that year. I did not work to the best of my ability, did not show neatness and care in assignments, did not cooperate with the group, and did not exercise self-control. About the only positive assessment was that I worked well independently. Of course: then as now, it was all that I could do.

Adopting a common attention spotlight, or joint attention, is something we use whenever we are in an instructional context, regardless of whether we adopt the role of teacher or student. If individuals are not proficient with joint attention, be it for reasons or ability or motivation, it can have a significant impact on their learning. This, of course, is not the same as saying that persons who grow up with different joint attention proclivities cannot learn. Indeed, Tim Page was probably one of the more capable learners in his classroom. He went on to a career reviewing classical music for *The Washington Post*, and is now a faculty member at a major West Coast university. The remarkable career of Temple Grandin in engineering and large-animal husbandry provides another illustrative example of this. In fact, decreased motivation for joint attention in the context of other well-developed cognitive faculties may enable people to be highly focused and even innovative with respect to their own ideas and observations. Nevertheless, there are likely to be important consequences for their experiences in classroom instruction as children and their social relatedness as adults.

Beyond the Spotlight Model of Joint Attention

The spotlight model may be too simple to fully capture the nature of joint attention. Rather than simply spotlighting one referent at a time, we often are required and able to attend to multiple points of focus, either simultaneously or in rapidly alternating succession. This ability to attend to more than one thing at a time probably builds on developments of short-term and working memory processes (Cowan et al., 2005), and it is critical to joint attention development.

Recall that joint attention development involves slow increments in the capacity to process at least three sources of information. During joint attention, we engage self-referenced information processing. This involves information that arises from within our minds and bodies that includes (but is not limited to) the spatial characteristics of our own attention, emotions evoked by attention to the stimulus, goals we may have relative to the stimulus, and memories of past relevant joint attention episodes. Second, we engage in processing information about one or more social partners, or other-referenced information. This includes information about at least one other person's direction of gaze or gestures, affect, and speech; the familiarity or novelty of the social partner(s); and the context of the joint attention episodes. Third, we also process information about the physical or mental object or event that is the common referent or with the common focus of attention (e.g., Adamson, 1995; Tomasello, Carpenter, Call, et al., 2005; Trevarthen & Hubley, 1978; Tronick, 2005). Thus joint attention is has been called *triadic attention* in seminal research (e.g., Bakeman & Adamson, 1984). It is a truly complex facility of the mind. Its demanding, triadic, referential information processing distinguishes it from cognitive functions specific to social orienting, face processing, and other dyadic forms of social interaction, including imitation.

To the degree that the foregoing basic task analysis is correct, it also guides our thinking about the nature of joint attention differences in autism spectrum development. It suggests at least three possible sources of these differences. Joint attention development in ASD may be affected by differences in the development of the ability or tendency to process external information about other people. It is also possible that joint attention is affected by differences in the development of the ability to process internal, self-referenced information. Finally, it may be that joint attention in autism spectrum development is affected by differences in the ability to coordinate or integrate self and other referenced processing. Historically, there has been a trend toward conceptualizing ASD as involving differences in the ability to orient to or process external, other-referenced information. However, both theory and data suggest that problems in self-referenced processing and the cognitive coordination of self- and other-referenced processing of information may be equally or more important in understanding the differences in joint attention development that characterize autism spectrum development (see Chapters 4, 5, and 7).

Joint Attention and Choice

In the study of attention, it is also wise to recognize that motivation plays a fundamental role in what we choose to consider in the world. Sometimes the external world exerts seemingly obligatory control over where or toward what we direct the spotlight of our attention. Noise, rapid movement, and especially the combination of collocated noise and movement will elicit a reflexive orienting reflex and information processing in most people (e.g., Bahrick & Lickliter, 2000). Alternatively, we can also spontaneously and volitionally direct the spotlight of our attention to an object or event of our choosing. Both types of processes are examined in the study of joint attention. This is because the development of joint attention involves practice with adopting two roles: that of initiating cues for social attention coordination, and that of following others' cues for such coordination. Motivation and reward processing are involved in both roles. However, research and theory suggest that motivation may play a more distinctive role in spontaneously initiating joint attention cues than in responding to such cues (e.g., Gordon et al., 2013; Schilbach et al., 2010). Hence, in the study both of typical joint attention and of joint attention in people with autism spectrum development, it is important to consider the role of motivation (Kasari, Sigman, Mundy, & Yirmiya, 1990; Mundy, 1995; Tomasello, Carpenter, Call, et al., 2005).

The role of motivation has most often been described in terms of three possibilities, and a fourth one has emerged more recently. First, individuals with ASD may engage in less attention to people and joint attention because the act of looking at people is aversive. To the best of my knowledge, this notion was first proposed by Tinbergen and Tinbergen (1972). However, evidence does not provide consistent support for an aversion model across all affected children (e.g., Wing & Ricks, 1977; Mundy & Sigman, 1989c). Another possibility is that attention to people and joint attention may be attenuated in ASD not because it is aversive, but rather because is not sufficiently intrinsically rewarding (e.g., Chevallier, Kohls, Troiani, Brodkin, & Schultz, 2012; Dawson, Webb, & McPartland, 2005; Mundy, 1995). Third, social attention and joint attention may be attenuated not because they are not rewarding, but because the rewards of social attention are trumped by the even greater reward value (prioritization) of looking at objects among people with ASD (e.g., Hughes & Russell, 1993; McCleery, Akshoomoff, Dobkins, & Carver, 2009). Finally, a relatively new hypothesis has emerged with the understanding that joint attention involves self-referenced processing. The perception of attention to ourselves may be rewarding and serve as an organizational pivot for early joint attention development (Farroni, Massaccesi, & Francesca, 2002), as well as its developmental disturbance in ASD (Reddy, 2003). The role of motivation is difficult to study in the typical and atypical development of joint attention, but it is perhaps singularly important to consider. Hence this book returns to discussions of the topic in Chapters 5–8.

Brains Are Made for Sharing

In a very real sense, the capacity for joint attention and reference is a very basic dimension of human cognitive neurodevelopment (Mundy, 1995). It is related to a superordinate function, which is to process external or *exogenous* information about environment, and then relate that to processing of internal or *endogenous* information about the physiological and mental status of the body. This allows people and animals to develop goal-directed behaviors that respond to environmental information in ways that best meet their internal physiological and mental needs. The neural circuits involved in this most basic function are likely to include a dorsal attention system for exogenous information processing, a default system for endogenous information processing, and a frontoparietal control system to regulate which type of information processing is needed at a particular time in maintaining an adaptive behavioral stance in the world (Spreng, Sepulcre, Turner, Stevens, & Schacter, 2013).

Much of evolution has involved one elaboration or another of this endogenous–exogenous information-processing function of brains. Rather than depending upon the singular processing abilities of one individual, one line of neurodevelopmental elaboration in more social animals has resulted in different ways and means by which brains can share information (Wilson, 1975). This line of elaboration reaches an apparent zenith in the information-sharing functions of the human brain.

To the extent that this assertion is true, we can envision two related, but also unique, developmental paths in human brain development. One developmental path involves the growth of people's ability for the processing and integration of endogenous and exogenous information in isolation. Another function involves the growth of people's ability for the processing of exogenous and endogenous information not in isolation, but with other people to adopt a socially shared spotlight on information in the world. This type of shared or joint processing of information enables two or more individuals to adaptively pursue goals related to the environment that cannot be accomplished without collaboration or cooperation. Joint attention and the cognitive capacity for diverse, referential information sharing develops in some other animals as a cognitive foundation for joint action and collaborative behavior, but not nearly to the same extent that it has developed as part of the evolution of the human brain (e.g., Povinelli & Eddy, 1996; Pack & Herman, 2006; Tomasello, 2008).

Certainly the most recognizable manifestation of the evolution of this shared information-processing function in people is the development of symbolic thinking and language. In this regard, though, both data and theory compellingly argue that advances in the cognitive capacity to attend jointly to a common point of reference provides a *necessary*, albeit not sufficient, foundation for the emergence of human language and symbolic representational abilities (e.g., Adamson, 1995; Bruner, 1977; Colonnesi et al., 2010; Tomasello, 2008; Tomasello & Carpenter, 2007; Werner & Kaplan, 1963). There is also evidence that specific neural networks support the development of the human capacity to attend jointly to a common point of reference, and that these networks are distinct from language-specific networks (e.g., Carlin & Calder, 2013; Elison et al., 2013; Gordon et al., 2013; Grossmann & Johnson, 2010; Mundy, 2003; Mundy, Card, & Fox, 2000; Mundy & Jarrold, 2010; Parise & Csibra, 2012; Redcay, Kleiner, & Saxe, 2012; Redcay, Dodell-Feder, et al., 2013; Saito et al., 2010; Schilbach et al., 2010; Williams, Waiter, Perra, Perrett, & Whiten, 2005). To the best of my knowledge, neither theory nor data make a similarly compelling argument for a strong association of the information-sharing functions of facial expression with human language or symbolic development (e.g., Karmiloff-Smith, 1995; Paterson, Heim, Friedman, Choudhury, & Benasich, 2006).

The evolution of the ability to attend jointly to a common point of reference is thought to be a *domain-general cognitive function*. That is, it may play a role in language development, but its role in human development is not singular to language development. Rather, the cognitive process of joint attention is essential to the broader capacity for human teaching and learning (Bruner, 1995) and for relatedness as well as social competence (Mundy & Sigman, 2006). Indeed, theory suggests that joint attention plays a pivotal role in the types of learning with and from other people that is necessary for the formation of culture (Tomasello, Carpenter, Call, et al., 2005).

This pivotal role of joint attention in learning is as important to autism spectrum development as is its role in social relatedness. Joint attention is essential to human social learning, but in a manner distinct from what is typically referred to as *social learning*. Most often, s*ocial learning* refers to acquiring new information by observing others as models and by imitating the goal-related behaviors of the models (Bandura, 1962; Meltzoff, 2007). Imitation allows people to acquire information about adaptive bodily actions for problem solving more quickly and directly than individual exploration alone often allows.

Joint attention complements and extends this type of modeled or imitative social learning. It literally extends social learning opportunities beyond the body: It reflects the development of a cognitive capacity to extend our attention and minds beyond the immediacy of our bodies, in order to share information socially or to engage cooperatively with an object or event in space (Butterworth & Jarrett, 1991). This information-sharing facility of joint attention enables a far greater range of signaling and instructional activity among people than does imitation or facial expression (cf. Tomasello, 2008). In some sense, then, joint attention may be conceived as a cognitive facility for an elaborated or higher-order type of social learning that we may call *referential social learning*. Differences in joint attention in autism syndrome development often rise to a level indicative of a *referential social learning disability* (Mundy, Sullivan, & Mastergeorge, 2009).

The phenotype of ASD is often primarily described in terms of differences in social-affective features of human interaction. However, the differences in social communication dimensions of the human mind, such as joint attention, that characterize ASD do not only affect moment-to-moment social interaction. They also have an important impact on the development of cognitive mechanisms of referential social learning (Mundy & Crowson, 1997). Others have begun to recognize the benefits and validity of the concept of social learning differences as defining features of the social phenotype of ASD. For example, Butterworth and Kovas (2013) categorize ASD as one of the specific learning disabilities in discussing how a deeper understanding of learning in neurodevelopmental disorders may improve education for all people. I agree with this assertion. One theme of this book is to argue that the social phenotype of ASD may be usefully divided into an axis that reflects the development of social affect and engagement, and an axis that reflects the development of social learning. See Figure 2.1 for an illustration of this division.

As an example of the usefulness of this perspective, let us consider the types of information acquired from mouse models of autism. These provide a range of irreplaceable data on the possible biological mechanisms behind autism behavioral development. The face validity of the

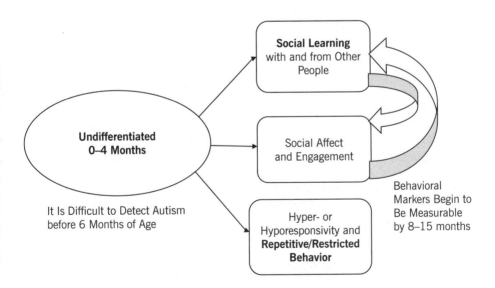

FIGURE 2.1. Illustration of the division of the social phenotype of autism into axes reflecting the development of behaviors and cognition involved in social learning and in social affect and engagement. The arrows illustrate the transactional or interactive nature of the two axes in development.

behaviors examined with mouse models often appears to be more closely associated with the social affect/engagement axis of the autism phenotype. However, we must keep in mind that dimensions such as social affiliation may only reflect part of the phenotype of ASD, and that other elements involved in the social learning axis of the phenotype may present additional targets and challenges for animal models. Similarly, when we conceptualize the neurodevelopment of autism, we may benefit from understanding more about how the neurodevelopment of the cognitive facility for reference fits in with other social brain processes, such as mentalizing about the thoughts of others, empathy, imitation, and the perception of animacy. My guess is that none of these dimensions is primary. Rather, all these dimensions may interact in the culmination of differences in the development of the social brain. We need to define and study the development of them all. If not, the internal validity of theory and research on a dimensional approach to ASD will be at risk. For example, if we do not recognize the distinct nature of joint referential cognition, how will we accommodate observations that problems in referential cognition and deictic shifting remain central to differences in social communication and learning among higher-functioning adolescents and adults with ASD (e.g., Mizuno et al., 2011; O'Connor & Klein, 2004)?

Cuthbert and Insel (2013) have acknowledged that no one approach, including the RDoC, is without problems. For example, the RDoC approach may lead to some investigations based on the availability of powerful concepts and paradigms regarding a dimension, rather than a clear link between a dimension and the central nature of the disorder. The probability of this type of error is multiplied when the connections between symptoms and critical underlying dimensions are not well understood. This, I think, is the case for the link between symptoms affecting joint attention in ASD and the dimension of the social-neurocognitive endophenotype that joint attention reflects in ASD. For example, although powerful concepts and paradigms exist for the study of face processing, they may be insufficient for the study of joint attention. To examine this assertion more critically, let us begin to consider the role of joint attention in ASD in more detail.

Joint Attention and the Evolution of the DSM Criteria for ASD

Although we have begun to look in many of the right places to describe the fundamental behavioral and psychological dimensions of autism, a profound understanding of what we have observed remains elusive. In no small measure, this is because the science of human social development is an emerging discipline. This is especially true for social-cognitive neuroscience and the science of early social development. Of course, a detailed understanding of the dynamics of early social development is critical if we want to understand the early-onset phase of autism.

As noted in Chapter 1, research in the late 1970s and early 1980s began to apply methods and concepts from the discipline of infant developmental psychology and psychiatry to uncover primary impairment dimensions associated with ASD in young children. For example, research led to the observations that imitation difficulties (Sigman & Ungerer, 1984) and the limited display of socially conventional object use in symbolic play (Wing, Gould, Yeates, & Brierley, 1977) were red flags for autism among preschool children. Imitation and play deficits were hypothesized to reflect an inability to mentally represent the actions of others and perhaps oneself in order to guide goal-directed behavior (e.g., Hobson, Lee, & Brown, 1999; Leslie, 1987; Rogers & Pennington, 1991; Ungerer & Sigman, 1981; Sigman & Ungerer, 1984).

The emergence of this information on early social development quickly began to have an impact on the diagnosis of autism. Soon after the publication of DSM-III (American Psychiatric Association, 1980), the criteria for autism underwent major changes in the publication of a revision (DSM-III-R; American Psychiatric Association, 1987). Some of these changes are illustrated in Table 2.3. DSM-III-R emphasized the social nature of autism by stipulating that affected individuals must display at least two symptoms of social impairment and at least one symptom of communication impairment to meet diagnostic criteria. The description of the social impairment of autism as a pervasive lack of responsiveness to others was also eliminated. Perhaps most importantly, multiple evidence-based social and cognitive symptoms were described for the first time, such as difficulties with imitation and symbolic play.

A more subtle change in the DSM-III-R criteria was that social and communication symptom items explicitly suggested that problems in initiating social communication behaviors, rather than just responsiveness to others, were also important to the nature of autism (see Table 2.3). This reflected observations that social initiations were especially problematic in, and even an important target of intervention for, children with autism (Koegel, Dyer, & Bell, 1987).

The increasingly rapid accumulation of new information on the social behavior of young children with autism led to additional changes in symptom descriptions with the publication of DSM-IV (American Psychiatric Association, 1994). Studies that had directly or indirectly begun to observe the presence and effects of social attention differences in infant development and in young children with autism were one powerful new

TABLE 2.3. The Evolution of the Social and Communication Symptoms of ASD in the American Psychiatric Association's DSM from 1980 to 2013

DSM-III: 1980

  B. Pervasive lack of responsiveness to other people (autism).
  C. Gross deficits in language development.
  D. If speech is present, peculiar speech patterns such as immediate and delayed echolalia, metaphorical language, pronoun reversal.

DSM-III-R: 1987

  A. Qualitative impairment in reciprocal social interaction . . . as manifested by the following: (1) marked lack of awareness of the existence or feelings of others . . . ; (2) no or abnormal **seeking** of comfort at times of distress . . . ; (3) no or impaired imitation . . . ; (4) no or abnormal social play . . . ; (5) gross impairment in ability to make peer friendships . . .
  B. Qualitative impairment in verbal and nonverbal communication and in imaginative activity . . . as manifested by the following: (1) no mode of communication, such as: communicative babbling, facial expression, gesture, mime, or spoken language; (2) markedly abnormal nonverbal communication, as in the use of eye-to-eye gaze, facial expression, body posture, or gestures to **initiate or modulate** social interaction . . . ; (3) absence of imaginative activity . . . ; (4) marked abnormalities in the production of speech, including volume, pitch, stress, rate, rhythm, and intonation . . . ; (5) marked abnormalities in the form or content of speech, including stereotyped and repetitive use of speech . . . ; (6) marked impairment in the ability to **initiate** or sustain conversation, despite adequate speech . . .

DSM-IV and DSM-IV-TR: 1994 and 2000

  A(1). Qualitative impairment in social interaction, as manifested by at least two of the following: (a) marked impairment in the use of multiple nonverbal behaviors such as eye-to-eye gaze, facial expression, body postures, and gestures to regulate social interaction; (b) failure to develop peer relationships appropriate to developmental level; (c) **a lack of spontaneous seeking to share enjoyment, interests, or achievements with other people (by a lack of showing, bringing, or pointing out objects of interest)**; (d) lack of social or emotional reciprocity.
  A(2). Qualitative impairment in communication as manifested by at least one of the following: (a) delay in or a total lack of the development of spoken language; (b) in individuals with adequate speech, marked impairment in the ability to **initiate** or sustain a conversation with others; (c) stereotyped and repetitive use of language or idiosyncratic language; (d) lack of varied, **spontaneous** social make-believe play or social imitative play appropriate to developmental level.

(continued)

TABLE 2.3. *(continued)*

DSM-5: 2013

   A. Persistent deficits in social communication and social interaction across
multiple contexts, as manifested by the following, currently or by history
(examples are illustrative, not exhaustive . . .): (1) Deficits in social-emotional
reciprocity, ranging, for example, from abnormal **social approach** and failure
of normal back-and-forth conversation; to **reduced sharing of interests,
emotions, or affect**; to failure to **initiate** or respond to social interactions. (2)
Deficits in nonverbal communicative behaviors used for social interaction,
ranging, for example, from poorly integrated verbal and nonverbal
communication; to abnormalities in eye contact and body language or deficits
in understanding and use of gestures; to a total lack of facial expressions
and nonverbal communication. (3) Deficits in developing, maintaining, and
understanding relationships, ranging, for example, from difficulties adjusting
behaviors to suit various social contexts; to difficulties in **sharing imaginative
play** or making friends; to absence of interest in peers.

Note. Words or phrases that are particularly applicable to the dimension of joint attention are
given in **boldface**.

source of information. For example, observations of what appeared to be
autism symptoms in children with congenital blindness had long indirectly
suggested that visual attention may play a role in the early expression and
development of ASD (e.g., Chess, 1977; Hobson et al., 1999). Research
also began to recognize the study of face processing as an important new
means for examining the social impairments of autism (Langdell, 1978;
Hobson et al., 1988). In addition to studies of visual attention, one study
of auditory attention raised the seminal hypothesis that the reward value
of orienting to people may also be different in children with ASD (Klin,
1991).

   This shift to the study of the role of attention and orienting in the
developmental etiology of ASD was consistent with the long-standing
notion that attention, especially visual attention, is a primary modality
of human social development (Bates et al., 1975; Rheingold, 1966; Robson, 1967; Scaife & Bruner, 1975). Infants increasingly gain volitional
control over their visual attention (display active vision) between 2 and
6 months of age (Canfield & Kirkham, 2001; Johnson, 1990, 1995). This
enables them to begin to exercise a goal-directed choice of information
to process, and to become aware of socially contingent responses to their
changes in their own line of regard. Infant gaze can, and often does,
elicit contingent social-behavioral responses from other people, such as
parental smiles, vocalizations, or gaze shifts. Infants' shifts toward and
away from other people are also among the first types of volitional actions

that infants use to control stimulation in order to self-regulate arousal and affect (Posner & Rothbart, 2007). By the end of the first year of life, aspects of social-cognitive development hinge on the information infants gather from processing the visual attention of others (e.g., Meltzoff & Brooks, 2008; Johnson et al., 2005), and on processing the responses of others to their own direction of gaze (Mundy & Newell, 2007).

Over the years, these lines of research have coalesced in the hypothesis that one essential dimension of autism reflects an early and abiding *neurodevelopmental disorder of social attention orienting* (e.g., Dawson et al., 2004; Klin, 1991; Klin, Jones, Schultz, Volkmar, & Cohen, 2002a; Mundy & Sigman, 1989a, 1989b; Mundy & Neal, 2000; Schultz, 2005). One of the first studies to *explicitly* study the frequency and duration with which children with ASD allocated visual attention to people *during social interactions* were studies of joint attention. This research began with the seminal observational study of Frank Curcio (1978), who reported that school-age children with autism regularly made eye contact and used gestures to make nonverbal requests directed to other people in a classroom. However, they rarely used eye contact and gestures to share experiences with others (e.g., to show objects to others).

These observations were quickly corroborated by four studies (Wetherby & Prutting, 1984; Loveland & Landry, 1986; Mundy, Sigman, Ungerer, & Sherman, 1986; Sigman, Mundy, Sherman, & Ungerer, 1986). The latter two studies included case controls for age, developmental disorder, and IQ. They indicated that 3- to 7-year-olds children with ASD displayed significantly lower frequencies of alternating eye contact (see Chapter 1, Figure 1.1, c1 through c3) to initiate sharing attention and experience with parents and unfamiliar testers. Children with ASD were also less adept at following the line of visual attention of other people who turned their head, shifted their gaze, and pointed to posters on a wall. However, analyses of the data suggested that problems with the tendency to initiate joint attention with alternating gaze were more powerful in discriminating children with ASD from children with other developmental disabilities than were problems in responding to joint attention (Mundy et al., 1986).

Curcio (1978) had also observed that children with autism did *not* display pervasive deficits in attention to other people. They would attend to others and engage in communicative acts when motivated to elicit aid in obtaining an object or event. On the other hand, they rarely did this to show an object to, or share their experience of an object or event with, others. Exactly the same pattern was observed in the subsequent structured observation of social interactions with younger children with ASD. Social attention disturbance was more pronounced when a child's goal was simply to look where others were looking, or to monitor whether others were sharing attention to objects or events that had captured the child's attention and interest. However, less evidence of a social attention disturbance was observed when children with ASD engaged in goal-related actions to initiate a request an object or event from another person, or to respond to a request from a social partner (Mundy et al., 1986).

Together, these five papers supported the hypothesis that a disruption in the development of the tendency to socially coordinate visual attention to objects and events, in order to share experiences with other people, was a central dimension of the early expression of autism (Curcio, 1978). As Chapter 3 describes, subsequent research indicated that joint attention measures were among the most sensitive behavioral markers for early identification of autism. Consequently, joint attention items have been included in the "gold standard" research-based diagnostic measures of ASD and experimental screening measures. Moreover, research suggested that the initiation of experience sharing in joint attention may be a stronger marker of ASD than is responding to joint attention, or gaze direction of other people (Mundy et al., 1986; Mundy, Sigman, & Kasari, 1994).

Whether or not this research was directly considered in the 1984 iteration of DSM is not clear. However, for the first time, a functionally specific description of a type of social symptom and dimension reflecting the initiation of joint attention was included in DSM-IV. Individuals affected by ASD were said to display a "lack of spontaneous seeking to share enjoyment, interests, or achievements with other people (e.g., by a lack of showing, bringing, or pointing out objects of interest)" (American Psychiatric Association, 1994, p. 70; see Table 2.3). The text of DSM-IV did not make an explicit connection between this symptom description and the dimension of joint attention. Nevertheless, this description of a lack of spontaneous seeking to share socially with other people "as indicated by a lack of showing . . . or pointing" was virtually an operational definition of the differences in initiating joint attention that characterize early autism syndrome development (Mundy, Sullivan, & Mastergeorge, 2009).

The most recent revision of the diagnostic criteria for ASD (DSM-5; American Psychiatric Association, 2013) has taken another step toward recognizing the role of joint attention in the development of autism. In the text on diagnostic features, DSM-5 states: "An early feature of autism spectrum disorder is impaired joint attention manifested by a lack of pointing, showing, or bringing objects to share interest with others, or failure to follow someone's pointing or eye gaze" (p. 54). This is the first explicit use of the term *joint attention* in the nosology. Moreover, the three new "severity levels for autism spectrum disorder" emphasize problems with initiation of social behaviors, from "difficulty initiating social interactions" to "limited initiation of social interactions" to "very limited initiation of social interactions, and minimal response to social overtures from others" (p. 52). Again, this is consistent with the observation that the initiation of experience sharing in joint attention may be a stronger marker of ASD than is responding to joint attention, or gaze direction of other people (Mundy et al., 1986; Mundy, Sigman, & Kasari, 1994).

Along with these advances in diagnostic description, however, it seems to me that the social communication criteria have become a bit less specific in DSM-5. Even though joint attention is noted in the text as an "early feature" of ASD, the succinct portrayal of that feature as "a lack of spontaneous seeking to share enjoyment, interests, or achievements with other people" has been deleted from the specific symptom description of ASD in DSM-5. Instead, it seems to have been incorporated into a compound criterion of "Deficits in social-emotional reciprocity, ranging, for example, from abnormal social approach and failure of normal back-and-forth conversation; to reduced sharing of interests, emotions, or affect; to failure to initiate or respond to social interactions" (p. 50; see Table 2.3).

Thus many of the changes in DSM-5 reflect possible advances in the diagnostic description of ASD. Yet the precise description of the social symptoms of ASD in the DSM is still an evolving process. The absence of any formal inclusion of joint attention as a distinct symptom dimension in DSM-5 illustrates that we have yet to reach consensus on the significance of this dimension of mental development in the science of ASD. Ironically, while DSM-5 was not yet clear on the role of joint attention, many of the "gold-standard" diagnostic and screening instruments for ASD emphasize joint attention measurement, at least among preschool children. The many studies on these instruments provide one line of compelling support for the validity of the joint attention symptom dimension in ASD, which is described in Chapter 3.

Joint Attention in Symptom Assessment and Risk Identification

One of the benefits of the NIMH RDoC system is that it emphasizes carefully establishing the construct validity of dimensions considered to be central to clinical differences in human mental health and development. *Construct validity* refers to the accumulation of clear evidence indicating that a dimension (1) can be accurately and reliably measured; (2) provides meaningful and distinctive information about the phenotype and/or course of a clinical difference in mental health and development; and (3) in the case of the RDoC system, reflects unique biological and psychological processes distinguishing it from other important dimensions of mental health and human development. This chapter considers the validity of the dimension of joint attention in autism spectrum development, with regard to whether it provides reliable and uniquely meaningful information for the diagnosis and identification of ASD. The degree to which joint attention reflects unique information about psychological and biological processes is considered to some degree in this chapter, but is examined in more detail throughout the remaining chapters of the book.

I begin this chapter by providing additional details about the history of the recognition of joint attention as a unique dimension of both human development in general and the human nature of ASD.

Joint Attention and Defining the Social Nature of Autism

Well before infants learn to use symbols and language to communicate with other people, they begin to share information spontaneously with others. One way they do this is by coordinating their visual–spatial attention, with another person, to an object or event. This seemingly straightforward task is characterized by a significant level of complex cognitive processing, especially for infants. Recall that it demands the development of the ability to (1) attend to and process the direction of visual attention of another person; (2) monitoring and control of one's own attention between the other person and the common visual referent (i.e., the object or event) somewhere in the environment; and (3) processing of information about the object or event. Because of the three elements, this task has often been referred to as *triadic attention* (e.g., Adamson, 1995). However, recall that attention is not just orienting to an object, event, or idea, but a means of facilitating information processing about a specific subset of information in the world or our minds. So joint attention may be best conceived as triadic attention *and* information processing (Mundy, Sullivan, & Mastergeorge, 2009).

Mastering each of these elements individually, and then functionally coordinating their rapid, unified implementation in social interactions, are not small tasks for infants. It takes years to develop the optimal cognitive control of this mental ability. Infants are not born with this ability, but its maturation begins early and rapidly between the second and eighth months of development (e.g., Gredebäck, Fikke, & Melinder, 2010; Elison et al., 2013; Mundy, 1995), and continues to play a role in human behavior and development thereafter (e.g., Böckler, Knoblich, & Sebanz, 2012).

The recognition of this cognitive dimension's development began with several fundamental empirical observations. Decades ago, research indicated that most infants probably learn to use eye contact, gaze direction, and gesture initiation to indicate or show objects, as well as to request objects or events, by 8–12 months of age (Bates, Benigni, Bretherton, Camaioni, & Volterra, 1979). A seminal study also indicated that infants' ability to follow the direction of gaze and head turns of a social partner increased systematically between 6 and 18 months of age (Scaife & Bruner, 1975). This particular observation was groundbreaking at the time. It was inconsistent with the prevailing notion of *egocentrism* (Piaget, 1952), or the cognitive hypothesis that infants could not differentiate or appreciate the dual perspectives of self and other until after the second year of life. Scaife and Bruner's (1975) observations suggested that infants begin to differentiate self- and other-attention very early in life. Moreover, this self–other cognitive differentiation is followed by their slow accrual of the ability to align their own visual perspective deliberately with another person's to an object or event in space (Butterworth & Jarrett, 1991).

Bruner (1975) proposed the term *joint attention* for this cognitive domain of infant development. He and his colleagues recognized that the ability of infants to *coordinate their attention with others* allows caregivers to direct the infants' attention more systematically. This in turn allows the caregivers to isolate and highlight a much wider range of environmental features than if the infants ignore the caregivers' attention-directing efforts. Hence Bruner and colleagues recognized that the emergence of joint attention ability allows infants and caregivers to adopt *co-reference* to the same object or event, and that this ability is pivotal to increased sophistication of social interaction, social information exchange (instruction), and caregivers' scaffolding of infants' learning (especially early vocabulary learning) (Bruner, 1995).

The aim of the research by Bruner and his team, that led to the recognition of joint attention, was to understand how infants learn. Instead of studying only how knowledge is acquired, however, Bruner's research group wanted to understand how the ability to *share acquired knowledge* develops, because this is essential to all forms of pedagogy (Bruner, 1995). Their work suggested that the emergence of joint attention marked a critical turning point in some then-unknown set of early cognitive processes that enabled infants to benefit more effectively from caregivers' scaffolding or instruction. Indeed, Bruner, along with others before him (e.g., Werner & Kaplan, 1963), understood that the development of the capacity to adopt a common point of view (*shared reference*) in the physical world might be necessary for the development of the human capacity to adopt a common point of mental reference, and hence for the development of symbolic thinking and of language.

Elizabeth Bates and her research team arrived at a very similar perspective on joint attention and its role in language development in a related set of studies (Bates et al., 1979). Bates and her collaborators were interested in the study of the development of *pragmatics*, or the functions of communication. They observed that the development of joint attention is expressed in different functional forms in infancy. Infants engage in joint attention in the service of declarative or imperative functions of social communication (Bates et al., 1979). In a declarative function, infants use their line of regard and gestures to *share their experience* of an object or event (e.g., their interest) with another person. The prototype of this declarative function is the *act of showing* to share the experience of an object or event with someone. The tendency of children to share what is of interest to them with others had also been recognized by Rheingold, Hay, and West (1976) as a distinct social communication function that dramatically increased in rate among children by 2 years of age. Bates's research group later recognized that, like receptive and expressive verbal communication development (Bates, 1993), joint attention ability develops as both expressive and receptive behaviors in infancy that are affected by common and distinct cognitive and motivational factors.

The Development of Clinical Measures of Joint Attention

Beginning in the late 1970s, structured observation measures of preverbal communication were created to assess development of both expressive (self-initiated) and responsive forms of the declarative functions of joint attention in infancy. One of the first systematic measurement systems was the Early Social Communication Scales (ESCS; Seibert, Hogan, & Mundy, 1982). The ESCS was designed to measure both *initiating joint attention* (IJA) and *responding to joint attention* (RJA). The ESCS also incorporated another distinction: In addition to being designed to measure joint attention (which serves to specify a referent in order to show or share information), it was also designed to measure children's capacity to coordinate attention to request assistance in obtaining an object or event, or to respond to such requests from others. Bates and her colleagues (1979) pointed out that the former serves a declarative function ("See that!") and the latter serves an imperative function ("I want that!"). They suggested that these very different nonverbal communication and cognitive functions are likely to reflect distinctly different facets of early social development (Bates et al., 1979). Differences between these behaviorally similar but psychologically different nonverbal joint attention and requesting behaviors have been illustrated in Chapter 1 (see Figure 1.1).

The ESCS was created by Jeff Seibert and Anne Hogan at a laboratory for translational research on infant attention at the Debbie School of the University of Miami Debbie Institute. The Debbie School served (and still serves) preschoolers with moderate to severe motor and cognitive impairments. Their motor impairments made the use of most available cognitive assessments and intervention approaches impractical, because almost all the assessments and interventions employed at the time required infants to manipulate objects. So Seibert, Hogan, and their graduate student (myself) began to develop an early assessment and intervention curriculum that focused on joint attention and preverbal communication skill development. This resulted in the ESCS, which organized precise and reliable observations of joint attention and social attention coordination into a measurement instrument that could also be used to guide to early intervention (Seibert et al., 1982). A lasting contribution of the ESCS, along with several related measures (see Stone, Coonrod, & Ousley, 1997; Wetherby, Allen, Cleary, Kublin, & Goldstein, 2002), was that joint attention assessment turned out to be especially powerful in the study of developmental disorders such as ASD.

Applications of Joint Attention Measures to the Study of ASD

As noted in Chapter 2, Frank Curcio (1978) was the first to observe that joint attention disturbance was characteristic of individuals with ASD. In a field observation study, he noted that 50% of a sample of elementary-school-age children with ASD systematically used eye contact and conventional gestures in their classrooms to express their requests. In contrast, few if any children with ASD displayed the use of eye contact or gestures to initiate nonverbal declaratives or joint attention bids. Curcio's observations were groundbreaking for at least two reasons. In particular, he deserves much credit for the origin of the hypothesis that impairments in the capacity to initiate joint attention and declarative communicative functions could be central to the nature of the social impairments in autism.

Following Curcio's observations, work in the laboratory of Marian Sigman at UCLA provided some of the first case-controlled comparative studies of joint attention in preschool children with ASD, age- and IQ-matched children with IDD, and mental-age-matched children with typical development. These studies indicated that the children with ASD displayed far fewer joint attention behaviors than the children in either control group did, regardless of whether these behaviors were assessed in structured ESCS administration with a tester (Mundy et al., 1986) or in observations of semistructured parent–child interactions (Sigman et al., 1986). Furthermore, replicating Curcio's findings, children with ASD did not display evidence of low frequencies of the use of eye contact and gestures to request objects or to take turns with social partners (e.g., to roll a car or ball back and forth), compared to the children with IDD (Mundy et al., 1986). This suggested that a specific functional disturbance of declarative, rather than imperative, referential cognitive development was a specific feature of ASD not observed in children with other developmental delays or differences.

In these studies, the children with ASD did not display pervasive differences from the children with IDD in eye contact or social communication behaviors. Instead, they displayed a more nuanced pattern of syndrome-specific strengths and weaknesses in their social behaviors. As noted, they displayed comparable levels of eye contact in requesting and turn taking. However, an eye contact difference specific to the children with ASD was clearly manifested in their diminished spontaneous use of alternating gaze to initiate sharing of experience of a mechanical toy with the tester. Again, this type of alternating gaze behavior has been illustrated in Figure 1.1.

We cannot yet definitively describe why a child does or does not engage in IJA during a social interaction. Nevertheless, ESCS testers often arrived at the impression that IJA behaviors signaled a child's desire (motivation) and/or goal (intent) to engage with an unfamiliar tester to share the experience of an object or event, or to elicit attention spontaneously to the child's own experience of an object or event. Consequently, in a subsequent study, it was not too surprising to observe that lower frequencies of IJA via alternating eye contact in young children were significantly related to parents' independent perceptions of their children's *social relatedness* on an ASD symptom checklist (Mundy et al., 1994). Interestingly, the evidence of a significant association between IJA and social relatedness was as strong for children with typical development as it was for children with autism spectrum development. However, other requesting-related eye contact measures were not associated with social relatedness.

This was the first report of a link between independent observations of joint attention and parent ratings of social symptoms in children with ASD. This observation was consistent with an idea proposed earlier (Mundy & Sigman, 1989a): We had suggested that measures of joint attention in young children with autism appeared to provide an operational definition of what Kanner (1943) had described as the cardinal impairment in relatedness and positive affective contact with others in ASD.

The idea that IJA might be related to a disturbance in positive social-affective contact in autism was more directly supported by research on the role of sharing affect during joint attention. Kasari et al. (1990) observed that about 60% of the IJA bids displayed by typical toddlers and preschool children with IDD involved the conveyance of positive affect to an unfamiliar tester on the ESCS. Alternatively, Kasari et al. (1990) observed that positive affect sharing was much less frequently part of the IJA behaviors displayed by children with autism. It was not the case, though, that the children with autism displayed significantly lower positive affect in requesting or turn-taking interactions than comparison children. Hence it was unlikely that the diminished positive affect in joint attention reflected a general aversion to social interactions or a pervasive decrease in the display of positive affect. Instead, this research suggested that an important component of IJA and its disturbance in ASD involved the preschool development of the tendency to share positive affect with other people.

Subsequent data confirmed that most of the IJA bids observed for typically developing infants on the ESCS involved sharing positive affect about the experience of an object. However, only a minority of initiating behavior requests did so (Mundy, Kasari, & Sigman, 1992). More recent evidence indicates that the onset of the systematic conveyance of positive affect in IJA bids begins to develop early in life, at about 8–10 months of age (Venezia, Messinger, Thorp, & Mundy, 2004), and is associated with later social outcomes in typical development (Parlade et al., 2009). Thus joint attention impairments in ASD, in part, reflect what are likely to be early-arising differences in the tendency to socially share positive affective experiences of objects or events. And thus motivation factors—specifically, sensitivity to the reward value of joint attention—may play a role in its disturbance in ASD (Mundy, 1995). I return to this idea in subsequent sections of this chapter and especially in Chapters 5 and 8.

The early research in the Sigman lab also revealed another important facet of joint attention development in children with ASD: The diagnostic differences in joint attention displayed by a group of 4-year-olds with ASD were stable over time. They were observed both at an initial assessment and then 12 months later at the follow-up assessment (Mundy, Sigman, & Kasari, 1990). Hence joint attention disturbance appeared to be a chronic feature of the preschool phenotype of ASD. Moreover, this observation demonstrated the test–retest reliability of observations of joint attention in research on ASD. Subsequent research has also documented the test–retest reliability of joint attention in preschool samples of children with typical development (e.g., Mundy et al., 2007).

The test–retest reliability observation was important, but the Mundy et al. (1990) study revealed something equally important about joint attention in autism spectrum development. The initial measure of frequency of joint attention predicted individual differences in language development 12 months later in the children with ASD. Other measures (measures of social turn taking, eye contact, and gestural request; initial language assessments; and initial IQ/mental age assessments) did not predict language development in that study of children with ASD.

Differences in RJA and IJA Development

By the early 1990s, research groups charged with developing more standardized and reliable research-based ASD diagnostic methods, such as the team led by Catherine Lord, considered joint attention to be one of several promising dimensions. This resulted in the inclusion of joint attention items in the development of the "gold standard" instruments: the Autism Diagnostic Interview–Revised (ADI-R; Lord et al., 1994), and the revised Autism Diagnostic Observation Schedule (ADOS-2; Gotham, Risi, Pickles, & Lord, 2007; Lord, Rutter, DiLavore, Risi, et al., 2002). These instruments include multiple items assessing joint attention items, and the revised ADOS has adopted the terms *IJA* and *RJA* from the ESCS to refer to some of the relevant items.

The inclusion of joint attention items in the ADI-R and revised ADOS-2 led to an important interaction of clinical and basic research information on the role of joint attention in ASD. Research indicated that that difficulty with RJA became less evident in children with ASD as their language or mental age level exceeded what was typically observed in 30-month-old children (Gillespie-Lynch, Elias, Escudero, Hutman, & Johnson, 2013; Mundy et al., 1994; Nation & Penny, 2008; see Figure 3.1). IJA differences, on the other hand, did not appear to begin to remit at 30 months. Instead, evidence of differences in IJA in children with autism continued to be observed through the preschool period and even through adolescence (e.g., Charman, 2003; Dawson et al., 2004; Hobson & Hobson, 2007; Mundy et al., 1986; Sigman et al., 1999). Since IJA and RJA are assessed in the ADOS, it became possible to test whether this dissociation in joint attention development was apparent in large samples of children with ASD. In their revision of the ADOS, Gotham et al. (2007) examined data from over 1,000 children with ASD and reported that both RJA and IJA were useful in the diagnosis of children with no words. However, once children developed the use of words, the validity of differences in RJA

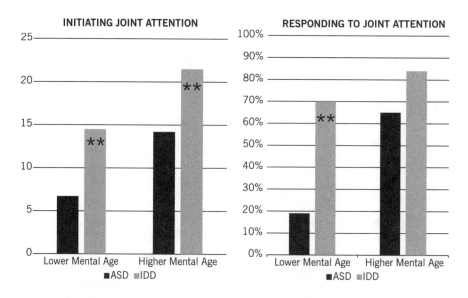

FIGURE 3.1. Differences in sensitivity of measures of IJA and RJA as characteristics of ASD in preschool children with different levels of mental development. The left panel shows that measures of IJA distinguished groups of 3- and 4-year-old children with ASD from children with IDD, regardless of whether they had lower mental ages (17 months, average) or higher mental ages (37.5 months, average). The right panel illustrates that measures of RJA distinguished the 3-year-old diagnostic groups with lower mental ages, but not the groups with higher mental ages. Data from Mundy, Sigman, and Kasari (1994).

decreased significantly, but the validity of IJA remained. (See further discussion of this below.)

This pattern of data does not suggest that RJA impairments are not important in the development of ASD. On the contrary, RJA impairments are critical to many aspects of development in children with ASD, not the least of which is early language development (e.g., Bono, Daley, & Sigman, 2004; Sigman & McGovern, 2005). However, early IJA deficits appear to tap into a somewhat different facet of the dimension of joint attention in ASD associated with evidence of developmentally chronic differences (Charman, 2003; Gangi, Ibañez, & Messinger, 2014; Kasari et al., 1990; Kasari, Freeman, & Paparella, 2007; Lord, Floody, Anderson, & Pickles, 2003; Mundy et al., 1994; Naber et al., 2008; Sigman & Ruskin, 1999).

The recognition of the differential development of forms of joint attention in ASD is consistent with studies of children with typical development. RJA and IJA display distinctively different patterns of growth, with RJA increasing with age and mental age between 9 and 18 months, and IJA displaying a flatter, less age-related pattern of growth (Mundy et al., 2007). IJA and RJA measures also have distinctly different patterns of correlates with measures of anterior and posterior cortical activity (Caplan et al., 1993; Henderson et al., 2002; Mundy et al., 2000; Redcay et al., 2012), attention and behavior inhibition and switching (Dawson et al., 2002; Griffith, Pennington, Wehner, & Rogers, 1999; Nichols, Fox, & Mundy, 2005; Vaughan Van Hecke et al., 2012), attention regulation (Morales, Mundy, Crowson, Neal, & Delgado, 2005), self-monitoring (Nichols et al., 2005), the expression of positive affect associated with social motivation (Kasari et al., 1990; Mundy, Kasari, & Sigman, 1992; Vaughan et al., 2003), and learning and reward sensitivity (Corkum & Moore, 1998; Nichols et al., 2005). These data indicate that IJA and RJA measure unique as well as common facets of the development of the dimension of joint attention (Mundy & Newell, 2007).

The differences in RJA and IJA growth create a challenge for how we study and explain joint attention in autism spectrum development. First, it may not be valid to study either RJA or IJA in isolation, and then draw wide-ranging conclusions about the nature of joint attention in ASD. Second, any explanation of causes of joint attention differences in ASD must rise to the challenge of explaining why RJA differences remit but IJA differences remain more chronic. For example, how does a primary disturbance in social orienting or face processing allow for RJA development, but more chronic effects on IJA? Similarly, how does the social-cognitive hypothesis of joint attention account for the dissociated patterns of RJA and IJA in the developmental phenotype of ASD?

The observation of the more chronic nature of IJA differences in ASD is very consistent with the long-standing observations from intervention research that a disturbance of the spontaneous generation of social behaviors—as much as, or more than, a disturbance of perception and response to the social behaviors of others—is central to ASD (Koegel, Carter, & Koegel, 2003). The importance of differences in the tendency to initiate social behaviors has also been observed in research on infant siblings of children with ASD (Zweigenbaum et al., 2005).

Recall from Chapter 2 that impairments in responsiveness were deemphasized and that the centrality of initiating deficits, such as IJA, was highlighted in the DSM-IV nosology (American Psychiatric Association, 1994). Unfortunately, though, the potential significance of the distinction between impaired responsiveness and impairment of the spontaneous generation of behavior, such as IJA, is still not fully appreciated in the field. Nevertheless, research on the dimension of joint attention in ASD emphasizes this observation, and the importance of joint attention as one of the defining dimensions of ASD has been emphasized in the research conducted to improve the diagnostic algorithms for the ADOS (Gotham et al., 2007). I now discuss this research in more detail.

The Joint Attention Factor in the Revised ADOS-2

As mentioned briefly above, the revised ADOS-2 includes both RJA and IJA items. More specifically, it includes both types of items in the diagnostic algorithms of Module 1 for younger nonverbal children, but includes only IJA items in Module 1 for children with some language and Module 2 for older or more developmentally advanced children. Hence the significance of the disturbance in IJA remains a focus of standardized diagnostic assessments such as the revised ADOS-2, at least as applied to children at the preschool level of development. Indeed, many of the items that make up the Social Affect (SA) factor-based scale assess the dimension of joint attention—so many that there may be a distinctive Joint Attention factor within many preschool assessments with the revised ADOS-2. To defend this assertion, we need to review some of the technical details of the analyses conducted to revise the ADOS.

A validation study of the ADOS-2 assessments of 1,191 children with ASD and 279 children with non-ASD delays (Gotham et al., 2007). These data were drawn from clinics at three different universities where Cathy Lord had worked, to the very significant benefit of children and families affected by ASD. Examinations of correlations among all items (factor analysis) revealed the now-familiar cluster of SA scale items and the cluster of Restricted, Repetitive Behaviors (RRB) items. These scales reflect what to many are the two superordinate behavioral dimensions of ASD.

It is instructive, however, to examine some of the details that arose in confirming that these two factors reflected the nature of ASD in children with preschool levels of development. The ADOS system uses different modules to assess children with different developmental levels. The younger two groups of children are assessed with Modules 1 and 2. The items in the SA factor for these modules are presented in Table 3.1. Remarkably, in analyzing the data for Modules 1 and 2, Gotham et al. (2007) reported that "a third factor called 'Joint Attention' also emerged from the data analyses" (p. 618). They continued, "This factor was comprised of pointing, gesturing, showing, initiating joint attention, and unusual eye contact in the *Module 1, Some Words [group]* and both *Module 2 groups, and* response to joint attention, gesturing, showing, initiating joint attention, and unusual eye contact in the *Module 1, No Words group*" (p. 618, emphasis added).

Gotham et al. (2007) reported that this factor was not included in the standard scoring of the ADOS-2 because the Joint Attention factor was not present in their analyses of Module 3 data. This may reflect a developmental change in the degree to which joint attention impairment is part of the phenotype of ASD in older and/or higher-functioning children. Alternatively, with the exception of the "shared enjoyment" item, there are no items in Module 3 that I recognize as clearly tapping the dimension of joint attention. So the lack of a Joint Attention factor in Module 3 probably reflects the lack of specific items scored for joint attention in this module.

The lack of joint attention items in Module 3 does not reflect an oversight on the part of this research team. Rather, it reflects the zeitgeist of recognizing joint attention as a milestone of early development, but not necessarily a feature of later development. This is an unfortunate and significant gap in the science of ASD, because it confuses the field about

TABLE 3.1. Joint Attention and the Social Affect Factor in the Revised ADOS

Module 1 (no words)	Module 1 (some words) and Module 2
• Gaze and other behaviors	• Gaze and other behaviors
• Facial expression	• Facial expression
• Frequency of vocalization	• Frequency of vocalization
• Quality of social overtures	• Quality of social overtures
• Shared enjoyment	• Shared enjoyment
• **Unusual eye contact**	• **Unusual eye contact**
• **RJA**	• **Pointing**
• **Gestures**	• **Gestures**
• **Showing**	• **Showing**
• **IJA**	• **IJA**

Note. Items loading on the Joint Attention factor are given in **boldface**.

the distinctive and important nature of the joint attention dimension. For example, Gotham et al. (2007) noted that the Joint Attention factor was consistent across Modules 1 and 2 of the ADOS, supporting the unique nature of this dimension in early diagnostic assessment. These authors also noted that this factor or dimension of the revised ADOS-2 may be of interest to some researchers and clinicians. However, at this writing, I could find no evidence of research with the revised ADOS-2 Joint Attention factor score. I think some of the most important applications of the revised ADOS-2 Joint Attention factor score may lie in what it has to offer genomic studies of ASD. I return to this idea in Chapter 8.

Of course, one study does not a scientific finding make, even if it is as large as the study described by Gotham et al. (2007). Gotham et al. (2008) have reported a partial replication of their 2007 observations. This second study was based on data from 1,068 children with ASD and 214 children with non-ASD delays, collected by independent research groups from multiple universities participating in two initiatives funded by the National Institutes of Health: the Collaborative Programs of Excellence in Autism (CPEAs) and Studies to Advance Autism Research and Treatment (STAART).

Gotham et al. (2008) reported that a distinct Joint Attention factor did not emerge in the analyses of Module 1 data. However, a Joint Attention factor was prominent and important in the analyses of Module 2 data. These analyses were conducted on a relatively young sample with some language and revealed that the expected two-factor solution, SA and RRB, did not emerge in the initial analyses. Instead, the SA factor emerged, but the RRB factor did not. Rather than the RRB factor, a second factor composed of pointing and IJA items was observed. So Gotham et al. (2008) examined the possibility that the Module 2 data for the revised ADOS would be best described by a three-factor model. This model turned out to be the best fit to the data: It included the expected SA and RRB factors, but also an "approximate joint attention factor" (p. 646).

These two large-scale factor-analytic studies of the revised ADOS-2 reveal several important facets of our current knowledge of joint attention as a unique symptom dimension in the development of ASD. First, joint attention items are included in the revised ADOS-2, and they appear to reflect a unique dimension of the phenotype of ASD relative to the SA and RRB dimensions. Second, the Joint Attention factor was observed in revised ADOS-2 modules that are applicable to children in the early preschool phases of language development. This may mean that joint attention only applies to ASD diagnostic assessment specific to this phase of development. Alternatively, it may mean that we are not yet well versed in how to assess this dimension in older children, but could benefit from research exploring this issue much more thoroughly than has been the case to date. The ways and means of assessing any dimension, such as joint attention, are likely to change over children's age and development. Evidence of this is provided by data indicating that infant RJA measures may be useful in assessing the Joint Attention factor in preverbal children, but not so useful in assessing this factor with more verbal Module 1 children and Module 2 children (Gotham et al., 2007).

Diagnostic Screening in the Second Year

Standardized measures such as the ADI-R and the revised ADOS-2 have become the "gold standards" for autism assessment because of evidence indicating that they have *high sensitivity*; in other words, they accurately identify children with ASD, with few missed cases (false negatives). There is also evidence of their *high specificity*, which means that they also accurately identify children with delays or typical development who are not affected by ASD. So these measures also lead to few false-positive identifications of ASD (Lord et al., 1994; Gotham et al., 2007, 2008). To reach their high levels of sensitivity and specificity, though, these instruments are comprehensive. The disadvantage of this feature is that they are relatively time-consuming to administer and demand systematic training for their accurate use. Therefore, their use for screening toddlers and preschoolers to promote the early identification of ASD is limited.

Early identification of specific types of developmental differences is challenging. Unfortunately, there are many children who display developmental delays in the first 2 years of life. One estimate indicates that as many 13% of all 9-month-olds exhibit some form of developmental delay (Rosenberg, Zhang, & Robinson, 2008). Not all of these children are affected by ASD. Indeed, recent prevalence estimates suggest that 1 in 68 children, or 1.4% of all children, are affected by ASD (CDC, 2014). So in the population of 9-month-olds who exhibit some form of developmental delays, perhaps as many as 10% may be affected by ASD. How can we efficiently identify this subset of children with symptoms of developmental differences equally well in all communities?

The solution is to develop instruments for children under 2 years of age that are quicker to administer and need less training than the ADI-R and revised ADOS-2 do, but that retain good sensitivity and specificity for identifying risk for ASD. Several such brief screening instruments have been developed. They contain 30 items or fewer and only require a modest amount of training for their appropriate use. Many of these screening instruments also include joint attention measures to identify young children with ASD and distinguish them from children who have developmental delays but not ASD. Among the first of these measures to be developed were the Checklist for Autism in Toddlers (CHAT; Baron-Cohen et al., 1996) and the Modified CHAT or M-CHAT (Robins, Fein, Barton, & Green, 2001). The latter is now widely used in research and clinical screening for symptoms of ASD in toddlers.

The CHAT was developed by a famous ASD research group at Cambridge University in the United Kingdom, led by Simon Baron-Cohen. It was a very brief (nine-item) parent report screening instrument, supplemented by five clinician or tester observations of a child. Baron-Cohen et al. (1996) reported that three items on the CHAT—the degree to which 18-month-olds engaged in gaze monitoring (RJA), protodeclarative pointing (IJA), and pretending—correctly identified 10 toddlers affected by ASD in a sample of 16,000 toddlers who were screened. At the time, this was a remarkable and truly seminal observation. It suggested that observations of joint attention skill development at 18 months could be a strong factor in the identification of ASD before the age of 2 years.

Robins et al. (2001) moved the development of early screening for ASD forward by modifying the CHAT. They eliminated the clinician/tester observations, expanded the parent report to include 23 items, and added a follow-up protocol by phone to clarify item responses for children who appeared from the initial screening to be at risk. Robins and colleagues also focused on screening at 24 months rather than 18 months. All of this was done in the hope of improving the instrument's sensitivity and specificity for the early identification of ASD.

The efforts of this research group paid off. Robins et al. (2001) screened 1,293 two-year-olds, of whom 139 (11%) were initially identified as at risk. The parents of these toddlers received the follow-up CHAT protocol, which eliminated the need to refer 74 of the at-risk children for more comprehensive assessments. Of the remaining 65 at-risk children, comprehensive diagnostic testing revealed that 39 were positive for ASD and that the remaining 19 were affected by a developmental disorder other than ASD. Finally, and most pertinently to the issue at hand, six items were identified as most powerful in the early identification of ASD. The six items pertained to three apparent dimensions of behavior: three "joint attention [items] (protodeclarative pointing, following a point, and bringing objects to show parent), [two] social relatedness [items] (interest in other children and imitation), and [one] communication [item] (responding to name)" (Robins et al., 2001, p. 141).

Numerous studies have subsequently replicated the validity of the M-CHAT for the early identification of ASD in toddlers from 16 to 30 months of age, across cultures and in large-scale community samples as well as in clinic-based research (e.g., Chlebowski, Robins, Barton, & Fein, 2013; Pinto-Martin et al., 2008; Roux et al., 2012; Ventola et al., 2007). Some limitations have been observed in its application in rural settings

(Scarpa et al., 2013) and in extremely-low-gestational-age infants with major motor, cognitive, visual, and hearing impairments (Kuban et al., 2009). However, in most applications, the M-CHAT and especially its joint attention measures enable the early identification of risk for ASD—and, equally importantly, the differential early identification of risk for ASD versus other developmental disorders.

The importance of joint attention to M-CHAT was emphasized in the report by Ventola et al. (2007), which provided a detailed examination of the items that best enabled the early differential identification of risk for ASD versus other developmental disorders. This research team took the important step of controlling for possible language differences among children, to provide a more precise estimate of the M-CHAT items that differentiated children at risk for these two types of disorders. When the researchers controlled for language, the specificity of the M-CHAT was based on three items involving joint attention (pointing for interest, following a point, and pointing to request) and response to name (see Ventola et al., 2007, p. 433).

Ventola et al. (2007) also examined the 1999 version of the ADOS items that best differentiated the two groups after language was controlled for: "All of the items from the reciprocal social interaction domain (eye contact, shared enjoyment, showing, initiation of joint attention, response to joint attention, and quality of social overtures) and one of the items from the communication domain (pointing) were found to significantly differentiate the groups" (p. 433). The authors went on to note that showing was the single most powerful individual item in discriminating the groups, and they concluded that joint attention items were especially important in differentiating young children with ASD from those with non-ASD developmental disorders. This is very much the same conclusion reached by several research groups in the 1980s (Loveland & Landry, 1986; Mundy et al., 1986; Sigman et al., 1986; Wetherby & Prutting, 1984).

Several other promising early screening or even early diagnostic instruments have been developed, and many if not all of these include joint attention assessments. For example, the Screening Tool for Autism in Two-Year-Olds (STAT; Stone, Coonrod, Turner, & Pozdol, 2004) may be sensitive for ASD in children as young as 14 months (Stone et al., 2008). The STAT measures four dimensions: social play, joint attention for requesting, joint attention for directing attention (IJA), and imitation. Another instrument, the Social Orienting Continuum and Response Scale (Mosconi, Resnick, Mesibov, & Piven, 2009), provides a method for more quantitative scoring from video recordings of revised ADOS-2 Modules 1 and 2. The derived scores include a Joint Attention dimension (IJA and RJA items), as well as Social Referencing (looking at faces), Social Smiling, and Responding to Name. However, to my knowledge, no research with either of these promising assessment approaches has yet provided data on the unique contribution of a joint attention dimension to early identification. Alternatively, two other studies have provided such data.

Cathy Lord and others have developed a Toddler Module along with the ADOS-2 for use with children ages 2 and under. Macari et al. (2012) provided a study of this module's utility with 12- and 24-month-olds. These authors reported that the reliable identification of ASD at 12 months is extremely challenging because of variable patterns of symptom emergence among children. Nevertheless, their analyses provided evidence that sharing experiences with others by using both showing and gaze to initiate joint attention, along with age-appropriate ability to regulate activity level and attention were positive indicators of developmental outcome by the end of infancy. In contrast, 86% of all infants who displayed mild to more serious delays or ASD by 24 months did not show all three behaviors at 12 months. Macari et al. (2012) concluded:

> Consequently, lack of early-emerging attention sharing behaviors should be considered a red flag with regard to risk of any kind of developmental problems in the second year (including language delays) both in high- and low-risk infants, indicating a need for closer monitoring. . . . Although developmentally- and language-delayed children 'catch up' with these social-communication behaviors in the second year of life, research on toddlers with ASD suggests that deficits in showing and initiating joint attention tend to persist and become some of the defining features of ASD in the 2nd and 3rd year . . . (p. 8)

Another informative set of observations comes from a total population screening of 3,999 toddlers attending well-baby evaluation clinics at 30 months of age in Gothenburg, Sweden (Nygren et al., 2012). This study compared the screening impact of the M-CHAT with that of a five-item observation scale of children's joint attention ability called the Joint Attention Observation Schedule (JA-OBS). The JA-OBS was developed by Nygren. The M-CHAT was conducted as a parent report checklist with follow-up interview, and the JA-OBS was used directly with children and parents by 139 clinical nurses at 44 clinics. The JA-OBS includes three specific measures of joint attention: (1) The child gazes at something that you point to in the distance; (2) the child uses index finger to point at something (e.g., in a book); and (3) during object play, the child uses eye contact to monitor that you are watching. The JA-OBS also includes measures to assess whether (4) the child tries to establish eye contact with you and (5) the child reacts to his or her name.

The screening identified 62 children as at risk for ASD and 78 children as at risk for language delays. Ultimately, follow-up assessments led to an

ASD diagnosis for 48 children. The *positive predictive value* of the M-CHAT was 92%. That is the proportion of children for whom the M-CHAT identified ASD risk who later received the diagnosis of ASD. The *sensitivity* of the M-CHAT identification, or the proportion of all children who ultimately received the diagnosis of ASD who were correctly identified, was 77%. The positive predictive value of the JA-OBS was also 92%, with a sensitivity of 86%. Both instruments combined had a sensitivity of 95.6%. Item analysis indicated that the three joint attention items and the "tries to establish eye contact" item were the best markers of ASD risk in the JA-OBS (see Figure 3.2). The "reacts to name" item was substantially less sensitive to ASD risk in this study. Hence it appears that clinical nurses can make systematic observations of joint attention and eye contact that can contribute to the early identification of ASD in medical clinics.

In summary, data from the revised ADOS-2 as a whole and its Toddler Module, the M-CHAT, and other early identification methods provide evidence consistent with the hypothesis that joint attention reflects

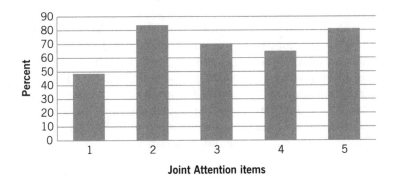

Does the child—
1. *react to own name (turns to person addressing the child)?*
2. *try to establish eye contact with you?*
3. *gaze at something that you point to further away in the room?*
4. *use his/her index finger to point at something (e.g., in a book)?*
5. *interact with you or parent in pretend play (e.g., during feeding a doll or putting the doll to bed; does the child use eye contact to monitor that you are watching)?*

FIGURE 3.2. An Illustration of the percentage of children who did not display joint attention behavior items who were identified as affected by ASD by nurses using the JA-OBS in a general population screening of 3,999 children age 30 months in Gothenburg, Sweden. From Nygren et al. (2012) Copyright 2012 by Elsevier/Pergamon Press. Reprinted by permission.

a unique latent dimension of social-behavioral development in preschool children. Moreover, this distinct dimension of development is sufficiently apparent that a wide range of parent report or clinician observations of this dimension in preschool children can assist in the early identification of ASD. The results of many studies using these instruments have provided compelling evidence for the long-standing hypothesis that joint attention, and especially IJA or the spontaneous sharing of experience with others, is a defining characteristic of the developing phenotype of ASD in the second and third years of life (e.g., Charman, 2003; Kasari et al., 1990; Kasari, Paparella, Freeman, & Jahromi, 2008; Mundy, 1995, 2003; Mundy & Sigman, 1989a, 1989b, 1989c; Mundy & Crowson, 1997; Mundy & Neal, 2000).

The research on the revised ADOS-2 reinforces the argument that joint attention is a significant and distinct feature of the ASD phenotype after the second year of life. However, little of the information reviewed so far speaks to whether joint attention is a clear and distinctive dimension of difference in the first year of autism spectrum development. The distinctiveness of the joint attention dimension could reasonably be called into question if other dimensions are more apparent in the first year of life, and if these predict joint attention development. With the advent of research on the very early signs of ASD in the infant siblings of children with ASD, there is now information that directly addresses this pertinent issue.

Risk Identification in Infant Siblings

It is difficult to know whom to credit with the innovative idea of examining the early development of infants with an older sibling affected by ASD. I do know that in a report submitted to the National Institutes of Health by a national Autism Working Group (Bristol et al., 1996), the section on Communication, Social and Emotional Development (written by Marian Sigman) noted "strong evidence that the capacity to share attention and emotion with others is specifically and universally impaired in autism" (p. 140). On the other hand, it noted:

> Simple recognition of facial expressions is intact in many individuals with autism. However, understanding that requires the person with autism to take the perspective of another is generally limited. This deficit is also manifested in serious difficulties in the functional use (pragmatics) of language by those individuals who acquire language skills. (p. 141)

This report went on to make numerous recommendations for future research. One of these was that "Measures of early social and communication functions (like imitation, joint attention and social orienting) could be administered either to children with suspected developmental difficulties . . . or to the infant siblings of children with autism. These children could then be followed to age 3–4 to validate the diagnosis" (p. 143). I believe that this was one of the first mentions (if not the first) of infant sibling research methods in the literature.

There are three reasons why infant sibling research has become important to the field. Since there is a *broad autism phenotype* or BAP (see Chapter 1), some evidence of early developmental tendencies associated with ASD may be present in many siblings, even though the majority do not go on to develop ASD. Second, although the current population rate for ASD is estimated to be 1 in 68, or about 1.5%, the recurrence rate of ASD in siblings is estimated to be higher, ranging from 3 to 19% (Ozonoff et al., 2011). This means that sibling research, when conducted collaboratively over multiple research centers, can provide observations of the early infant development of sizable numbers of children who ultimately go on to receive the diagnosis of ASD. This provides not only the opportunity to learn about the earliest dimensions of the phenotype of ASD, but also the potential for providing early intervention for affected children (Rogers et al., 2014).

Initially, the hope was to identify a behavioral or biological marker of ASD that could be used to identify ASD in the first 12 if not 6 months of life. However, after nearly 15 years of effort, this line of research has not revealed a clear marker of ASD in the first half of the first year (Rogers, 2009). This is not a problem that is specific to ASD research. Rather, it is endemic to attempts to identify behavioral markers of clinical syndromes in the first 12 months of life.

For example, before the efforts to identify the early social-behavioral markers of ASD began, researchers spent decades attempting to identify the early cognitive markers of IDD. This led to the influential observation that attention and rate of encoding in neonates and infants from 2 weeks to 12 months old was significantly associated with individual differences in childhood intelligence (e.g., Colombo, 1993; Rose, Feldman, Wallace, & Cohen, 1991; Sigman, Cohen, & Beckwith, 1997). Surprisingly, though, neonates who looked longer at visual stimuli tended to have lower intellectual outcomes. The longer looking reflected slower stimulus encoding and/or poorer state and early attention regulation ability (Sigman et al., 1997; Bornstein & Sigman, 1986). Nevertheless, even though early infant measures of visual attention provided some insights about the nature of the processes leading to risk for IDD in groups of infants (Bornstein &

Sigman, 1986), they were not as valid as researchers hoped for identification of risk in individual infants.

The problem was that all the studies indicated that the *estimates of measurement error* of the visual attention measures in young infants were moderate to large. As a consequence, individual measures were (and are) psychometrically powerful enough to provide identification of group-level but not individual-level risk for IDD, especially for children under 12 months of age (e.g., Fagan & Detterman, 1992; Colombo, Mitchell, & Horowitz, 1988). For example, Colombo et al. (1988) reported that the test–retest reliability of infant visual information-processing performance across similar tasks in one assessment session was .20 for 4-month-olds and .24 for 7-month-olds. These are relatively low reliability indicators, and the lower the reliability, the higher the measurement error is assumed to be. Colombo and colleagues also reported moderate-strength test–retest reliabilities of .54 and 48 for the number of visual fixations of pictures infants displayed at 4 and 7 months, respectively. However, the 3-month longitudinal stability of individual differences in fixations from 4 to 7 months was a more modest .33, indicating the likelihood of significant measurement error even in this "older" age range of assessment.

These observations should give us pause when we interpret the infant sibling research. First, we need to remember that according to a significant research literature, measures of dimensions of visual attention in infant siblings are *as likely to be sensitive to risk for IDD as they are to risk for ASD*. Therefore, we must look for infant sibling research designs that control for this possible confound. Second, we must know and understand the internal consistency and test–retest reliability of the measures used in infant sibling research. This certainly applies to those measures of infant visual attention that are scored in terms of number or duration of stimulus fixations. Research reports from the infant sibling literature do not yet provide enough (or, in many cases, any) information on the age-related test–retest reliability of many of the measures used in these studies (Jones, Gliga, Bedford, Charman, & Johnson, 2014). Most often, reliability reports in infant siblings research address interrater reliability; this is important, but by no means the only type of reliability that needs to be examined in these studies.

These omissions are understandable, due to the vicissitudes, complexities, and very considerable effort involved in recruiting infant sibling samples and collecting meaningful data with these infants and their families. However, the long-term value of information stemming from this research may well hinge on our ability to address both of these basic issues of research methodology in the near future.

Social Orienting and Risk at Birth

One way to handle the problem of measurement error is to use longitudinal data collection and multiple assessments of the change or growth in attention across age (Jones & Klin, 2013). The use of multiple measures tends to offset the measurement error in any one measure to a significant degree. Indeed, using this method, Jones and Klin (2013) have provided some of the first clear evidence of differences in social orienting in the first 6 months of life for at-risk infant siblings. However, the results challenge ideas about the primacy of a deficit in social/face orienting in autism spectrum development.

Jones and Klin's (2013) seminal paper[1] reported a set of observations using eye tracking to characterize the development of social attention between 2 and 6 months of age in a sample of infant siblings who were later diagnosed with ASD. Compared to infant siblings who did not go on to receive an ASD diagnosis, those who did displayed a steep decline in looking to the faces and eyes of videos of caregivers over the 2- to 6-month developmental interval. The ASD-positive infant siblings also displayed an increase in object engagement, compared to infants who did not receive a diagnosis. These observations were very much in line with the social orienting hypothesis. However, the data also indicated that the infants who received the diagnosis of ASD actually started off with *greater* levels of eye contact at 2 months. As a group, the ASD-positive infants only reached lower levels of eye contact than the comparison siblings by 6 months. This attention growth pattern was inconsistent with the social orienting hypothesis, which holds that ASD is characterized by significantly less looking to people's faces and eyes from birth (Jones & Klin, 2013).

Of course, developmental science has long observed that infants with typical development also show a decline in fixed attention to faces in the 2- to 6-month period (Johnson, Dziurawiec, Ellis, & Morton, 1991). With increasing frontal control of attention, neonates begin to disengage from face looking and begin looking more widely throughout their environments. However, typical infants also tend to return to looking at faces frequently, in conjunction with visual exploration of objects in their world. This alternation between nonsocial and social looking emerges between 2 and 4 months of age and is thought to demark the beginning of the neurocognitive capacity for joint attention, or at least for RJA (e.g., Farroni et al., 2004; Elison et al., 2013). The infants with ASD in the Jones and Klin (2013) study may not have as clearly shown this developmental shift to

---

[1]This paper was recognized for advancing the field by the national Interagency Autism Coordinating Committee's review of ASD research published in 2013.

alternating between social and nonsocial looking. Once the early period of high levels of social orienting diminished, infants at highest risk for ASD did not alternate social with nonsocial orienting. Consequently, they gradually began to display more object looking between 2 and 6 months, relative to comparison infants.

How should we interpret this observation? Does it reflect a difference in the maintenance of social orienting in children with ASD, or a difference in the initial development of the integrated self–other–object processing of joint attention? My guess is that it reflects both. In my view, the extent to which human infants continue to display social orienting as the frontal control of attention increases after 2 months of age is fully intertwined with the functional, adaptive development of the dimension of joint attention. However, this is just a guess at this point.

What I am sure of is that we cannot currently accept a social orienting "explanation" of joint attention disturbance in autism, based on current data. However, we probably now know how to resolve this issue: We need to engage in detailed studies of the 2- to 8-month period in both typical development and autism spectrum development before we can definitively understand the causal sequence of social orienting and joint attention development. (See Chapter 5 for a related discussion.)

Joint Attention and Risk

Although the hypothetical relations between social orienting and joint attention remain unclear, several observations suggest the use of joint attention methods for infant sibling research.

We do know that joint attention measures displayed a moderate level of longitudinal test–retest reliability over 3-month assessment intervals between 9 and 18 months of age in a typical sample of 95 infants (Mundy et al., 2007). This observation, along with evidence of its diagnostic sensitivity, argues for a focus on the dimension of joint attention in infant sibling research.

Specifically, the Mundy et al. (2007) paper reported that individual differences on both the IJA and RJA scales of the ESCS were reliable from 9 to 12 months, from 12 to 15 months, and from 15 to 18 months. In particular, the reliability of 9-month IJA and RJA data for the prediction of 12-month data suggests that measurement error may be low enough for both of these measures to be useful in identifying risk in the second half of the first year. It is also informative to note that IJA scale reliability was carried by the alternating gaze item rather than by the pointing or showing items. This IJA behavior may thus be especially useful in early risk identification. Measures of requesting that also involved joint attention behaviors, such as pointing to request, displayed significant reliability from 9 to 12 months but not thereafter. So measures of requesting forms of joint attention have appropriate psychometric characteristics for early risk identification.

It is also noteworthy that individual differences on the IJA scale at 9 months in the Mundy et al. (2007) study were significantly associated with IJA differences at 18 months (see Figure 3.3). Figure 3.3 reveals two interesting facets of IJA behaviors in typical infants. First, the differences in the typical tendency to share experience by alternating eye contact in reference to an active toy ranged from about 10 to 40 bids in a 20-minute assessment. Yet these very considerable differences displayed significant stability over a 9-month developmental interval, speaking to the coherence of the dimension of IJA in this development period. Second, by 9

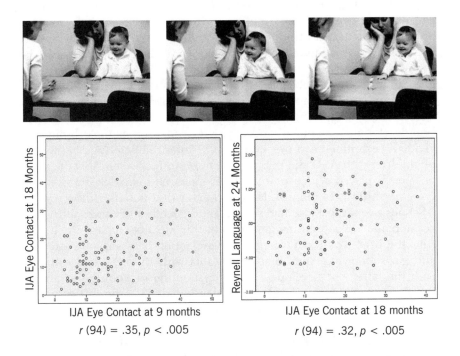

FIGURE 3.3. Scatterplots illustrating the reliability and meaning of individual differences in infants' tendency to initiate joint attention by using alternating eye contact between an active wind-up toy and an unfamiliar tester. The left panel illustrates the developmental continuity of differences in this IJA behavior (IJA-EC in the figure) from 9 to 10 months of age in 95 infants. The right panel illustrates developmental continuity between this IJA behavior at 18 months and combined scores for the Reynell Expressive and Receptive Language Scales at 24 months for the same sample of infants. Data from Mundy et al. (2007).

months all infants displayed multiple alternating eye contact IJA bids, *suggesting that this behavior was well enough developed by 9 months of age to enable it to be a sensitive marker for typical and atypical development.* Moreover, data indicated that this was true for the 32 infants in this sample with slower rates of cognitive development at 18 months, as assessed on the Bayley Mental Development Index (mean MDI = 77, standard deviation = 5.05), as well as for the 63 infants with typical rates of cognitive development (mean MDI = 98.9, standard deviation = 8.9) (Mundy et al., 2007). So this aspect of joint attention development may be resistant to the potential confound of differences in cognitive development between infant siblings with and without ASD.

Given these characteristics of early joint attention development, it is not surprising to find that several studies provide evidence of the sensitivity of RJA and IJA to risk for ASD in infant siblings. This may also be the case for measures of joint attention for requesting. There are, however, also inconsistencies in findings across studies, which make drawing conclusions from this literature challenging. Nevertheless, studies of at-risk infant siblings have begun to illuminate our understanding of the nature and timing of the disturbance of the joint attention dimension in ASD.

Several studies have focused on the possibility that a delay in the development of RJA is an early marker of atypical social and communication development among infants at risk for ASD. For example, Sullivan et al. (2007) examined RJA in a sample of 51 infant siblings (age 14 months) of children with ASD. Siblings who went on to receive an ASD diagnosis or later displayed evidence of the BAP appeared to be delayed in following gaze shifts at 14 months. However, many (but not all) children in the ASD-positive sample also had significant difficulty when gaze shifts were accompanied by a pointing gesture, but this was not true for the infants with the BAP. These data suggest a dissociation between joint attention and gaze following, such that the infants with the BAP had difficulty with the latter but developed an understanding of pointing as a referential cue. For the infants who later developed ASD, the difficulty with responding to cues of reference was exhibited across face and gestural cues.

Sullivan et al. (2007) also examined one facet of the reliability of performance across different types of RJA measures at 14 and 24 months. The "looking and pointing" experimental measures and the ADOS RJA measure displayed a strong internal consistency reliability coefficient at 24 months (.73), but relatively little evidence of internal consistency was observed at 14 months, especially in the samples with later ASD and the BAP. It may not be surprising, then, that infant sibling studies have been inconsistent in observations of the utility of RJA measures before 24 months, with several studies failing to observe effects. However, other data consistently indicate that RJA measures, especially the use of multiple measures, can contribute to the identification of risk for ASD before 24 months of age.

Presmanes, Walden, Stone, and Yoder (2006) compared 46 at-risk siblings (ages 12 and 23 months) with 35 siblings of children with typical development. This study used a 10-item measure of RJA. The results indicated that 28 out of 46 children in the ASD risk sample (68%) scored at or below the 20th percentile on the RJA measure, compared to 12 out of 35 (43%) of the sample without ASD risk. This study also examined possible factors involved in the group differences, but found no evidence that attention disengagement ability, the tendency to orient to the face of the tester, or visual–spatial problem solving explained the group differences in RJA. Unlike the Sullivan et al. (2007) study, however, this study found group differences on RJA trials involving gaze following, but not gaze following accompanied by pointing.

The British Autism Study of Infant Siblings research team at King's College London has provided another important facet of information about early RJA disturbance in infants at risk for ASD (Bedford et al., 2012). Seventy-three infants were administered an eye-tracking, gaze-following measure of RJA at 7 and 13 months of age. Thirty-five of these were at-risk infant siblings, and 38 were low-risk siblings of children with typical development. Notably, the measure of gaze following per se was not sensitive to ASD risk status differences at either 7 or 13 months. However, by 13 months, looking time to stimuli indicated by gaze following was significantly lower for the at-risk group. This observation is very important. It emphasizes that many children at risk for ASD may display gaze following, but still may be affected by a difference in joint attention development. This is because RJA does not just involve socially guided orienting to a stimulus; it involves cueing to become engaged in shared information processing of the stimulus with another person (Mundy, 2011; Mundy et al., 2009). If children with ASD orient to gaze at cued referents, but don't engage with the stimulus and process information, they could potentially experience significantly different developmental benefits of the practice of RJA. (See Chapters 4, 5, and 6 for more on information processing during joint attention.)

Different Measures of Joint Attention and Risk

Several other studies have examined the utility of both IJA and RJA measures for the early identification of risk for ASD. These studies have also obtained variable patterns of results. Nevertheless, they illustrate that research methods involving a deeper conceptualization of the nature of joint attention, especially IJA, may be valuable in research on risk identification in ASD. This is particularly true of a study by Cornew, Dobkins, Akshoomoff, McCleery, and Carver (2012).

This research group used a measure of *social referencing* to examine IJA with an adult in 44 lower-risk 18- to 21-month-old infants and 38 higher-risk age-matched infant siblings of children with ASD. Infants were presented with a potentially emotionally evocative ambiguous stimulus, such as a remote-controlled mechanical spider or a battery-operated randomly bouncing ball. The tendency of each infant to (1) look to the caregiver and a tester and (2) react to the adults' positive or negative affect to regulate approach or withdrawal from the ambiguous toy was rated.

The study revealed three potentially important findings. First, there were group differences in the tendency to spontaneously look to an adult after initial toy presentation. In the low-risk group, 21% did not reference adults; in the group with higher risk but without ASD diagnosis (HR-NDX), 40% failed to reference adults spontaneously; and in the higher-risk ASD group with an eventual ASD diagnosis, 67% did not reference. This pattern of evidence suggested that this social referencing measure might reflect something of the BAP, but not necessarily something specific to ASD onset within the high-risk sample.

The second contribution of the study was the observation that that higher-risk infants who met criteria for ASD at 36 months of age sought information more slowly (latency to look from toys to adults) than either low-risk infants or higher-risk infants who did not go on to receive an ASD diagnosis. This finding is consistent with the notion that joint attention impairments in young children with ASD may reflect slower speed of information processing or greater executive effort (see Chapters 5 and 7). However, differences in speed of processing may also be explained by differences between the groups in IQ.

Finally, the results indicated that although higher-risk ASD-positive infant siblings displayed evidence of impairment in the joint attention component of social referencing, this was not so clearly the case for the behavior regulation component of social referencing. *No group differences were observed in the tendency of the infants to react to toy approach or withdrawal in response to the positive affective cues of the adults.* Thus, compared to the attention measures, the facial and vocal affect-processing measure of the social referencing paradigm was not a sensitive marker of risk group differences in this study. These results are consistent with studies of older children, which show that children with ASD who engage in some social referencing respond typically to the facial and vocal affect of adults (Sigman, Kasari, Kwon, & Yirmiya, 1992), and that attention to affect is related to joint attention but does not mediate the relations of joint attention to communication outcomes in affect children (Dawson et al., 2004). Thus this study also provided some information about the relative sensitivity of social orienting and face processing in the early identification of ASD.

In an influential study, Rozga et al. (2011) noted that previous research had reported that measures of joint attention for sharing experiences and requesting may be sensitive markers of risk between 14 and 24 months. However, these authors also noted inconsistencies in the ages and types of measures for which risk sensitivity was observed across these studies. To arrive at a better understanding of joint attention and risk identification, they worked with a large sample of 98 infant siblings. Seventeen infants later received confirmed diagnoses of ASD, and the other 81 siblings did not go on to exhibit the syndrome of ASD. The researchers gathered ESCS data at 12 months for all children, and dyadic mother–child interaction data at 6 months for many of these children. The study also included a sample of 60 infants with typical development.

Few if any 6-month behaviors were significant predictors of risk for IJA diagnosis in this study. The results, however, did reveal that the RJA measure, the requesting measure, and (to a lesser extent) the IJA measure at 12 months were associated with infant risk status. Regarding the latter finding, the association with risk was limited to pointing and showing behaviors; it did not include the measure of alternating eye contact. An interesting methodological facet of this report was that it was conducted across two university sites. Significant study site effects were observed for the IJA and RJA measures, but not the requesting measures. Although the cause and implication of these site effects in the measurement of RJA and IJA were not discussed in this paper, they may have affected the pattern of data in this study. The site effects may indicate that more efforts (such as this book) are needed to achieve a fuller and more coherent understanding of the nature and measurement of the joint attention dimension within the field.

Like Jones and Klin (2013), other researchers have begun to explore the power of longitudinal growth measures in the study of infant siblings. Yoder, Stone, Walden, and Malesa (2009) were among the first to do this with joint attention measures. They examined the degree to which an RJA and IJA measure could predict diagnostic outcome in at-risk siblings from about 15 to 34 months of age. The children received four repeated assessments of RJA, using the methods described by Presmanes et al. (2007). They received four IJA-related assessments of unprompted *triadic communication,* defined as "the use of gestural, vocal, gaze, and/or symbolic communication that shows attention to the message recipient and the physical referent of communication" (p. 1385). Functionally, this operational definition is consistent with an IJA measure, albeit one that includes language as well as nonverbal behaviors. The IJA/triadic communication measure used was from the STAT, discussed earlier in this chapter.

The results revealed that the RJA of 14- to 15-month-olds (but not RJA growth), and the index of growth of triadic communication (IJA) over four repeated measures (but not initial IJA), were both significant predictors of ASD diagnosis among the at-risk infant siblings. This study was also one of the very few to control for the effects of initial differences in language development in predicting outcomes in infants sibling research. When the authors controlled for language development, the evidence for the links among RJA, IJA/triadic communication, and later ASD diagnosis was reduced. However, the likelihood that this study revealed true effects of RJA and IJA/triadic communication was still greater than 90%.

Two recent risk studies illustrate several important, but less well-recognized, facets of joint attention development. Ibañez, Grantz, and Messinger (2013) provided a longitudinal study of RJA, IJA, and requesting at 8, 10, 12, 15, and 18 months for 35 at-risk infant siblings of children with ASD and 21 infants with typically developing siblings. The original version of the ADOS was used to assess ASD symptoms and confirm diagnostic status with the infants at about 30 months of age. This study revealed that infants' initial status of IJA and RJA at 8 months distinguished between the at-risk and not-at-risk samples. For requesting, it was an index of growth across the repeated measurements that distinguished the two samples. Data also indicated that within the at-risk sample, the initial status of IJA and the growth of requesting were significant predictors of which at-risk infants did or did not receive the diagnosis of ASD. However, RJA was not a significant predictor in this study.

When the IJA and requesting measures were considered together, to determine which (if either) exhibited *unique* predictive validity for ASD diagnosis, only IJA was associated with predictive validity. Indeed, the predictive model with 8-month IJA intercept term correctly identified 6 of 9 at-risk infants who received the diagnosis of ASD (sensitivity = 67%) and correctly identified 25 of 26 at-risk infants who did not receive the diagnosis of ASD (specificity = 96%). The data in this study were collected with the ESCS; therefore, it is likely that the alternating gaze item of the ESCS made a contribution to the predictive sensitivity and specificity of the 8-month IJA measure in this study.

This study also illustrated the problem of comorbid language disabilities and IDD in infant sibling research. At 3 years of age, the at-risk infants in this study who received the diagnosis of ASD had significantly lower language abilities (specifically, receptive language abilities) than those of at-risk infants who did not receive an ASD diagnosis. So it is difficult to appreciate whether the joint attention measures in this study were sensitive to ASD outcome, language outcome, or both.

Be that as it may, this study also provided a unique comparative view of the development of joint attention in at-risk and not-at-risk infants. This useful perspective on joint attention development is illustrated in Figure 3.4. The patterns of development that characterized IJA versus RJA and requesting were different. Both RJA and requesting increased steadily with age. RJA appeared to increase at the same rate in risk and not-at-risk infants, but with an earlier starting point for at-risk infants (8 months). On the other hand, infants had the same starting point for requesting, but the at-risk infants increased requesting at a slower rate than the not-at-risk infants did. What may be more revealing to many, as well as surprising, is that IJA did not display a steady increase with age from 8 to

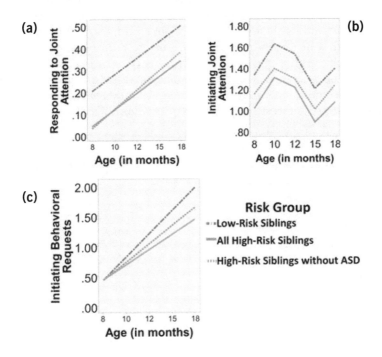

FIGURE 3.4. Illustration of the growth curves of RJA (a), IJA (b), and initiating behavioral requests (c) in low-risk and at-risk infants. Panel a indicates that regardless of diagnostic outcome, high-risk infants scored uniformly lower in correct RJA responses across repeated assessments from 8 to 18 months. Panel b indicates that unlike the linear growth patterns of RJA and initiating behavioral requests, a nonlinear cubic pattern of growth characterized IJA development in both low-risk and high-risk infants. Moreover, the frequency of IJA bids was lowest in the high-risk sample that included children who went on to receive the diagnosis of ASD. Panel c illustrates the linear divergence of initiating behavioral requests by 15–18 months across the groups of low-risk and high-risk infants. From Ibañez, Grantz, and Messinger (2013). Copyright 2013 by Lawrence Erlbaum Associates, Inc. Reprinted by permission.

18 months. Instead, it increased from 8 to 10 months, then declined significantly through 15 months, and then rebounded with maturation to 18 months. This pattern was apparent for both the at-risk and not-at-risk infant samples.

This comparative pattern of up-and-down IJA expression across development after 10 months is not only evident in this study, but has also been observed elsewhere. In the Mundy et al. (2007) study, the longitudinal ESCS data on 95 infants revealed very similar growth patterns between 9 and 18 months, with a decline in IJA also noted between 12 and 15 months (see Figure 3.5). Sheinkopf, Mundy, Claussen, and Willoughby (2004) observed a similar development pattern of second-year decline in IJA, although at 15–18 months, in a sample of at-risk preschool children with a history of prenatal exposure to cocaine. Little is known about the factors that may contribute to this pattern of development in IJA. It may be related to the development of walking, with ambulatory independence creating a new developmental challenge in spontaneously seeking to share interests regarding a proximal object or event with a

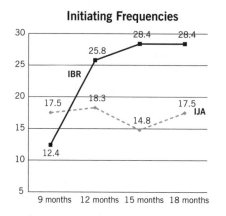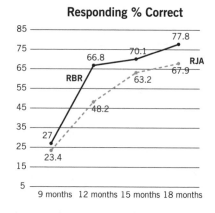

$N = 95$

FIGURE 3.5. Illustrations of the differences and similarities in IJA, RJA, initiating behavior requests (IBR), and responding to behavior requests (RBR) growth patterns in typical development between 9 and 18 months of age. The left panel illustrates the difference between the linear quadratic growth pattern for IBR and the nonlinear quadratic pattern that characterizes IJA growth in typical development. Figure 3.4 displays a similar nonlinear cubic growth pattern for IJA observed in the development of at-risk infants. The right panel illustrates the similar linear quadratic growth patterns observed for RJA and RBR in typical development. Data from Mundy et al. (2007).

distal social partner. However, this is speculation at best. What is not speculation is this: Growth pattern data from three studies suggest that the factors involved in the development of IJA are different from those involved in RJA and requesting. We would do well to understand these factors better as we delve further into the role of joint attention in ASD. So, in addition to understanding the development of joint attention and social orienting in the 2- to 8-month period, these data speak to the need to understand the 8- to 18-month period more fully as well.

Affect Sharing in Joint Attention

Recall that the conveyance of affect may be one important feature that distinguishes the growth and development of RJA, requesting, and IJA. Kasari et al. (1990) conducted a detailed study of the confluence of affect with different types of joint attention behaviors in three groups of children. One group included young children with ASD; a second group included children with IDD, but not ASD; and a third group included children with typical development. Kasari et al. (1990) hypothesized that the conveyance of positive affect might be integral to IJA development, but not necessarily a feature of RJA or requesting. A corollary of this hypothesis was that an attenuation of the tendency to share positive affect might be integral to the nature of IJA developmental differences in autism spectrum development.

Kasari et al. (1990) coded the emotional facial expressions of 18 children with ASD (50 month olds), 18 children with IDD (age- and IQ-matched), and 18 typically developing children (mental-age-matched at 22 months) from video recordings of ESCS testing of the children. The results of the study were informative. The proportion of looks that conveyed positive affect to the adult tester during IJA was far greater in the groups with typical development and IDD than in the group with ASD (see Figure 3.6). However, this pattern was specific to IJA bids. The conveyance of smiles on requesting trials was much lower and did not differ across the groups with typical development and ASD. It should be noted that there were no reliable group differences on the proportion of looks to objects that were associated with positive affect. Thus differences in a general disposition to express positive affect did not account for the findings. These results suggested the hypothesis that the difference in ASD involves processes associated with sharing the affective experience of a common referent with another person, and not just socially coordinating visual attention to the referent.

Subsequent research indicated that sharing affect was truly part of IJA development in children with typical development. Greater frequency of sharing positive affect was observed in each type of ESCS IJA

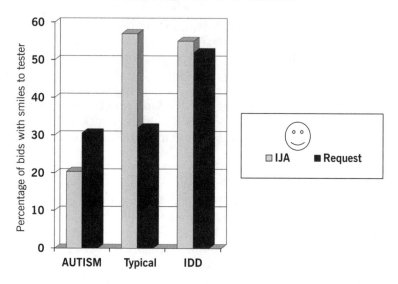

FIGURE 3.6. Illustration of the association of positive affect (smiling) with IJA compared to initiating behavior requests (Request). The lighter shaded columns in the figure represent the percentage of IJA bids that were displayed with smiles to the tester by children with ASD, typical development, or IDD. Comparison of these lighter shaded columns illustrates that children with ASD displayed smiles with IJA bids far less often than did children in either of the other groups. The darker columns in the figure illustrate Requesting bids accompanied by smiles to the tester. Comparison of these darker columns illustrates that there were no differences between the ASD and typically developing groups of children on smiling to testers while requesting. The figure also illustrates that the children with IDD tended to smile more often during requesting than did children with ASD or typical development. Only the IDD group smiled equally often during requesting and IJA. Data from Kasari, Sigman, Mundy, and Yirmiya (1990).

bid (eye contact, alternating eye contact, pointing, and showing), relative to comparable ESCS requesting behaviors such as eye contact, reaching plus eye contact, giving, and pointing (Mundy et al., 1992). However, our understanding of this affective component was truly propelled forward at the University of Miami by the expertise of Daniel Messinger and his research group on emotional development in infancy. Venezia et al. (2004) examined the development of infants at 8, 10, and 24 months in order to understand whether infants truly *conveyed* positive affect to testers in IJA. The alternative possibility was that infants alternated looking from and object to a tester and then smiled in response to looking at the face of the tester; this could be called a *reactive smile*. Alternatively, if infants smiled first at an object, and then turned to a tester, this could be considered an act of conveying affective experience and could be called an *anticipatory smile.*

Venezia et al. (2004) observed that 22 of 24 infants displayed IJA alternating gaze *at all three ages.* Neither the frequency of IJA bids nor the proportion of bids associated with smiles changed across these three ages. However, the number of infants who displayed anticipatory smiles increased from 7 infants at 8 months, to 15 infants at 10 months, and to 16 infants at 12 months.[2] These data suggested the presence of a developmental shift in processes associated with the conveyance of positive affect during IJA between 8 and 10 months of age in typical development. This is important for our understanding of the nature of joint attention and its study in ASD. When we are talking about development up through 8–10 months, sharing affect may be primarily a dyadic process. However, after 10 months, sharing affect increasingly becomes a triadic process and an important facet of the joint attention dimension.

Affect Sharing, Joint Attention, and ASD Risk Identification

This program of research on affect in joint attention set the stage for a potentially important set of observations from the infant sibling research literature. Remember that Ibañez et al. (2013) reported that 8-month IJA was a significant individual level predictor of 30-month ASD outcome in a sample of infant siblings. As a follow-up, Gangi et al. (2014) examined the degree to which the diagnostic predictive validity of 8-month IJA for ASD risk could be explained in terms of its associations with anticipatory or reactive smiling. This study produced several findings of note.

First, the rates of IJA bids displayed with anticipatory smiling per minute on the ESCS distinguished at-risk from low-risk infants. Moreover, the rates of IJA with anticipatory smiles were more powerful in this regard than the rates of either IJA with reactive smiles, or IJA bids without smiles (see Figure 3.7). This raises the possibility that the measurement of the tendency to share positive affect in IJA may be part of the expression of the BAP in at-risk infants. This finding also reminds us that we may want to be careful when we treat sharing positive affect and joint attention as measures of different domains of assessment in risk research. Whenever infant IJA measures are used for ASD risk assessment, some observations will include sharing positive affect with others, and vice versa.

---

[2] Ratings of anticipatory smiles were conservative. At 12 months, 6 infants displayed *indeterminate smiles*, which may be a prelude to anticipatory smiling (see Venezia et al., 2004, for details).

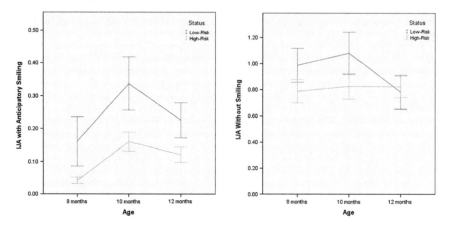

FIGURE 3.7. Anticipatory smiling during IJA in low- and high-risk infants. The left panel illustrates the tendency of high-risk infants to display less positive affect to testers during IJA trials than low-risk infants at 8, 10, and 12 months of age. The right panel illustrates the difference between high- and low-risk infants on the display of IJA without smiles at 8 months, which was predictive of later ASD diagnostic status. From Gangi et al. (2014). Copyright 2014 by Springer Science+Business Media. Reprinted by permission.

Gangi et al. (2014) also reported a surprising observation. They had hypothesized that the measure of IJA with anticipatory smiles would also be the best early individual-level predictor of ASD diagnostic outcome within the sample of at-risk infant siblings. The results, however, indicated that the best individual-level predictive indicator of ultimate ASD status was the measure of IJA without smiles. Gangi et al. (2014) recognized that since IJA with smiling occurred at a lower frequency than IJA without smiling, it was possible that the measurements of the former were less reliable than those of the latter. If so, this could explain the lack of association between IJA smiling and diagnostic outcomes in this sample of at-risk infants.

From a more conceptual point of view, Gangi et al. (2014) raised another possibility in their discussion of this pattern of the results. They noted that time spent in neutral affect in interaction with others has been linked to better language learning in infants with typical development. Gangi et al. (2014) went on to suggest that joint attention initiated without positive affect may be related to the social learning functions of joint attention. These functions, rather than those associated with affect sharing, may be most closely associated with ASD diagnosis development in at-risk infants. Moreover, variability in the tendency to share positive affect may reflect a moderator effect on joint attention symptom expression in

ASD. Recall that evidence of a relative bias toward behavioral activation may be associated with later symptom clarity in ASD (Burnette et al., 2011; see Chapter 1), and that behavioral activation is related to the affective expression of positive "approach" emotions (e.g., Van Honk & Schutter, 2006).

This line of argument is speculative. Nevertheless, it is speculation that also fits with a very similar pattern of data reported in an exemplary longitudinal study by Landa, Gross, Stuart, and Faherty (2013).[3] This research team examined the relative growth of language, joint attention, and affect sharing between 6 and 36 months in a group of 204 infant siblings of children with ASD and 31 low-risk infant comparison controls. Fifty-four of the at-risk infant siblings went on to receive the diagnosis of ASD at 36 months. A unique element of this study was that the research group used an experimental application of the original ADOS and were able to identify a subset of these 54 at-risk infants who displayed clinical levels of ASD symptoms at 14 months. So the study was able to compare the growth of early-identified and later-identified infants and toddlers with that of a group without ASD.

Data on growth before 12 months did not demonstrate diagnostic outcome group differences. Analyses of growth after 12 months, however, revealed significant differences among the three groups (infants with early-onset ASD, later-onset ASD, and no ASD) on IJA, sharing positive affect, language, and speech (Figure 3.8). Although the groups differed in absolute levels of language and speech development at 14, 18, and 24 months, the patterns of growth on these dimensions were similar across the three groups. Alternatively, the groups not only displayed wide disparities in IJA and shared-affect at 14 months, but also distinctly different patterns of growth (see Figure 3.8).

IJA and shared affect were assessed with the Communication and Symbolic Behavior Scales Developmental Profile (Wetherby & Prizant, 2002). Unlike the ESCS, this instrument provides a measure of "smiling paired with eye contact" apart from IJA behaviors. Thus this measure was defined in terms of social orienting or mutual gaze accompanied by positive affective. Figure 3.8 reveals that at 14 months, both the groups with ASD (early-onset and late-onset) displayed less IJA than the group without ASD. This effect, though, was more pronounced for the early-onset group, but between 14 and 18 months the difference in IJA development became more pronounced in the late-onset group. In part, this convergence seemed to be because of negative growth on IJA between 18 and 24 months for this group.

---

[3] This paper was also recognized for advancing the field by the national Interagency Autism Coordinating Committee review of ASD research published in 2013.

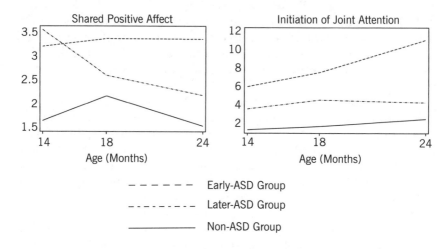

FIGURE 3.8. Comparative illustration of the differences in the degree to which shared positive affect and IJA distinguished three groups of risk infants. Both shared positive affect and IJA measured on the ECSB discriminated the development of toddlers at 14, 18, and 24 months who went on to develop ASD. However, toddlers with later onset of ASD symptoms displayed more shared positive affect on ECSB than the group without later ASD at 14 months of age. From Landa, Gross, Stuart, and Faherty (2013). Copyright 2013 by Blackwell Publishing, Inc. Reprinted by permission.

In contrast, the pattern of development on shared affect was quite different across the groups with early- and later-identified ASD. The later-identified group displayed as much smiling paired with eye contact as the controls without ASD did at 14 months, and much more than the early-identified group. However, the frequency of sharing affect declined in the later-identified group sharply between 14 and 18 months and between 18 and 24 months, to levels similar to (but still in excess of) those for the early-onset group. As I look at this pattern of data, it is difficult to see how it is consistent with the hypothesis that disturbances in social orienting, face processing, or facial affect lead to joint attention differences in children with ASD. Of course, it is possible that a measure of social orienting *without affect* would have revealed significant differences in the development of both groups with ASD at 14 months. However, without that information, the data of Landa et al. (2013), along with the data from Jones and Klin (2013), suggest that the social orienting hypothesis of joint attention differences in ASD requires much more scrutiny before it can be accepted. Alternatively, the data in the studies of Landa et al. (2013) and Gangi et al. (2014) indicate that by 8–14 months, IJA—perhaps especially IJA without the conveyance of affect—is a significant indicator of high risk for the syndrome of autism spectrum development.

Again, these sets of data are consistent with several inferences. Shared affect, mutual gaze, and IJA reflect related, but distinctive, dimensions in the early development of ASD. IJA is an indicator of ASD onset at 8–14 months of age. Sharing affect with eye contact may be part of the BAP, but not all children with autism spectrum development display clear differences in this dimension in early development (also see Ozonoff et al., 2010). The utility of measures of social orienting and affect sharing in early identification is currently less well supported than the utility of joint attention measures.

One admittedly provocative possibility that may explain this pattern of findings is that sharing affect reflects a moderator dimension of ASD, not a syndrome-specific dimension. In particular, relative behavioral activation bias may be associated with a greater tendency to express "approach" emotions with the expression of positive affect. Recall from Chapter 1 that some, but not all, children with ASD display EEG patterns associated with behavioral activation. Also recall that retrospective data indicated that parents became aware of the symptoms of these children later in development (Burnette et al., 2011). This leads me to wonder whether EEG asymmetry measures of behavioral activation bias, which may be used by 10 months of age, could be used in future infant sibling studies to examine the degree to which differences in early sharing of affect reflect a moderator process in symptoms.

Of course, the astute reader may be aware of a certain circularity in all this. The data indicate that joint attention predicts the diagnosis of ASD in at-risk infants. At the same time, the diagnosis of ASD is often confirmed with the ADOS or ADOS-2, which contains a Joint Attention factor in one of its two primary assessment dimensions (Gotham et al., 2007, 2008). Sharing affect may not be so well measured in the ADOS. It is possible, then, that studies tend to confirm the utility of early joint attention measures in infant risk studies because joint attention is also primary to diagnostic confirmation. Rather than a criticism, this observation is meant to point out an opportunity. Since the ADOS includes a Joint Attention factor, it offers numerous opportunities for more closely examining the continuity in existing data between early symptom onset and the specific dimension of joint attention. For example, was the decline in growth in social orienting at 2 to six-months observed by Jones and Klin (2013) specifically predictive of the Joint Attention factor score in the subsequent assessments with the ADOS? Was the early identification of ASD at 14 months by Landa et al. (2013) influenced by the ADOS Joint Attention factor? Was joint attention at 8 months predictive of the ADOS Joint Attention factor in the Gangi et al. (2014) database? Many questions of this type can be asked and answered through recourse to the ADOS Joint Attention factor in currently available archival data sets. Better yet, with increased awareness of the Joint Attention factor score in Modules 1 and 2 of the ADOS, many new questions about the dimension of joint attention in ASD may be addressed prospectively in future studies.

Joint Attention in Other Conditions

Up to this point, evidence for the validity of the joint attention dimension has been based on appraising its sensitivity for diagnosing or identifying risk for autism spectrum development in young children. However, there are groups of children with other clinical conditions that exhibit significant differences in early social development. Indeed, often children in these clinical conditions may appear to exhibit the symptoms of ASD, such as children with fragile X syndrome or Williams syndrome? Does joint attention help us to understand common and distinctive features of ASD relative to the social development differences in these other syndromes? This chapter concludes with a brief discussion of this issue.

Fragile X Syndrome

Fragile X syndrome (FXS) is a relatively rare (1:4,000 males) single-gene disorder on the X chromosome that is associated with IDD and, in some cases, symptoms of ASD. These associations have led many to describe FXS as the most common inherited cause of IDD *and* the most common known cause of autism (*www.fraxa.org/fragilex*, retrieved April, 8, 2014). However, there have been relatively few detailed comparisons of the similarities or differences in the symptom patterns that give rise to the ASD diagnosis in children with FXS versus children with idiopathic autism. Nevertheless, at least four recent studies have provided comparative information on joint attention in children with ASD and children with FXS who were comorbid for ASD symptoms (FXS + ASD).

Wolff et al. (2012) compared 23 four-year-old boys with FXS + ASD to 38 age- and IQ-matched boys with ASD only. Many children in both groups were affected by moderate to severe levels of IDD. The group with FXS + ASD displayed a mean IQ of 30.2 with a reported IQ range of 8.9–60.8, and the group with ASD displayed a mean IQ of 38.4 with a range of 14.2–92. Analyses that controlled for variance in IQ revealed the most pronounced differences between the clinical groups on responsive social behaviors on the ADOS (including RJA, Social Smiles, and Facial Expressions), and on initiation behaviors that involved gaze integration and quality of social engagement.

A second study (Hall, Lightbody, Hirt, Rezvani, & Reiss, 2010) used parent report of symptoms from the Social Communication Questionnaire (SCQ) to examine the social phenotype of children with FXS + ASD. The SCQ is a brief version of the "gold standard" ADI-R (Rutter, Bailey, & Lord, 2003). The study included data on 120 individuals, ages 5–25 years, with FXS. The results reported reflected findings from the subsample of 73 males with FXS. These individuals had a mean IQ of 46 with a range of 40–74, and a mean SCQ rating of 17 with a range of 3–39. Of the sample of 73, 44 met criteria for ASD on the SCQ (60%), and 19 of 37 who were administered the ADOS met criteria for ASD (51.4%).

Hall et al. (2010) reported that parents endorsed problems on 7 of the 13 items of the Communication domain of the SCQ significantly less often for the males with FXS, compared to the SCQ's reference sample with ASD. These items included the IJA item of pointing to express interest, as well as imitation, gesture, and conversation items. Parents of the sample with FXS endorsed 12 of 16 items on the Social Interaction domain less often than parents of children with ASD in the SCQ's reference sample. These included the IJA items of showing, directing attention, and offering to share enjoyment, as well as items involving gestures, friends, social smiling, range of facial expressions, interest in other children, and attention to voices.

Data were also provided on the ADOS for the 19 boys who met ASD criteria on this instrument. Here Hall et al. (2010) reported that the sample with FXS + ASD received better symptom ratings than the ADOS autism reference sample on 4 of 9 items of the Communication domain, including the joint attention item of pointing, as well as conversation, gestures, and stereotyped words. The sample with FXS also received better symptom ratings on 8 of 13 items in the Social Interaction domain, including the joint attention items of showing (IJA), shared enjoyment (IJA), and RJA, as well as items for spontaneous initiation, quality of social overtures, amount of reciprocal social communication, quality of rapport, and empathy.

One recent study compared the contribution of joint attention to language learning in samples of 7-year-olds with mild to moderate IDD and ASD or FXS. McDuffie, Kover, Hagerman, and Abbeduto (2013) presented participants with the opportunity to learn nonsense word labels (e.g., "Look, it's a *modi*") for novel objects. During novel object–word pairings, testers attempted to establish joint attention with participants by exaggerating their head turns and gaze direction to the novel objects, as well as pointing and saying, "Look!", before providing the nonsense labels. This type of fast referential mapping of a nonsense word onto an object provides a measure of young children's use of joint attention in early language learning. The results indicated that both groups responded above chance levels with respect to learning labels in this referential mapping study. However, the boys with FXS outperformed the boys with ASD, despite lower levels of cognitive development. Moreover, word learning in the fast referential mapping task was more strongly related to an independent test of language development in the children with FXS than in the children with ASD. This study provided suggestive evidence of differences in the role or impact of joint attention on language learning in children with FXS and children with ASD. However, many questions still need to be asked and answered with this potentially useful information paradigm, to arrive at a clear picture of these possible differences.

Finally, a study conducted by Rogers, Hepburn, Stackhouse, and Wehner (2003) also provides data on differences in the social phenotypes of children with ASD and children with FXS. This study compared the imitation skill development of 24 children with ASD (ages 2–4 years) with that of 18 chronological- and mental-age-matched children with FXS and 20 children with other developmental disorders. The results indicated that the children with ASD were more impaired in imitation development. Moreover, imitation development was strongly associated with a pointing measure of IJA in the sample with ASD, but not in the other samples. The authors did not report group comparative data on the joint attention measure. However, they interpreted their data to suggest that the clustered pattern of dyadic and triadic social skill development (imitation and joint attention) distinguished the impairment in the social phenotype of children with ASD from that of children with FXS and other developmental disorders.

Like any good research, these studies raise as many questions as they answer because of study limitations that were well described by the authors of each paper. For example, McDuffie et al. (2013) and Rogers et al. (2003) did not provide separate data on the subgroup of children with FXS in their samples who met diagnostic criteria for ASD. If the group comparisons had been limited to those children with FXS who were most affected, the patterns of results might have been different. With that caution in mind, these reports do provide convergent evidence that the social phenotypes, and associated social-neurodevelopmental endophenotypes, of ASD and FXS may be significantly different (also see Hazlett et al., 2009; McDuffie et al., 2013, 2015). Level or intensity of joint attention disturbance appears to be one of the main axes of differences in the developing social phenotypes of children with ASD and with FXS + ASD symptoms, and imitation may be another. These differences are of sufficient import to lead Hall et al. (2010) to caution that ASD treatment protocols may not be the referrals of choice for children with FXS. Of course, the reverse may also be true: Innovative and effective therapies developed for

FXS may not necessarily target processes essential to the social nature of ASD.

Murphy and Abbeduto (2005) have provided a relevant and insightful account of joint attention disturbance in FXS. According to these authors, the level of joint attention disturbance observed in children with FXS may be a secondary outcome of their arousal modulation difficulties, perhaps associated with the inhibitory/anxious temperament that may be primary to the nature of social disturbance in FXS. In Murphy and Abbeduto's account, joint attention disturbance contributes to subsequent language development difficulty in children with FXS, but joint attention disturbance is not so robust as to be a diagnostic characteristic of the disorder. The research of Hall et al. (2010) and Wolff et al. (2012) suggests that joint attention impairment is not a robust part of the symptom picture even among children with FXS + ASD.

The results of joint-attention-related research accord with a contemporary hypothesis that the underlying cognitive neurodevelopment of FXS and ASD leading to differences in social development in both groups may be unrelated in substantial ways (e.g., Hall et al., 2010; McDuffie et al., 2015). These, though, are tentative conclusions that call for more work on making very careful comparisons of the developing phenotypes of children affected by ASD and FXS.

Williams Syndrome

Williams syndrome (WS) is another relatively rare disorder (1:10,000 individuals) caused by the spontaneous deletion of region q11.23 of chromosome 7, which includes more than 25 genes. WS involves cardiac, auditory, facial–cranial, visual, and neurodevelopmental differences. Like children with ASD, children with WS often exhibit delayed language development in the first 3 years. They also exhibit symptoms of attention deficits in childhood and a wide range of intellectual outcomes, from moderate IDD to high intelligence. However, unlike children with ASD, many children with WS display typical to heightened social engagement, dyadic social attention (e.g., eye contact), face processing, empathy, and a desire to engage in social interactions and/or conversations (Asada & Itakura, 2012; Järvinen-Pasley et al., 2008). Children with WS have also been observed to be more likely to imitate facial affect and vocalizations than other children with developmental delays (children in mixed comparison groups). People with WS also tend to use speech that is rich in emotional descriptors and high in prosody, such as exaggerated rhythm and emotional intensity (Mervis & Becerra, 2007).

On the other hand, many children with WS who exhibit what appears to be age-appropriate language development may use idiosyncratic terms and idioms, and may have difficulty with converging on or maintaining a common point of reference in conversations with other people (Stojanovick, Perkins, & Howard, 2006). That is, their referential skills in language appear to be different. This observation is consistent with the finding that many children with WS share a disturbance of joint attention development with children with ASD. Paradoxically, then, even though children with WS may be regarded as highly social, research suggests that they also may display symptoms of ASD.

Klein-Tasman, Mervis, Lord, and Phillips (2007) used Module 1 of the original ADOS (prior to its revision) in an assessment of ASD symptoms in 29 children with WS with mental age equivalence estimates between 12 and 35 months (mean = 22.29 months, standard deviation = 6.07). Within what was then referred to as the Communication domain of the ADOS, more than 50% of the children with WS were rated as abnormal on the joint attention item of pointing and the related item of gestures. Within the original ADOS Social Interaction domain, more than half of the children with WS showed abnormality on three joint attention items (showing, IJA, and RJA), as well as four other items (giving, integration of gaze with other behaviors, unusual eye contact, and response to name). However, very few participants showed any abnormality in shared enjoyment or requesting. This pattern of impairments was sufficiently robust that 14 of the 29 children with WS in this study met criteria for ASD on the original ADOS.

In the same year, Lincoln, Searcy, Jones, and Lord (2007) published a direct comparison of ADOS scores for a sample of 20 children with WS between 27 and 58 months old, and 26 age- and IQ-matched children with ASD. The results were very consistent with those of Klein-Tasman et al. (2007). Lincoln et al. (2007) reported that 50–80% of the children with WS displayed abnormalities in pointing, showing, and IJA, as well as imaginative play, while more than 90% of the sample with ASD displayed abnormalities on each of these items.

In an earlier study, Laing et al. (2002) used the ESCS to examine social communication development in 13 toddlers with WS with a mean mental age of 14 months, and 13 mental-age-matched typical controls. Because of the more detailed (and time-consuming) quantitative coding of joint attention and social behaviors on the ESCS versus the ADOS, this study revealed nuances about joint attention development in children with WS. As in the research described above, the children with WS in this study displayed a deficit in IJA. However, the Laing et al. study also revealed a deficit in ESCS request behaviors and an advantage for the WS children on ESCS social interaction behaviors. The ESCS items involved in this pattern of results were revealing.

On the IJA scale, the children with WS displayed a deficit in pointing, but no evidence of a deficit in alternating eye contact between an active mechanical toy and a tester. Both the typical sample and the sample with WS displayed alternating eye contact more frequently than any other IJA item in this study. This relatively high frequency of alternating eye contact was also evident on the ESCS with over 100 infants tested longitudinally between 9 and 18 months (Mundy et al., 2007). Indeed, it is the most reliable IJA item on the ESCS. Moreover, it is the ESCS item that is most sensitive to the IJA impairments of children with ASD (Mundy et al., 1986, 1994; Kasari et al., 1990). Alternating eye contact behaviors appear to emerge and consolidate in development by no later than 9 months of age, before the use of pointing for IJA, which increases in frequency after 12 months of age (Mundy et al., 2007).

This raises the possibility that many children with WS and ASD display comparable second-year joint attention deficits in pointing and showing, but not developmental differences on earlier aspects of joint attention, which are specific to children with ASD. Why might this be the case? It may be that the cognitive processes that give rise to joint attention problems in ASD and WS are different. In particular, differences in spatial processing may have an impact on joint attention development in children with WS, but this may not be the case in ASD,

In an early article titled "What Minds Have in Common Is Space," Butterworth and Jarrett (1991) pointed out that joint attention development is likely to involve visual–spatial analytic abilities. Children with WS are prone to impairments in visual–spatial cognitive development (Kaplan, Wang, & Francke, 2001). This is less clearly the case in children with ASD (e.g., Bertone, Mottron, Jelenic, & Faubert, 2005). It may be that that vulnerabilities in different neurocognitive systems are at play in the development of joint attention and children with ASD and WS. Regardless of the veracity of this conjecture, it seems possible that a more in-depth comparative examination of joint attention development in ASD and WS may be revealing with respect to the nature of the social communication differences that characterize each syndrome.

In summary, research with FXS suggests that differences in joint attention development may exist between children with ASD and children with FXS + ASD. If so, this would suggest that the dimension of joint attention may contribute to an understanding of what distinguishes the expression of the syndrome of ASD from the comorbid presentation of some symptoms of ASD in other disorders, such as FXS.

The validity of joint attention items for discriminating primary ASD from ASD symptom presentation in WS is less clear. In some ways the findings on joint attention in WS are more intriguing and potentially informative than those in FXS. In Chapter 2, I have briefly discussed the need for greater operational precision in measuring and conceptualizing what is meant by the social impairments or social phenotype of ASD. The data on WS extend this admonition to the need for greater precision in defining what we mean by *joint attention*. This term has often been equated with the development of pointing and showing, which for the most part blossom in the second year of development. However, as we have seen, the behavioral, cognitive, and neurodevelopmental features of the dimension of joint attention do not begin (or end) with the development of pointing and showing. The goal of the next chapter is to deepen the understanding of the nature of this dimension by more fully considering its role in human learning and social cognition.

Chapter 4

Joint Attention, Learning, and Social Cognition

The conceptualization of joint attention in the initial version of the NIMH RDoC as singularly a measure of face processing (see Chapter 2) seems incongruent with the account of joint attention as a major axis in the diagnosis and screening of autism (see Chapter 3). This incongruence is illustrative of the differing interpretations of joint attention in the science of autism that were alluded to in the Preface. An important perspective on these differing views has been provided in a recent, cogent research review by Catherine Lord and Rebecca Jones (2012). These authors embody unparalleled expertise in translating theory on the nature of ASD social processes into reliable, efficient, and clinically valid measurement of dimensions of ASD.

Among their many observations, Lord and Jones (2012) noted that

> empirically defining mechanisms that traverse age and development to underlie these unique patterns of behavior [the social behavior difficulties in ASD] has been a challenge. Many of the most theoretically important constructs proposed, such as theory of mind . . . , joint attention . . . , and social motivation . . . are striking in their presence at some ages and in some individuals, but [either] not observable in very young children or no longer present in significant numbers of older children or adults . . . These findings call out for broader cognitive theories to underlie dimensions of social deficits across development that might unite important, but often age and language-related constructs such as

joint attention and theory of mind, as well as ways of measuring concepts that span these theories (Hobson, 2002). (pp. 494–495)

The observations of Lord and Jones (2012), as well as the earlier thoughts of Hobson (2002), point to a fundamental challenge in identifying and studying the diagnostic, phenotypic, and endophenotypic dimensions of ASD. The challenge is that we must concertedly adopt and maintain a developmental perspective in our science, in order to understand a neuro*developmental* disorder such as ASD. The human nature of autism is such that it develops from infancy to adulthood. Just as the social-cognitive and emotional endophenotypes and phenotypes of all people change significantly from infancy to adulthood, the mental (cognitive and emotional) nature of autism's effects on people must be expected to change significantly with age, development, IQ, and a host of other factors. At a minimum, then, we must think about and search for *developmental continuities* across seemingly distinct behaviors in order to capture the reality of the dimensional nature of autism. This recognition of the *developmental complexity of social dimensions* is not yet fully inculcated in the RDoC system, at least not within the work to date on the Systems for Social Processes domain.

Advances in developmental research on joint attention, though, have begun to provide the outline of a broad cognitive theory of a primary dimension of autism. In this theory, the constructs of social motivation, social orienting, joint attention, and social cognition may all be viewed as expressions of primary, developmentally continuous dimensions of ASD across age and IQ. To support this assertion, this chapter addresses theory and research on the continuities between the development of joint attention and that of social cognition. In so doing, the chapter also discusses the role of joint attention in social, cognitive, and learning development beyond infancy. This is important, because if joint attention does not have construct validity and measurable impact in significant numbers of older children or adults, then its utility as a dimension of ASD may be significantly limited (Lord & Jones, 2012). To address this issue the chapter begins with a detailed description of the developmental continuity between infant joint attention and lifespan social cognition. The possibility of sex differences in joint attention development is also discussed. The chapter then concludes with a discussion of how joint attention during childhood and adulthood may be readily assessed with measures of language, cooperative and collaborative behavior, and information processing. Subsequently, Chapter 5 addresses the developmental continuities among social orienting, social motivation, and joint attention, together with the nettlesome problem of whether these are orthogonal or overlapping dimensions of development.

Joint Attention, Mentalizing, and Autism

The weight of evidence over the last three and a half decades indicates that atypical social-cognitive development is one of the most robust features of the childhood phenotype of ASD (e.g., Pellicano, 2010). The term *social cognition* is most often used to refer to the ability to imagine or "mentalize" the thoughts, beliefs, intentions, and emotions that guide another person's behavior. Mentalizing other people's thoughts or intentions, however, is not the same as mind reading. Rather, it is the cognitive means by which we rapidly estimate another person's internal mental, emotional, or goal-related status. This estimation is based on an our appraisal of our observations or memory of what the other person has seen, heard, and felt during one or more events, or in one or more particular episodes and contexts. We engage in this type of estimation of other people's mental status fluidly and frequently each day. Moreover, we all learn that our estimations of others' thoughts, goals, and feelings can at times be extremely accurate, but at others regrettably error-prone. In autism, and in other forms of psychopathology such as schizophrenia (Couture, Penn, & Roberts, 2006) and ADHD (Uekermann et al., 2010), the level of error in estimating others' mental status is unusually high in many affected individuals.

Research on social cognition is rarely conducted in the midst of social interactions. Rather, research participants are presented with information about other people's experiences through the use of storyboard or video portrayals of another person's experience; brief language or text that presents information about another person's experience or emotional status; and/or pictures or video of another person's facial expressions of emotion

For example, one early prominent paradigm used a storyboard to examine whether children could separate their own perceptions of the location of a hidden object from the mistaken or false belief about the object's location held by a character portrayed on the storyboard. Most often, correct or incorrect responses on such social-cognitive tasks are scored and interpreted as evidence about what the research participant knows or can mentalize about the beliefs, intentions, or emotions of another person. That is, these paradigms are thought to measure the epistemic or knowledge status of an individual. However, these paradigms are seldom designed to precisely measure the types of information processing that children might need to use in order to separate self-referenced information from other-referenced information, and then to estimate what another person is likely to know or not to know. Hence the possible joint attention/social-information processing demands of these social-cognitive tasks have rarely been considered.

I think that this oversight may have impeded recognition of the role played by internalized mental joint attention in the development of knowledge about the human nature of people's minds. When we think about the content of other people's minds, we often consider our own observations or mental representations of what the other persons have attended to, experienced, and are likely to remember, in order to estimate their thoughts, intentions, or emotions. At the same time, though, we must develop the capacity to keep these representations of other people's available information cognitively "tagged" as *other-referenced information*, in order to keep our own minds' histories of attention, experience, and encoded knowledge separate and distinct (Leslie, 1987). At times, we must also draw upon our own funds of memories about our own and others' reactions to similar information and experiences, in order to estimate the likely thoughts, feelings, or goals of other people. To the degree that the latter is true, we would expect working memory to be involved in social cognition (cf. Kiyonaga & Egner, 2014).

To illustrate this information-processing approach to social-cognitive measurement, let us apply it to the Sally–Anne task, which is depicted in Figure 4.1. This was one of the first tasks used to reveal the presence of conceptual social-cognitive impairments in ASD (Baron-Cohen et al., 1985). A task analysis of the Sally–Anne measure illustrates the role that internalized joint attention is hypothesized to play in social cognition. In this task, children observe five panels in a storyboard. In the first panel, a child sees Sally and Anne, a marble, a box, and a basket. Next, the child sees Sally place the marble in the basket. Third, he or she sees Sally "leave for a walk." In the fourth panel, the child witnesses Anne moving the marble into the box. In the final panel, Sally has returned, and the child research participant is asked, "Where will Sally look for the marble?"

The child research participant has to "mentalize" Sally's false belief that the marble is in the box in order to answer this question correctly. What are the steps involved in this mentalizing process? According to joint attention theory, the child has to represent (recall) what he or she experienced with Sally (what they saw together), and distinguish that from what the child saw with Anne, *but not with Sally*. That is, the child must internally represent, compare, and distinguish episodes of the different experiences (joint visual information) shared with Sally and Anne, in order to process the social information that leads to mentalizing that the false belief will guide Sally's choice behavior.

This account raises the possibility that internalized or mental joint-attention-related information processing constitutes a cognitive dimension that is engaged in many types of social-cognitive problem solving in later childhood and across the lifespan. The suggestion here is that internalized mental joint attention process are integral to what is referred to as

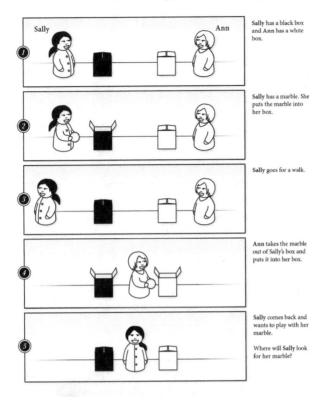

FIGURE 4.1. Schematic illustration of the Sally–Anne (Ann, in this study) false-belief theory-of-mind task. From Byom and Mutlu (2013). Reprinted in accord with the open-access guidelines of the *Frontiers in Human Neuroscience* journal.

"mentalizing" in the current literature on social cognition. This hypothesis, as we will see, is consistent with observations (detailed in Chapter 7) that there is a very considerable overlap between the cortical activation patterns elicited by joint attention and social-cognitive task performance in children, adolescents, and adults. In this chapter, the developmental and cognitive basis for the neurocognitive overlap of joint attention and social cognition is described. This is achieved by examining three ideas that are central to joint attention theory in the study both of typical development and of ASD.

One hypothesis of joint attention theory is that *knowledge about the minds of other people* does not lead to joint attention (e.g., Mundy & Newell, 2007). Rather, practice with the self–other information processing that is intrinsic to joint attention provides a type of input that is necessary for social-cognitive knowledge development to occur (e.g., Adamson,

Bakeman, & Deckner, 2004). The second premise is that *conceptual social cognition*, such as the knowledge that others have intentions, does not replace joint attention in the course of typical or atypical development. Instead, internalized mental joint attention remains an active executive component of many aspects of social cognition throughout the lifespan (Mundy, 2003; Mundy et al., 2009). Third, the factors that affect joint attention development are not limited to social-cognitive processes, and the domain of human social cognition is not limited to knowledge about the minds of other people. For example, human social cognition involves phenomena associated with facilitation of information processing in social groups, the ability and desire to cooperate and collaborate with other people, and the awareness of a sense of relatedness to individuals or groups (e.g., Bayliss et al., 2013; Boothby, Clark, & Bargh, 2014; Kim & Mundy, 2012). I argue that all of these social-cognitive phenomena are also linked to joint attention throughout the lifespan.

The Social-Cognitive Hypothesis of Joint Attention

To some extent, the field once considered social-cognitive differences to constitute the starting point of social impairments in ASD. Now, however, social-cognitive disturbance in ASD is viewed from a more transactional point of view. That is, social-cognitive disturbance may both influence social development and be *influenced by* other dimensions of development, such as language and executive function development in ASD (Hale & Tager-Flusburg, 2003; Hughes & Leekam, 2004; Milligan, Astington, & Dack, 2007). Nevertheless, the significance of social-cognitive impairment in ASD remains well supported.

Pellicano (2010), for example, reported an instructive 3-year longitudinal study of the development of 37 higher-functioning children with ASD and 31 comparison children, all of whom were 4–7 years old at the beginning of the study. She examined the development of three sets of cognitive abilities—*theory of mind*, *executive functions*, and *central coherence*—in these children. The term *executive functions* refers to measures of planning and attention-shifting abilities, and *central coherence* refers to measures of the tendency to be able to integrate details of a stimulus (pictures, sentences, stories) into an integrated whole, rather than to perceive the separate components but not the whole. A tendency to do the latter is called *weak central coherence*.

At the beginning of the study, 73% of the 4- to 7-year-old children with ASD displayed evidence of a theory-of-mind difficulty in combination with other deficits, relative to the comparison group. Sixty-five percent of the children with ASD also displayed evidence of executive functioning problems in combination with other impairments, and 100% of the children with ASD displayed evidence of weak central coherence, either alone or in combination with other problems. Three years later, some features of this pattern of problems in the children with ASD had stayed the same, and some had changed. The proportion of 7- to 10-year-old children who displayed evidence of theory-of-mind problems was virtually the same, at 70%. However, the proportion of children who displayed weak central coherence dropped precipitously (to 48%), and the proportion with executive functioning problems dropped moderately (to 54%). The number of children who did not display significant evidence of deficits on any of these three dimensions increased to 13%.[1] These results suggested that with development, symptom presentation changes in children with ASD. However, in this study, theory-of-mind disturbance displayed the most consistent evidence of a role across the early and late elementary-school-age developmental period of children with ASD.

The prominence of social-cognitive difficulties in school-age children, and of joint attention difficulties in preschool children, has long raised questions about the link between the two dimensions in research and theory on ASD. The first explicit hypothesis about this relationship was that a disturbance of social cognition explains joint attention difficulties in children with ASD (Baron-Cohen, 1989). Just as joint attention problems in ASD were first being described by Curcio (1978), Premack and Woodruff (1978) described methods to evaluate whether primates were capable of thinking about the mental intentions of other primates. Wimmer and Perner (1983) soon followed with the translation of the Premack and Woodruff methods to the study of cognitive development in children. Wimmer and Perner developed what became known as the *false-belief* paradigm.

Very quickly thereafter, other research groups in London began to apply Wimmer and Perner's false-belief paradigm to the study of autism. This led to a truly seminal sequence of observations that children with autism appeared to have more difficulty solving the false-belief problem, as presented in measures such as the Sally–Anne paradigm, than did comparison children (e.g., Baron-Cohen et al., 1985; Leslie & Happé, 1989; Frith, 1989). Furthermore, children with ASD seemed to have more difficulty with this type of social-cognitive problem solving than with analogous nonsocial problem solving. Children with ASD also tended to display more difficulty with social-cognitive problem solving than did children

---

[1] It is not clear if all children remained clearly symptomatic at Time 2. Nevertheless, Pellicano (2010) reported that the follow-up ADOS scores (mean = 12.62, standard deviation = 4.98) suggested that many if not all the children displayed clinical elevations of ASD symptoms at Time 2.

with other forms of developmental disorders. So social-cognitive problem solving appeared to be a defining feature of autism.

Outside research for autism, theory had begun to link the development of joint attention to the emergence of social cognition. Bretherton (1991) built on Baldwin's (1894) ideas of the emergence of subjectivity and infants' attribution of subjectivity of others. Bretherton suggested that "9- to 12-month-olds already possess the ability to intentionally recruit and guide a partner's attention through well-timed and well directed gestures. . . . Thus, during the preverbal and early verbal periods, infants' understanding of mind can be best inferred from how they communicate" (p. 50).

Tomasello and Call (1997) subsequently suggested that young children could only consistently and meaningfully respond to joint attention or initiate joint attention if they understood that attention of other people was goal directed or intentional. Hence infants needed to have some understanding or concept of intentionality in others to engage in joint attention. The intuitive nature of this supposition was compelling for many, and the ideas of Baron-Cohen et al. (1985), Bretherton (1991), and Tomasello and Call (1997) converged to form a very solid basis for the social-cognitive model of joint attention disturbance in ASD.

According to this model, infants need to become cognizant of their own and others' intentional capacity to coordinate attention and share information before they can be truly said to engage in joint attention (Tomasello, Carpenter, Call, et al., 2005). Similarly, joint attention impairments in ASD are thought to occur because social-cognitive modules, or a dedicated neural network that enables children to be cognizant that others have intentions, has broken down (Baron-Cohen, 1989). As noted previously, though, there are several joint attention developmental phenomena that this type of univariate causal model fails to address, be it a social-cognitive or social orienting/face-processing model.

Joint Attention, Developmental Dissociations, and Timing

Recall that infants display a wide range of individual differences in the development of joint attention (see Chapter 3, Figure 3.3). A study of 100 typically developing 9-month-olds indicated that the infants displayed from about 10 to 40 alternating gaze bids to initiate joint attention in a 20-minute interaction with an unfamiliar tester (Mundy et al., 2007). These differences did not occur by chance. Rather, individual differences were significantly correlated across the first and second years of life. This observation suggested that individual variations in joint attention development reflect stable and meaningful differences in mental processes in infants between 9 and 18 months of age—differences that are subsequently associated with later language development.

Nothing in the social-cognitive or theory-of-mind model of joint attention accounts for individual differences of the kind displayed by these 9- to 18-month-old infants (Mundy et al., 2007). This does not mean that we should discard the social-cognitive hypothesis. It simply means that the social-cognitive hypothesis does not provide a comprehensive explanation of joint attention development and differences in human nature. No mechanism is described in the social-cognitive model that clearly comports with observations of stable differences among infants in the tendency to display more or less joint attention in interactions with others. This is because social-cognitive models largely explain social cognition in terms of all-or-none development, rather than in terms of factors related to more or less expression of joint attention across development.

Two social-cognitive models are illustrative of this issue. Baron-Cohen (1995) described social-cognitive development in terms of the sequential maturation of cognitive modules. These include a dedicated cognitive facility that attributes goal-directed behavior to objects or people, called the *intentionality detector*, and the *eye direction detector*, which senses and processes information about eyes. These combine to form the *shared attention mechanism*, a joint attention cognitive module that represents self and other as attending to the same referent. This module also serves to attribute volitional states (intentionality) to other people's direction of gaze. As infancy ebbs, the theory-of-mind mechanism replaces the shared attention mechanism; it enables representation of the full range of others' mental states and enables us to make sense of others' behaviors. This model clearly recognizes several types of functions involved in joint attention and social cognition. It does not, though, describe the types of actions and information processing (or input) that may be necessary to the adequate maturation of these modules. This is because modules, by their very nature, are thought to arise inherently and without the need to consider an infant's active engagement with the social world, information processing, or learning.

A second model, proposed by Michael Tomasello and colleagues (Tomasello, Carpenter, Call, et al., 2005), explicitly describes joint attention development in terms of three stages of the development of what infants know about people, based on interpretations of astute experimental tests of their behavioral capabilities. In the first stage, *understanding animate action*, the model accepts that 3- to 8-month-old infants can perceive contingencies between their own animate actions and emotions, and the animate actions and affective expressions of others. However, they cannot know or represent the internal mental goals of others that are associated with these actions.

In the next stage, *understanding of pursuit of goals*, 9-month-olds become capable of shared action and attention on objects (e.g., building a block tower with parents). Tomasello, Carpenter, Call, et al. (2005) suggested that this stage involves joint *perception* rather than joint attention, because the social-cognitive capacity to represent others' internal mental representations (which is necessary for true joint attention) is not available at this stage of development.

The incipient awareness of others' internal mental emerges between 12 and 15 months, in the third stage, *understanding choice of plans*. This stage is heralded when infants' behavior indicates that they become systematically active in attempts to initiate episodes of joint engagement by alternating their eye contact between interesting sights and caregivers (Tomasello, Carpenter, Call, et al., 2005). This shift to active alternating gaze is thought to indicate infants' dawning appreciation that others make mental choices about the allocation of their attention. Infants also now know themselves (have self-awareness) as agents who initiate collaborative activity based on their own goals. Hence the development of "true" joint attention at this stage is revealed in the capacity to flexibly adopt and shift between two perspectives analogous to the roles of speaker and listener, or of signal sender and signal receiver.

I think that the model espoused by Tomasello and colleagues is a very well-developed and valid model of joint attention development. It seems to me to be more informative than describing joint attention development in terms of modules, because it includes more details about the interaction between an infant's behaviors and the constructivist roles these may play in social-cognitive development. Moreover, the elegant experimental studies of the Tomasello et al. three-stage model provide relatively clear evidence for the emergence of the third stage (understanding choice of plans) by 12–15 months of age (e.g., Behne, Liszkowski, Carpenter, & Tomasello, 2012).

The three-stage model, however, does not necessarily claim to provide a comprehensive explanation of joint attention development in human nature. It does not anticipate or explain the observation that meaningful (e.g., predictive) individual differences in joint attention behaviors emerge in development by 9 months of age (Mundy et al., 2007). This is not an oversight, but rather a design feature of the model. The three-stage model of Tomasello and colleagues is designed to describe the early emergence of social-cognitive conceptual knowledge, in much the same way that Piaget's sensorimotor stage model was designed to chart the early development of nonsocial conceptual knowledge. In many ways, the Tomasello et al. model has been equally successful in generating a body of evidence on social-cognitive conceptual development in childhood.

When it comes to the clinically relevant study of joint attention (such as in ASD), though, understanding the processes that give rise to individual differences in development is of primary interest. Why do some infants engage in a lot of joint attention bids at 9, 12, 15, and 18 months, and others consistently engage in some but fewer joint attention bids across this period of development? This is a critical question. In clinical developmental science or developmental psychopathology, we want to understand the factors that give rise to the normal range of individual difference in a dimension, in order to identify factors responsible for the extremes of typical variation that characterize clinical conditions. The science is less concerned with the ordinal stages of development than it is with the factors contributing to the quantitative differences in development that characterize neurodevelopmental disorders (e.g., Kasari et al., 2008; Mundy et al., 1990; Senju, 2013).

Can stage models help us to understand the factors that lead to more or less, better or worse utilization of joint attention in typical or atypical development? I'm not sure. However, I do think that it is difficult to explain the range of individual differences we observe in infant joint attention simply in terms of whether or not the infants have knowledge of other people's minds. For example, some infants and toddlers may consistently display lower frequencies of IJA alternating bids, and some may display higher frequencies of this IJA behavior. How do these differences relate to the children's social-cognitive knowledge? Do these differences indicate that young children differ meaningfully in the *amount or strength of knowledge* about others' intentional behavior? Perhaps, but I think not. To explain these individual differences, and to reach a full understanding of the human nature of joint attention, we need to look beyond stage models of social cognition and consider factors other than knowledge about people's intentions (Mundy et al., 2007).

Similarly, can we explain the dissociation of IJA and RJA in development in terms of a dissociation in the social-cognitive knowledge they represent? Both RJA and IJA are useful in the early identification and diagnosis of autism, but RJA impairments become less evident with advances in preschool cognitive development (e.g., Mundy et al., 1994, Lord et al., 2000; Nation & Penny, 2008). IJA deficits, on the other hand, remain diagnostic into the school-age period of development, *and* IJA is a better discriminator than RJA between children with autism and children with other developmental disorders (e.g., Charman, 2003; Dawson et al., 2004; Hobson & Hobson, 2007; Mundy et al., 1986; Sigman et al., 1999). No explanation that I am aware of has yet been presented from the perspective of the social-cognitive model for this phenomenon of joint attention development in ASD.

Evidence for this dissociation in development is perhaps best illustrated by a comparison of the patterns of growth that characterize IJA, RJA, and nonverbal requesting behaviors in typical infants. When IJA is measured in terms of frequency of occurrence, it displays a remarkably flat profile of minimal change or growth across the 9- to 18-month-period. This is all the more remarkable, compared to clear evidence of age-related growth in the frequency or consistency of requesting behaviors and RJA behaviors across ages in typical infants (see Chapter 3, Figure 3.5).

If social cognition is the essential mechanism for all of joint attention development, what social-cognitive factor accounts for observations of the dissociation of IJA and RJA in typical and atypical development? Moreover, if IJA follows a pattern of growth marked by a qualitative change in social cognition at 12–14 months, why doesn't it display an age-related change comparable to that in RJA and other forms of joint attention behavior across 12–18 months of development (Mundy et al., 2007)? These types of questions are not addressed in the stage-based social-cognitive models, just as they are not clearly addressed by social orienting, face-processing, or imitation explanations of joint attention development. This is not a critique of stage-based models. It is simply the observation that they were not developed to offer an explanation of the factors that contribute to variation in the human nature of joint attention development. However, understanding these factors is a primary goal of the science of developmental psychopathology.

Conceptual stages of development are often thought to arise incrementally from significant periods of constructive engagement with the environment (e.g., Piaget, 1952). So one important path to explaining individual differences may be to understand the nature of the incremental constructive engagement with the environment that leads to joint attention and social-cognitive development. Indeed, the first stage (understanding animate action) of the Tomasello, Carpenter, Call, et al. (2005) model speaks directly to the nature of this constructivist activity. In this stage, as noted earlier, 3- to 8-month-olds can perceive contingencies between their own animate actions and emotions, and the animate actions and affective expressions of others. *However, they cannot know or represent the internal mental goals of others that are associated with these actions.* This last assumption of the model suggests that perceiving contingencies between self and other relative to a common referent is an important milestone in the development of joint attention, but one that is surpassed later by attainment of knowledge about others' intentions.

Alternatively, the model espoused here suggests that perceiving contingencies between one's own animate actions and emotions, and the animate actions and affective expressions of others, relative to a common reference point is the information-processing essence of joint attention. It begins to develop in the 2- to 8-month period and becomes more rapid and efficient thereafter. With increasing efficiency and speed of processing, it becomes possible for children to include information from memory to deepen the nature of the comparative information processing of self–other relative to a common referent that occurs in joint attention. This contributes to social-cognitive development, but is not replaced by social-cognitive development. The comparative processing of self- and other-information relative to a common referent remains a defining information-processing feature of joint attention. It becomes an element of information processing that is central to social-cognitive problem solving. According to this model, the factors that contribute to the consistency and efficiency of self–other information processing are what give rise to human variation in joint attention development.

This logic leads to the assumption that experience and practice with joint attention in the first year of life (2–12 months) are likely to contribute along a constructive path of development to social cognition and its differences in autism spectrum development (Mundy & Sigman, 1989a, 1989b). Numerous studies have subsequently provided data consistent with the idea that joint attention contributes to social-cognitive development, as much as (or more than) social-cognitive development leads to joint attention. Let us consider the innovative sequence of studies provided by Meltzoff and Brooks as an example.

Brooks and Meltzoff (2002) observed that 12-month-olds often followed the head turn and gaze direction of testers, even if the testers' eyes were closed. After 12 months, though, infants only followed the gaze of testers whose eyes were open; they did not follow the head turning and eye direction of testers whose eyes were closed. This suggests that infants' understanding of the intentional meaning of the eye gaze of others may improve in this period, leading older infants to be more discriminating in their practice of joint attention. They inhibit attention following in eyes-closed conditions (Brooks & Meltzoff, 2002). It also means that infants 12 months of age or younger may engage in joint attention with a less discriminating social-cognitive conceptualization of others.

To better validate and understand this phenomenon in joint attention development, Meltzoff and Brooks (2008) conducted an experimental intervention. They replicated their previous observations, but this time, instead of an eyes-closed condition, they had the testers wear blindfolds. They then provided 12-month-olds with the opportunity to wear blindfolds that occluded their own lines of sight. After gaining that experience, 12-month-olds did not follow the head turns of blindfolded testers, but did follow the head turns and gaze of nonblindfolded testers. In another clever experimental manipulation, Meltzoff and Brooks also provided

18-month-olds with experience with blindfolds that looked opaque but were transparent when worn. After this condition, the 18-month-olds reverted to following the gaze of blindfolded social partners. The pattern of the results suggested to Meltzoff and Brooks that the infants constructed social-cognitive awareness about others' gaze behavior, based on the self-referenced processing of their own practice with gaze behavior and experience.

Of course, even if the foregoing is true, it still could be the case that joint attention behaviors deficits only emerge in ASD after practice with these behaviors fails to trigger social-cognitive development in the second year. In this case, we might expect to see a relatively typical path of joint attention development in the first year of life for children affected by ASD. After that, joint attention might decline because of a failure specific to the social-cognitive stage of development in the second year. Recall, however, the Ibañez et al. (2013) study described in Chapter 3 (see Figure 3.4). This study revealed that IJA at 8 months of age was a unique predictor of confirmed ASD diagnosis at 30 months among at-risk infants. The predictive model with the 8-month IJA variable correctly identified 6 of 9 at-risk infants who received the diagnosis of ASD on the ADOS (sensitivity = 67%), and correctly identified 25 of 26 higher-risk infants who did not receive the diagnosis of ASD (specificity = 96%). These data suggest one of two things relative to current stage models of joint attention. The onset of joint attention differences may occur in children with ASD before the mentalizing of intention in others is expected to emerge in typical development; moreover, the onset of these differences at 8 months in some children with ASD may make a causal contribution to subsequent social-cognitive developmental perturbations. On the other hand, these data may indicate that the development of understanding of intentionality in others has a much earlier onset in development than was previously imagined.

We do not yet have evidence on hand that would enable us to choose between these alternatives. Nevertheless, they suggest why a precise understanding of the relations between joint attention development and social-cognitive development is one of the more important goals for the developmental science of ASD. The developmental continuity between these two domains of disturbance remains one of the most profoundly informative characteristics of the cognitive phenotype of ASD (Charman, 2003). Other types of disorders may be characterized by vulnerability to social-cognitive disturbance, especially face and emotion processing (Cohen et al., 1998; Couture et al., 2006; Uekermann et al., 2010). However, evidence to date suggests that only ASD is characterized by a continuous sequence of development differences in joint attention and social-cognitive development from infancy to adulthood.

An Alternative Theory of Joint Attention and Social Cognition

One alternative to the stage model approach is to describe the continuity between joint attention and social-cognitive growth in both typical and autism spectrum development in terms of a *parallel and distributed processing model* (PDPM) (Mundy et al., 2009). A PDPM is based on neurocognitive connectionist theory, which attempts to describe information processing in the way it appears to take place in the brain (McClelland, Rumelhart, & Hinton, 1986). Accordingly, information processing occurs across distributed brain networks, rather than in isolated brain regions. Second, memory and knowledge resulting from information processing is stored, in part, in the pattern of connections between neural networks activated during information encoding. Finally, learning and cognitive development occur incrementally, partly in terms of changes in connection strength across nodes of neural networks.

The types of issues addressed by a PDPM have applications to neurodevelopmental disorders, including (1) identifying the types of information processing that are central to the cognitive and behavioral phenotypes of various conditions; (2) describing how these types of information processing change over time in typical and atypical development; (3) understanding how these types of information processing are instantiated in neural networks; and, finally, (4) postulating why differences in processing and neural networks occur in clinical conditions.

Our initial publication of a PDPM of ASD (Mundy et al., 2009) described joint attention and social-cognitive development as resulting from the interactive flow of triadic information processing across a neurocognitive network involved in self-referenced processing of information about attention, processing of information about the status of another person's attention, and processing information about some third object or event. On the basis of then-current knowledge, it also suggested that the mature human joint attention network involves primary nodes found in the prefrontal, insula, cingulate, temporal, and parietal cortices (see Chapter 7 for details). The PDPM of joint attention emphasizes the cortically multidetermined nature of human cognition, because of the "massively parallel nature of human brain networks and the fact that (cognitive) function also emerges from the flow of information between brain areas" (Ramnani, Behrens, Penny, & Matthews, 2004, p. 613), not just from isolated neural networks.

The PDPM of joint attention also suggests that cognitive development need not be construed only in terms of changes in discontinuous stages of knowledge. It can be usefully modeled as a continuous change in the speed, efficiency, and combinations of information processing that give rise to knowledge (Hunt, 1999). Specifically, the PDPM envisions joint attention development in terms of increased speed, efficiency, and complexity of processing of the following: (1) internal information about self–referenced visual attention; (2) external information about the visual attention of other people; and (3) the neural networks that integrate processing of (a) self-generated visual attention information, (b) mutual gaze and the gaze direction of other people, and (c) spatial, temporal, and ultimately sematic information about a common focus of reference (Mundy, 2003; Mundy & Newell, 2007).

The notion that *true* joint attention does not emerge until requisite social-cognitive knowledge emerges at 12–15 months (Tomasello, Carpenter, Call, et al., 2005) is not especially germane to the PDPM. Instead, based on a growing empirical developmental literature, the PDPM holds that the joint processing of attention information about self and others relative to a common point of reference begins to be practiced by infants by 2–4 months of age (e.g., D'Entremont, Hains, & Muir, 1997; Farroni, Csibra, Simion, & Johnson, 2002; Hood, Willen, & Driver, 1998, Morales, Mundy, & Rojas, 1998; Striano, Reid, & Hoel, 2006; Striano & Stahl, 2005). Moreover, incipient mechanisms associated with an attentional bias to look where others' eyes look may be observed in the first week of postnatal life (Farroni, Massaccesi, Pividori, & Johnson, 2004). Moreover, the types of active alternating gaze behaviors thought to mark the onset of true joint attention at 12–15 months (Tomasello, Carpenter, Call, et al., 2005) develop no later than at 8–9 months of life, and quite possibly earlier (Mundy et al., 2007; Venezia et al., 2004).

Equally important, the PDPM assumes that *joint attention is not replaced by the subsequent development of social-cognitive processes.* No evidence of which I am aware indicates that phenomena specifically associated with joint attention cease at some age to be active and essential phenomena of the human mind. For example, data indicate that the frontoparietal parallel distributed processing systems stipulated to support joint attention (Mundy, 2003; Mundy et al., 2009) are elicited in adults by joint attention tasks (Redcay et al., 2012; Schilbach et al., 2010; Williams et al., 2005; see Chapter 7). There is burgeoning evidence that the experience of joint attention is associated with change and enhancement of information processing in adults, just as it appears to be in infants (e.g., Kim & Mundy, 2012). Indeed, there is even evidence that the aging social-cognitive systems of older adults may be characterized by a breakdown in joint attention (Slessor, Phillips, & Bull, 2008). Rather than being replaced, joint attention remains an active system of information processing that supports cognition through adulthood (Mundy & Newell, 2007).

Symbolic Development

As an example of joint attention's lifespan nature, consider the relations between joint attention and human symbolic development. Werner and Kaplan (1963) were among the first to suggest that a cognitive foundation for the capacity to imbue an abstract symbol with a common meaning across people (i.e., symbolic thinking) was provided in the infant–caregiver *primordial sharing situation*. The primordial sharing situation occurs when infants and caregivers coordinate their senses (visual or tactile) in order to process the same information about the same object at the same time. Werner and Kaplan (1963) were describing infant–caregiver practice with joint attention (Adamson, 1995). Their claim was that many episodes of infant–caregiver practice with sharing information in joint attention lead to the development of a cognitive mechanism for sharing information that is necessary for symbolic thinking.

Tomasello, Carpenter, Call, et al. (2005) provide a more detailed explication of how joint attention scaffolds symbolic development. Recall that in Tomasello and colleagues' view, true joint attention development is indicated when infants become truly active in initiating episodes of joint engagement by alternating their eye contact between interesting sights and caregivers. This shift to active alternating gaze indicates infants' appreciation of others as self-aware agents who make mental choices about alternative actions that affect their attention. At this stage, infants also know themselves (have self-awareness) as agents who initiate collaborative activity based on their own goals and attention. Hence the development of "true" joint attention comes with the capacity to flexibly adopt and mentally shift between two perspectives analogous to those of speaker and listener.

The capacity to adopt two perspectives is also assumed to be an intrinsic characteristic of symbolic representations. In this regard, Tomasello, Carpenter, Call, et al. (2005) raised a seminal hypothesis that symbolic thought is a developmental conversion of joint attention. This differed from Werner and Kaplan's (1963) claims that joint attention provides a foundation for symbolic thought. Tomasello, Carpenter, Call, et al. (2005) suggested that *symbolic thinking involves joint attention*, at least as I read these authors. Symbols serve to coordinate internal mental attention socially, so that the intention or shared focus of attention of the listener aligns with that of the speaker. In other words, linguistic symbols both lead to and are dependent upon the efficient social coordination of covert mental attention to common abstract representations among people.

This is not to say that joint attention in and of itself gives rise to symbolic thinking. The primary foundation of symbolic thinking is likely to involve advances in cognitive representational capacity. Symbolic thinking, though, may arise in human ontology and phylogeny via the interaction of advances in representational ability and joint attention with advances in speed of information processing and memory. The hypothesis here is that for a cognitive representation to take on shared meaning (symbolic quality), it needs to become associated with properties that elicit awareness of shared reference. In the second and third years of life, practice with adopting consensual meanings for abstract representation, such as making a doll "walk" as if it were animate, becomes a primary activity within joint attention episodes. That is to say, symbolic development and adopting consensual meaning for representations is scaffolded in the context of joint attention (e.g., Adamson et al., 2004). According to the PDPM, during this scaffolding process neural networks associated with a specific cognitive representation become coactivated with neural networks involved in joint attention and joint references, to yield the developmental onset of a hybrid form of mental representation we call *symbolic thinking*. In other words, symbolic thinking involves neural network joint attention activation patterns that imbue mental representations with information about their shared reference or *signal value*.

Let me unpack this notion a just bit more. Just as 12-month-olds can shift eye contact or use pointing to establish a common visual point of reference with other people, 4-year-olds can use symbols to establish common points of reference to covert mental representations with other people. Symbolic representations are often, if not always, initially encoded during the joint processing of information about the overt attention of self and of others directed toward some third object or event (Adamson et al., 2004; Baldwin, 1995; Werner & Kaplan, 1963).[2] The PDPM combines this hypothesis with the connectionist notion that "representations can take the form of patterns of activity distributed across processing units" that *occur during encoding* (Munakata & McClelland, 2003, p. 415). Together, these two ideas lead to the PDPM's assumption that *early symbol acquisition incorporates the distributed activation of the joint self-attention and other-attention neural processing units, which were engaged during encoding, as part of their functional neural representational that supports the shared meaning of the symbol.* Hence the distributed joint attention processing system may be activated as network encoding that contributes to the initial conscious awareness of a sense of shared attention and meaning (intersubjectivity), which may be necessary for the development of symbolic cognition.

---

[2]Presumably, adult scaffolding of the development of symbolic play demands referencing acts of play with objects while interacting with infants or children. As such, scaffolding of play with young children (or any other early intervention target) also involves cultivating joint attention with infants. This observation is consistent with the finding that the play component of JASPER (see Chapter 6) increases joint attention, but the joint attention component, which does not involve reference to symbolic play acts with objects, does not necessarily advance symbolic play skills (Kasari, Freeman, & Paparella, 2006).

In infancy, the distributed joint attention processing system is initially effortful (Gredebäck et al., 2010; Vaughan Van Hecke et al., 2012). However, thousands of episodes of practice allow the joint information processing of self- and other-attention to become efficient, less effortful, and even automatically activated in social interactions. Hypothetically, as this occurs, joint attention becomes a social-executive "subroutine" that supports the capacity to maintain the necessary level of shared focus of attention for adopting common meanings in social interactions. Thus the distributed neural activation associated with joint attention can be thought of as an enduring stratum of a more *continuous spiral* of human social-neurocognitive development—a spiral that supports, if not enables, later-emerging human symbolic, linguistic, and social-cognitive facilities (see Figure 4.2).

Inside-Out Processing

The PDPM may be distinguished from other models of social-cognitive development by its overtly constructivist perspective on development. Rather than focusing on the age at which behavior implies changes in

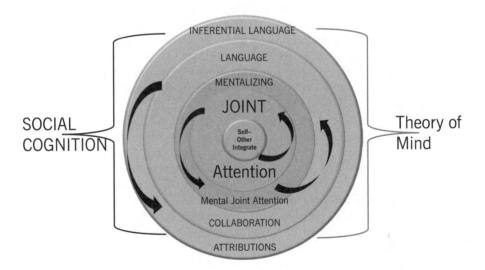

FIGURE 4.2. An illustration of the continuous nature of joint attention development. Development is modeled as a spiral in which the initial acquisition of the capacity for integrated processing of information about self- and other-attention (joint attention) remains an active but deeper layer of cognitive activity throughout life that supports symbolic thought, language, and cultural social exchange. From Mundy, Sullivan, and Mastergeorge (2009). Copyright 2009 by John Wiley & Sons, Inc. Reprinted by permission.

knowledge *about other people*, the PDPM focuses on how infants become aware of their own intentional visual behavior in joint attention and social-cognitive development (Mundy, Sigman, & Kasari, 1993). The assumption here is that neonates and young infants receive greater quantities and fidelity of information about intentional action through proprioceptive processing about their own volitional actions than they do through external information processing of the actions of others. In other words, infants have the opportunity to learn as much or more about intentionality from their own actions as they do from observing other people. This assumption may be recognized in a hypothesis suggesting that joint attention is a form of embodied action that helps shape cognition and the mind (Feldman & Narayanan, 2004; Mundy, Gwaltney, & Henderson, 2010). The development of joint attention comprises, if not epitomizes, an embodied constructivist process that involves perception of self-action as a foundation for the attribution of meaning to the perception of others' behaviors. We have dubbed this embodied cognition hypothesis the "inside-out" processing assumption of the PDPM (Mundy & Vaughan Van Hecke, 2008).

The general tenor of this constructivist assumption is nothing new. Bates et al. (1979) suggested that a sense of self-agency is basic to joint attention. More generally, Piaget (1952) argued that infants do not learn through the passive perception of objects (or others) in the world. Rather, infants take actions on objects and learn from these (causal) actions. They then modify their actions, observe changes in causal relations, and learn new things about the physical world. Thus Piaget viewed the processing of self-initiated actions on objects as a singularly important fuel for the engines of cognitive development.

The constructivist viewpoint is not only central to the PDPM; it is also a mainstay of contemporary connectionist biological principles of typical and atypical neurocognitive development (e.g., Blakemore & Frith, 2003; Elman, 2005; Mareschal et al., 2007; Meltzoff, 2007; Quartz, 1999). The vast number of functional neural connections made in early postnatal brain development is thought to be too great to be specified by genes alone. Instead, genes specify relatively wide channels of potential neurodevelopmental architecture (e.g., Quartz, 1999). Within these prescribed channels, the specifics of important functional connections in the developing nervous systems are shaped by our experience. Since the vast majority of people experience more similar than dissimilar environments and experiences in early life, developmental brain organization displays significant similarities across most people (Mareschal et al., 2007). Greenough, Black, and Wallace (1987) refer to the similar outcomes of gene-by-environment interaction over varied but largely similar milieus as "experience-expectant" neurodevelopment.

Greenough et al. (1987) also explicitly observed that *infants' genera-tion of actions, and observations of social reactions, are likely to play a role in experience-expectant processes specific to neurodevelopmental basis of human social behavior.* So just as Piaget envisioned that infants learn about the physical world from their self-generated actions on objects, it is reason-able to think that a significant portion of what infants learn about the social world comes from their self-generated actions with people. One type of self-generated action that may be developmentally key in this regard is active vision.

Active Vision

One of the first and most vitally informative types of actions infants take involves the self-control of their looking behaviors, or *active vision*. The sci-ence of vision has moved away from the study of "seeing," or passive visual perception, to the study of "looking," or intentional, active vision and attention deployment (Findlay & Gilchrist, 2003). Active vision in infancy begins to be observed at 3–4 months of age (e.g., Canfield & Kirkham, 2001; Johnson, 1990, 1995). Active vision involves the goal-directed selec-tion of information to process, and can elicit contingent social-behavioral responses from other people, such as parental smiles, vocalizations or gaze shifts. It also is one of the first types of volitional actions that infants use to control stimulation to order to self-regulate arousal and affect (Pos-ner & Rothbart, 2007).

Vision and looking behavior have unique properties. Vision pro-vides information regarding the spatial location of ourselves, and our own spatial location relative to other people. Moreover, direction of gaze conveys the distal and proximal spatial direction of our attention to oth-ers, and vice versa. Comparable information on the spatial direction of attention is not as clearly available from the other senses. The importance of visual–spatial information for the development of joint attention was emphasized by Butterworth and Jarrett (1991) in their influential article "What Minds Have in Common Is Space."

In some sense, primate eyes are specialized for *social* spatial attention processing (e.g., Tomasello, Hare, Lehman, & Call, 2006). Frontal bin-ocular eye positions allow for enhanced spatial processing and depth of perception through parallax perception. Intricate musculatures allow for rapid visual focus on objects that are far or near. Equally important, pre-cise information about the spatial direction of attention is available from human eyes because of the sharp contrast of the dark coloration of the pupil and iris with the light to white coloration of the sclera. These obser-vations have led to the suggestion that the ease of processing the direction of attention of other people's eyes contributed to the human phylogenetic and ontogenetic development of social cognition (e.g., Tomasello et al., 2006).

It is also the case, though, that these characteristics of the human eye allow the saccades of infants to be readily observed by other people. Consequently, infant saccades can effectively act as elicitors of contingent social feedback. When infants shift attention to an object, their parents may pick up and show them the object. When infants shift attention to their parents' eyes, they may also receive a vocal, affective, or physical parental response. Thus, just as the characteristics of eyes make it easier for infants to perceive the attention of others, the signal value of eyes makes the active control of vision a likely nexus of infants' own early-developing sense of agency.

The notion that active vision has primacy in social development relates back to the time-honored observation that visual behavior is at least as important to human social development as physical contact (Rheingold, 1966; Robson, 1967). However, the importance here is in the dynamic of infants' processing information about their own control of vision, as well as about the vision of other people. The contemporary literature on social-cognitive development, however, emphasizes only the importance of the latter (e.g., Johnson et al., 2005). It neglects the potential importance of the information infants process about their own active vision, and of socially contingent mutual gaze. For example, caregivers' reactions to young infants' intentional attention shifts and the eye contact effect (Senju & Johnson, 2009) may help guide the dynamic process of joint attention development.

Senju and Johnson (2009) proposed that typical infants exhibit positive cognitive arousal to caregiver eye contact via a fast-acting neural network. Being the object of social attention of others—whether this occurs through infant-directed speech or infant-directed visual attention—may have a positive impact on infant arousal (Kim & Johnson, 2014). If so, it is plausible that contingent gaze and speech to infants may be an especially important spur to promoting infants' awareness of the impact of their own intentional attention shifts on the world. The corollary is that this spur to the development of awareness of self-directed attention may well be muted in some children, contributing to vulnerability to autism spectrum development. The novel ideas of Senju and Johnson (2009) will be discussed in more detail in comparing the joint attention and social orienting models of autism in Chapter 5.

Of course, it is also the case that *any type of disruption of early alerting and orienting responses* could have an impact on social joint attention development in children with ASD (Mundy, 2003; Sacrey, Armstrong, Bryson, & Zwaigenbaum, 2014). It is important to keep in mind that we have not yet done the concerted types of research that would permit a confident conclusion that a disturbance of *social* attention, as opposed to more general attention disturbance, is primary in autism. In this regard, it is useful to consider how the active vision hypothesis in the PDPM of joint attention may be informed by the role of visual development in social attention in ASD.

The work of several research groups indicates that basic mechanisms of visual control may play a role in autism (Brenner, Turner, & Muller, 2007; Landry & Bryson, 2003; Johnson et al. 2005). Brenner et al. (2007) have noted that one of the essential issues for this line of research is to understand precisely "how an ocular-motor system that is over-specialized for certain tasks and under-specialized for others early in life might affect later development in [social] domains such as joint attention" (p. 1302). The PDPM offers a guide in this regard. First, it encourages the research community to recognize the possibility that joint attention may not be a "later" development, but one that begins as part of the development of volitional visual attention control by the fourth month of life, at the latest. In addition, the PDPM provides means for understanding how significantly altered early visual preferences could have a cascading effect on the development of intentional joint attention and autism (Mundy, 1995). In this regard, consider the following two studies.

McCleery, Allman, Carver, and Dobkins (2007) observed that magnocellular visual processing might be atypically enhanced in a sample of 6-month-old infant siblings of children with autism. Similarly, Karmel, Gardner, Swensen, Lennon, and London (2008) observed visual attention patterns consistent with a magnocellular bias in 6-month-olds in neonatal intensive care who received the diagnosis of autism at 3 years of age. The magnocellular visual system contributes to orienting based on movement and contrast sensitivity (related to small achromatic differences in brightness). This system dominates early visual orienting. However, by 2–4 months visual orienting is increasingly influenced by the parvocellular system, which contributes to orienting based on high-resolution information about shape or low-resolution information about color and shades of grey. The studies of Karmel et al. (2008) and McCleery et al. (2007) raise the possibility that a delay in the developmental shift from the magnocellular to the parvocellular visual system could alter what children with autism choose to attend to early in life.

Hypothetically, the maintenance of a magnocellular bias may lead to a relatively long-standing visual preference for stimuli or objects characterized by movement or achromatic contrasts, such as surface edges, power lines, spinning objects, the outlines of faces, or mouth movement. Reciprocally, the decreased influence of the parvocellular system could lead to developmental delays in the emergence of a visual attention bias to targets that are socially informative, but that involve differentiation based on high resolution of shape and color information, such as distal processing of eyes and facial expressions. Thus the alteration of visual preferences during early critical periods of development could degrade the establishment of the dynamic system of internal information processing about active looking, relative to contingent social feedback and to information about the attention of other people (Mundy, 1995; Mundy & Burnette, 2005). Moreover, if magnocelluar guidance bias and connectivity impairments are orthogonal processes, combinations of varying levels of their effects could present as phenotypic differences in joint attention processing and social symptom expression in autism.

The message here is that any or many types of processes that affect visual orienting and alerting in the first months of life may disrupt joint attention development and the types of social learning that follow (Mundy, 2003; Jones & Klin, 2013). However, recall from Chapter 4 that processes associated with attention regulation, such as stimulus disengagement or length of fixations, are well known to vary with general cognitive or intellectual development (e.g., Sigman et al., 1997). So we must use careful methods in studies of the early development of attention in research on ASD. We need to determine what types of attention differences may be specific to autism, and what types may be better explained by the elevated risk for IDD associated with ASD. Both types of differences may be important. There may be specific factors (such as the eye contact effect), nonspecific factors (such as the slower rates of stimulus disengagement associated with IDD), or other processes entirely that disrupt attention development in ASD. Any combination of these factors may result in a cascade of effects that disrupt joint attention and its embodied social learning impact on language and social cognition in autism spectrum development. Let us begin to consider some of the evidence and dynamic processes that may be involved in the developmental cascade of joint attention disturbance in the social phenotype of ASD.

Dynamic Systems and Integrated Processing

The PDPM emphasizes inside-out processing, constructivism, and the role of active vision in the development of joint attention. However, it does *not* maintain that the inside-out processing of self-attention is more important for social-cognitive development than the outside-in processing of other-attention. This is because the PDPM incorporates the long-standing idea that social meaning and conscious self-awareness cannot be derived from processing either self-attention or other-attention in isolation (cf. Baldwin, 1995; Decety & Sommerville, 2003; Keysers & Perrett, 2004; Vygotsky, 1962). Ontogeny may be best viewed as a dynamic system that, through interactions of multiple factors over time and experience, coalesces into higher-order integrations, structures, and skills (e.g., Smith & Thelen, 2003). The development of joint attention, or the joint processing of the attention of self and other, is such a dynamic system. Indeed, the pertinence of joint attention for human development derives in no small part from the unique synthesis that arises from of the rapid, parallel processing of self-attention and other-attention across distributed neural networks. Practice with this type of parallel processing is most constructive when experience is derived from the dual perspectives of drawing attention to self and directing others' attention (IJA), and of being sensitive to the attention of others and joining with their line of regard (RJA). Consequently, it is not possible to account for the role of joint attention in typical or atypical development with research or theory that focuses on only one role (attention to others *or* attention to self) in what amounts to the dialogical process of joint attention.

The dynamic, dialogical system of joint attention begins to synergize as frontal executive functions increasingly enable infants to attend to multiple sources of information during the second through sixth months of life. According to one definition, executive functions involve the transmission of bias signals throughout the neural network to selectively inhibit comparatively automatic behavioral responses in favor of more volitional, planned, and goal-directed ideation and action in problem-solving contexts (Miller & Cohen, 2001). These bias signals act as regulators for the brain, affecting visual processes and attention, as well as other sensory modalities and systems (those responsible for task-relevant response execution, memory retrieval, emotional evaluation, etc.). The aggregate effect of these bias signals is to guide the flow of neural activity along pathways that *establish the proper mappings among inputs, internal states, and outputs needed to perform a given task more efficiently* (Miller & Cohen, 2001). According to this definition, joint attention development may be thought of as reflecting the emergence of frontal bias signals that establish the proper mappings across (1) outside-in, posterior cortical (temporal–precuneous–superior colliculus and amygdala) processing of inputs about the attention behaviors of other people; and (2) rostral–medial–frontal (Brodmann's area [BA] 8–9, anterior cingulate, and insula cortex), inside-out processing of internal states and outputs related to active vision (e.g., Mundy et al., 2009; Senju & Johnson, 2009). This mapping results in the integrated development of a distributed anterior and posterior cortical joint attention system. The beginnings of this mapping may be evidenced in recent imaging data at 5 months of age (Elison et al., 2013).

It is conceivable that the early establishment of this mapping of the joint processing of attention is formative with respect to the shared neural network of self- and other-representations that Decety and Grèzes (2006) suggest is essential to social cognition. It also may a play a role in what Keysers and Perrett (2004) have described as a "Hebbian" learning model of social cognition. Neural networks that are repeatedly active at the same time become associated, such that activity (e.g., re-presentation) in one network triggers activity in the other (Hebb, 1949). Keysers and Perrett suggest that *common* activation of neural networks for processing self-generated information and information about conspecifics is fundamental to understanding the actions of others. This Hebbian learning process is fundamental to the hypothesized functions of simulation (Gordon, 1986) and mirror neurons (i.e., Decety & Sommerville, 2003; Williams, 2008), which are commonly invoked in current models of social-cognitive development.

The PDPM is not only consistent with these interrelated ideas, but suggests that Hebbian mapping in social cognition begins with integrated rostral–medial–frontal processing of information about self-produced visual attention and parietal–temporal processing of the attention of others (Mundy, 2003). Moreover, the PDPM specifically operationalizes the study of development of this dynamic mapping system in terms of psychometrically sound behavioral measures of early joint attention development (Mundy et al., 2007). IJA assessments may be relatively powerful in research on social-cognitive development and autism, because they provide a means to measure variance in the whole dynamic system in social interaction, rather than only one part of the system at a time (see Chapter 7).

Once well practiced, the joint processing of attention information requires less mental effort. As basic joint attention processing is mastered and the necessary effort to engage in it decreases, it can become integrated as an executive function that contributes to the initial development and increasing efficiency of social-cognitive problem solving. Thus joint attention development may be envisioned as expanding from *learning to* do joint attention from 2 to 9 months, to *learning from* joint attention in the second year of life (Mundy & Vaughan Van Hecke, 2008; Mundy et al., 2009; see Figure 4.3). In the study of ASD or other neurodevelopmental disorders, it is important to recognize that the learning-to phase may be longer. Consequently, joint attention may remain more effortful for years beyond infancy. Children with ASD may be able to engage in joint attention, but may not be able to benefit fully from joint attention in social learning opportunities. The amounts of effort required to engage in and maintain joint attention are likely to vary across children affected by ASD, and this variance may contribute to syndrome heterogeneity. If this set of assumptions is valid, it suggests that a goal for future research is to measure variance in the effort required for joint attention or the

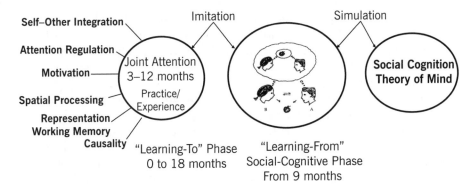

FIGURE 4.3. A multiprocess model of joint attention. In the first year, the development of joint attention involves the *learning-to* integration of executive, motivation, and imitation processes to support the routine, rapid, and efficient (error-free) execution of behavior patterns that enable infants to coordinate processing of overt aspects of visual self-attention with processing of the social attention of other people. In the latter part of the first year and the second year, infants can better monitor their own experience and integrate it with information about the social partners during joint attention events. This provides a critical multimodality source of information to the infants about the convergence or divergence of their own and others' experience and behavior while sharing information in social interactions. Theoretically, this provides the basis for the *learning-from* phase of joint attention development. In this stage, infants can control their attention to self-organize and optimize information processing in social learning opportunities. The integration of anterior and posterior self- and other-attention processing provides a neural network that enriches encoding in social learning. The internalization of the overt joint processing of attention to the covert joint processing of attention to representations is part of an executive system that facilitates symbolic development and the social cognition. Both symbolic thought and social cognition may be characterized by a transition from learning to socially coordinate overt attention to the capacity to socially coordinate covert mental representations of the attention of self and others. From Mundy, Sullivan, and Mastergeorge (2009). Copyright 2009 by John Wiley & Sons, Inc. Reprinted by permission.

benefits provided by joint attention among people with ASD. Looking further ahead, and well beyond my expertise, I wonder whether differences in mitochondrial dynamics (Safiulina & Kaasik, 2013) within neural networks could be at play if joint attention is truly more effortful for many people with ASD.

In the learning-from phase, the capacity to attend to multiple sources of information in triadic attention deployment becomes more common (Scaife & Bruner, 1975). Triadic attention contexts provide infants with rich opportunities to compare information gleaned through processing internal states associated with volitional visual attention deployment and the processing of the visual attention of others in reference to a common third object or event. Through simulation (Gordon, 1986), infants may begin to impute that others have intentional control over their looking behavior that is similar to their own.

The role of simulation in the learning-from phase of joint attention development is well illustrated by the sequence of elegant experimental studies provided by Meltzoff and Brooks, as described earlier in this chapter. Recall that 12-month-olds often follow the gaze direction of testers even if their eyes are closed. After 12 months, though, infants discriminate and follow the gaze of testers whose eyes are open but not closed. This suggests that infants' understanding of the meaning of the eye gaze of others may improve in this period, leading older infants to inhibit looking in the eyes-closed condition (Brooks & Meltzoff, 2002). Meltzoff and Brooks (2008) showed that infants can develop evidence of this understanding from their own experience in joint attention episodes. After 12-month-old infants were provided with the experience of blindfolds that occluded their vision, they acted as though they had learned that blindfolds occluded the vision of testers who attempted to get the 12-month-olds to follow their line of visual regard. Meltzoff and Brooks also provided 18-month-olds with experience with blindfolds that looked opaque but were transparent when worn. After this condition, the 18-month-olds followed the gaze direction of a tester's line of regard. This suggested that their own experience guided their social-cognitive, or at least social-perceptual, interpretation of a blindfold on a tester.

The observation that infants use their own experience with visual attention to make an attribution about the impact of the environment on the intentional visual acts of others has recently been corroborated (Senju, Southgate, Snape, Leonard, & Csibra, 2011). Woodward (2003) has also reported that responding to joint attention behavior (i.e., gaze following) in 7- to 9-month-olds does not as clearly involve understanding of the perception of others (social cognition) as it does in 12-month-old infants.

Gender Differences and Joint Attention

Another issue in the dynamic systems approach to the science of joint attention concerns whether culture and gender have significant impacts on its patterns of growth. It is not clear whether cultural variation in joint attention development is pertinent to research on ASD. Research on gender differences in joint attention development, on the other hand, is more clearly relevant. This is because the sex of a child influences behavioral neurodevelopment (Cahill, 2006; Fausto-Sterling, Coll, & Lamarre, 2012a). Moreover, ASD, like many other neurodevelopmental disorders, occurs more frequently and/or clearly in boys than in girls.

In early typical development, little consistent evidence has been reported of gender differences in the IJA or RJA development of 9- to 18-month-olds in interaction with a tester (e.g., Mundy et al., 2007; see Rogoff, Mistry, Goncu, & Mosier, 1993, for a contrasting point of view). However, a study of joint attention in interactions with parents provides evidence that 2-year-old girls may display more joint attention bids with mothers than do boys (Saxon & Reilly, 1999).

A greater proclivity to engage in joint attention in girls has also been reported in a study of young school-age children. Gavrilov, Rotem, Ofek, and Geva (2012) reported observations of IJA in a sample of 5- to 7-year-olds that included 33 boys and 29 girls. The frequencies with which children directed or redirected an adult's attention to an aspect of a toy were recorded. Observations were conducted when children played with three types of toys: more social (dolls), moderately social (Legos with miniature figurines), and less social (a construction set). Girls and boys displayed more joint attention with the more social toys than with the moderately social toys, and higher rates of joint attention with the moderately social toys than with the less social toys (see Figure 4.4). Girls, however, displayed a much higher frequency of IJA bids in play with the more social toys than boys did. No gender differences were noted in play with the other types of toys. Interestingly, all children showed more symbolic play and positive affect with the more social toys, and the IJA bids were related to sharing experiences with the social partner in the context of symbolic play.

A study of differences in adult male and female joint attention reported by Bayliss, Pellegrino, and Tipper (2005) was motivated by the *extreme male brain* (EMB) theory of autism (Baron-Cohen, 2002). The EMB theory holds that autism involves an extreme and maladaptive expression of a typically male cognitive bias to engage in detail-oriented, systematizing thought processes, and/or a diminution of a typically female cognitive bias to engage in empathizing (Baron-Cohen, 2002). *Systematizing* refers

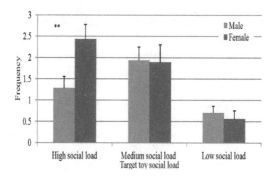

FIGURE 4.4. Joint attention behaviors as a function of gender and social load.
**$p < .05$. From Gavrilov, Rotem, Ofek, and Geva (2012). Reprinted in accord
with the open-access guidelines of the *Frontiers in Human Neuroscience* journal.

to a tendency to note the characteristics that lend themselves to organizing objects, events, or ideas according to a rule or set of rules. *Empathizing* refers to the ability to understand and share the feelings of another
person.

The assumptions underpinning the EMB theory may not have over-
whelming support in the basic developmental science of gender differences (Fausto-Sterling et al., 2012a). Moreover, it may be that a typically
male cognitive style tends to be associated with any disorder that that is
expressed to a greater extent in males than in females, such as ADHD or
dyslexia. Nevertheless, the EMB theory led Bayliss et al. (2005) to under-
take an informative study on gender and joint attention.

Bayliss et al. (2005) observed that both men and women responded
equally quickly to gaze when it correctly indicated where in space to look
for a stimulus target. That is, they exhibited equivalent RJA latencies.
However, when gaze direction was incongruent with the target spatial
location, it led to longer RJA latencies to look correctly at the target in
women than in men. This result suggested that gaze exerts a more powerful influence on orienting in women than in men. To the extent that following gaze either is not part of systematizing or is part of empathizing,
this pattern of results was considered consistent with expectations based
on the EMB theory. However, Bayless et al. conducted a critical clarifying
experiment, which indicated that the same pattern of gender differences
was observed when an arrow, instead of eye gaze, was used as a congruent or incongruent cue for target location. This indicated that the gender
effect in this study was not specific to joint attention. Rather, the results
suggested that men respond to noninformative spatial cues differently

(less powerfully) than women, regardless of whether they involve joint attention or a nonsocial directional signal. In other words, men may display a weaker tendency to coordinate attention with *any* directional signal, be it social or nonsocial. One might even say that men display a greater degree of *field independence* (Witkin, Moore, Goodenough, & Cox, 1977) with respect to the influence of both social and nonsocial orienting cues.

The EMB theory may not apply to the study of joint attention, because the development of the human tendency to engage in joint attention does not clearly stem from processes associated with either empathy or systematizing cognition. However, the EMB perspective does raise the question about whether some set of gender-related factors may make boys more vulnerable than girls to joint attention disturbance during infant development. I don't believe that this possibility has ever been directly examined in the developmental science of infancy or the applied science of the early identification of risk for ASD. Nevertheless, the possibility of gender-related vulnerability to joint attention disturbance is supported by evidence presented in two outstanding recent papers on developmental dynamic systems and gender differences (Fausto-Sterling, Coll, & Lamarre, 2012a, 2012b).

Fausto-Sterling et al. (2012b) summarize some of the differences associated with the early development of social interaction and communication of boys and girls in the first 6 months of postnatal life. Neonatal boys and girls start with different levels of cortical mass and cortical maturity associated with sensory (girls) and motor (boys) development (see Figure 4.5). More to the point, Fausto-Sterling et al. (2012b) examined research on communication patterns observed during the first 6 months of life. This involved a review of studies that observed the development of three states of dyadic mother–infant interaction: (1) *symmetrical patterns*, where both partners were mutually engaged; (2) *asymmetrical patterns*, in which one partner actively tried to engage a passively attentive pair member; and (3) *unilateral patterns*, which occurred when one partner tried by a variety of means to engage the attention of a socially disengaged pair member.

The studies reviewed indicated that, on average, boys had a harder time self-regulating and required a longer period of development to make the transition from predominantly unilateral patterns to symmetrical patterns of mutual engagement with mothers (see Figure 4.5). For boys, such mutual engagement was still developing from 3 to 9 months. However, mutual engagement seemed to stabilize at an earlier point in development in many mother–daughter dyads (Fausto-Sterling et al., 2012b). Why this gender difference in development of facility with mutual engagement

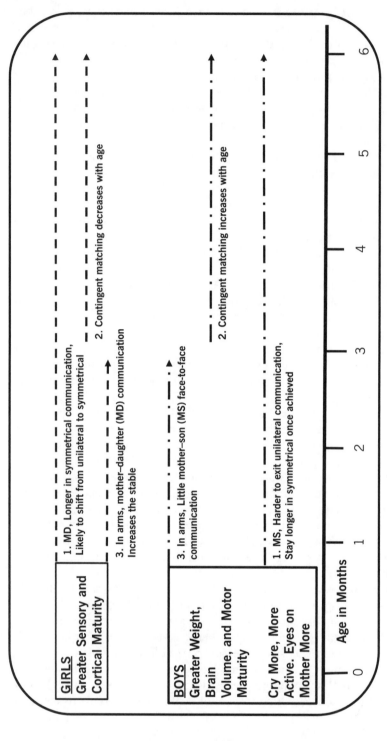

FIGURE 4.5. Differences in male and female development during the first 6 months following birth. Dashes represent early dimensions of behavior. Abbreviations: MS, mother–son; MD, mother–daughter. From Fausto-Sterling, Coll, and Lamarre (2012b). Copyright 2012 by Elsevier/Pergamon Press. Reprinted by permission.

occurred is not clear, at least to me. However, if these observations are validated and expanded with additional research, they would have numerous implications for the science of ASD.

First, there is some very real likelihood that a more precise understanding of the biobehavioral factors at play in gender differences in the development of mutual engagement in the first 9 months of life would be informative with respect to the study of ASD. Second, the observation of gender differences in mutual engagement calls into question the assumption that social attention and engagement are well established, or equally well established, for all typical infants in the first 9 months of life. Third, the typical variation in the development of consistent mutual engagement, especially among boys, is likely to contribute to the challenges of identifying early behavioral markers of ASD. Fourth, males do display relative independence from the influence of orienting cues (Bayliss et al., 2005); this phenomenon may be related to the longer period of development required by male infants to consistently adopt periods of mutual engagement with the attention of caregivers.

It is also interesting to note that the research reported by Fausto-Sterling et al. (2012b) suggests that caregivers may need to work harder or more persistently across a longer period of development to cultivate joint engagement with boys. Likewise, joint attention interventions for ASD (e.g., JASPER; see Chapter 6) provide methods for caregivers or professionals to work more persistently and effectively on the cultivation of joint engagement in young affected children. If ASD involves an extreme expression of the infant male tendency to be less affected by social influences on attention and orienting, then perhaps JASPER may provide an evidence-based model for the development of targeted caregiver–infant sibling intervention methods for ASD risk reduction in the first 12 months of life.

Longitudinal Studies of Joint Attention and Theory of Mind

In addition to research that focuses on the infant development of joint attention, a small vital set of studies provides evidence of a longitudinal continuity between variance in infant joint attention and later social cognition. This evidence is critical if we are to entertain the validity of the hypothesis that joint attention information processing plays a role in social cognition. In perhaps the first research to address this issue, Charman et al. (2000) examined the relations between imitation and a task that assessed IJA alternating gaze at 20 months with language and theory-of-mind development in a longitudinal study of a small sample of 13 children. They observed that the imitation task at 20 months was a significant predictor of language development, but that the IJA task was a significant predictor of theory-of-mind performance, at 44 months.

A fundamental recent study has corroborated the observation of the significant predictive validity of infants' initiating joint attention behaviors for social-cognitive processes in the fourth year of life. Kühn-Popp, Kristen, Paulus, Meinhardt, and Sodian (2015) assessed joint attention pointing and pointing to request in 32 fifteen-month-old infants. When the children were 48 months of age, they were asked to play with bear figurines. After 5 minutes of play, the children were prompted to tell a story about the "bear family." Scores for total word count and total terms referring to the characters' mentalizing, such as *think*, *know*, *guess*, or *believe*, were obtained for each bear family narrative. Longitudinal analyses indicated that joint attention pointing (and nonverbal IQ), but no other variables, displayed significant, unique predictive associations with individual differences in the 4-year-olds' use of mental state terms.

Other studies have focused on the connections between responding to joint attention tasks and subsequent theory-of-mind development. Kristen, Sodian, Thoermer, and Perst (2011) reported that RJA at 9 months in a sample of 88 infants predicted intention-based imitation at 15 months, and the use of mental state language (words about thinking, intentions, or desires) at 24 and 36 months. A similar finding has been reported by Brooks and Meltzoff (2015), who observed 32 children and found that gaze following at 10 months was associated with higher rates of mental state productive language at 2.5 years, which in turn was associated with greater success on a theory of mind battery at age 4.5 years. Importantly, significant evidence of this longitudinal continuity was observed after the investigators controlled for general language development, maternal education, and nonsocial attention performance. Another recent study has reported that RJA at 9 months was significantly associated with theory-of-mind performance at 4 years of age in a sample of 28 children with typical development (Abreu, Cardoso-Martins, & Barbosa, 2014).

Using a different paradigm, Nelson, Adamson, and Bakeman (2008) have also reported that observations of more frequent periods of joint attention of 42 children in interactions with caregivers at 18–20 months and 27–30 months predicted false-belief theory-of-mind performance assessed at 43 and 54 months of age. Again, this predictive association was observed after the researchers controlled for language development. Neither IJA nor RJA is separately measured or necessarily measurable in this type of joint engagement paradigm.

Of course, although significant predictive associations between joint attention and social cognitive development have been observed, the strength of these associations has been modest (as one might imagine). Indeed, the investigators in these studies have often needed to use thoughtful and well-informed data-analytic approaches to make these observations (e.g., Nelson et al., 2008). Modest effect size is a bane of the translational science of developmental psychopathology. For one thing, it nearly ensures the presence of inconsistent findings in a literature. For example, Camaioini, Perucchini, Bellagamba, and Colonnessi (2004) reported that pointing to initiate joint attention, but not pointing for requesting, at 12 months of age predicted understanding of intentions at 15 months of age in 40 infants. However, in a similar study of 35 infants, Colonnessi, Rieffe, Koops, and Perucchini (2008) were unable to replicate this observation. Nevertheless, there are now five independent observations of significant longitudinal continuity between infant joint attention and subsequent evidence of social-cognitive development in children.

Two additional studies are noteworthy in connection with this small but important literature. One attests to the ongoing role of joint attention in social cognition after the second year of life. Lee, Eskritt, Symons, and Muir (1998) have reported that that 2- to 3-year-olds use information processing of the gaze direction of other people (RJA) in making inferences about their intentions under conditions of ambiguity. Finally, Schietecatte, Roeyers, and Warreyn (2012) examined the relations between joint attention and understanding the intentions of other people in 23 three-year-old boys with ASD. This study employed measures of both IJA and RJA, as well as general cognitive development, general attention shifting, intention understanding, and preference for attending to social or nonsocial stimuli. In a finding consistent with those of many other studies of RJA, Schietecatte et al. reported that RJA ability was related to the understanding of intentions in this sample of children with ASD. However, a dissociated pattern of correlations was observed for IJA: Children with ASD who were more capable on the IJA measures were faster at disengaging from a central visual stimulus on the attention-shifting task. However, the correlation between IJA and understanding of intentions only approached a conventional level of significance.

The model of learning-to and learning-from phases of joint attention helps us understand the process and importance of targeted early interventions for joint attention such as JASPER (Kasari et al., 2006, 2008), discussed in Chapter 6. According to joint attention theory, some set of factors inhibits the learning-to phase of joint attention development in infants at risk for ASD. This phase typically begins in the first 4 months of life. We do not have clear evidence that inhibition of the learning-to phase occurs at this time or later. However, there is evidence that some children with ASD display deficits in joint attention by 8–12 months (Chapter 4), a time when evidence suggests that the learning-from phase of joint attention development is just beginning.

Left untreated, a developmental cascade ensues, with the dearth of opportunity to engage in typical learning from joint attention degrading language and social-cognitive development in affected children. Comprehensive treatments such as the Early Start Denver Model (ESDM; see Chapter 6) may effectively interrupt this transactional developmental impairment in early social learning in children with ASD. At present, though, the only direct evidence for effective treatment comes from research on early interventions that target joint attention. The current research on these interventions (Kasari et al., 2008; also described in Chapter 6) provides especially comprehensive evidence that they may interrupt the cascade of joint attention disturbance as it relates to early (lexical) language-learning problems in children with ASD. Thus, even with a delayed learning-to phase, targeted intervention seems to enable to children with ASD to learn from joint attention. However, we do not yet know whether early joint attention intervention has a direct effect on vulnerability for the subsequent development of social-cognitive deficits in children with ASD.

An axiom of the theory unfolding in this book is that joint attention is a faculty of mind that plays a vital role in learning and social relatedness well beyond the infant and toddler phases of development (e.g., Mundy & Sigman, 2006). It is important to understand the role of joint attention in later childhood, because this may improve the understanding of the continuity in social communication and social cognition across the preschool and school-age phases of development. This understanding in turn may spur thinking about the development of targeted joint attention interventions for older children with ASD. The next section of this chapter considers dimensions that may be related to joint attention research across preschool and school-age development in ASD. Specifically, I discuss research on language, collaboration, cooperation, and reading that may help inform longitudinal studies of how joint attention unfolds in typical development throughout childhood.

Joint Attention in Childhood

This chapter has begun with the observation by Lord and Jones (2012) that the lack of a clear appreciation of joint attention's continued impact on child development beyond infancy may limit the application of this dimension in the science of autism. However, this limitation may be more of a limit in our conceptualization of joint attention than it is a limit in the true impact of this dimension on development beyond infancy. An evidence-based argument can be made that joint attention continues to influence language development, the development of cooperative and collaborative behavior, and information processing, as well as readiness to benefit from instruction, into childhood and across the lifespan. Some of the evidence for this assertion is considered in the final sections of this chapter.

Joint Attention and Language Development in Childhood

One of the more important lines of developmental continuity involves the role of joint attention in language development. As alluded to earlier, there is considerable correlational and experimental evidence for joint attention's contribution to early lexical or vocabulary development (e.g., Beuker, Rommelse, Donders, & Buitelaar, 2013). This evidence is described in some detail in the next two chapters. However, its significance notwithstanding, it does not clearly provide support for the extended role of joint attention in childhood beyond the early preschool period. This is because the development of language extends far beyond the period of early vocabulary acquisition, as do the problems in language development experienced by many children with ASD. So the question arises: Is there evidence that joint attention contributes to phases of language development beyond early lexical acquisition? Far too little information is currently available to enable us to answer this question definitively. However, currently available information suggests that the answer may be yes: Joint attention does continue to play a role in language and social communication development well after infancy.

One important aspect of childhood language development involves understanding indirect communication. For example, a child may ask, "Can I play outside?", and the child's caregiver may respond, "We have to go shopping soon." Some research has suggested that children may often not be capable of correctly interpreting this type of indirect communication until 5–6 years of age. Schulze, Grassmann, and Tomasello (2013), however, reported an elegant set of studies indicating that 3- to 4-year-olds are capable of this type of sophisticated communicative inference when the communication is naturally imbedded in an ongoing interaction *and supported by joint attention.* Tribushinina (2014) recently extended this type of research by demonstrating that 30- to 42-month-olds are more capable of drawing correct inferences from the adult use of adjectives in speech when supported in a joint attention condition compared to a condition without joint attention.

With respect to mature adult language, Shockley, Richardson, and Dale (2009), in an edifying review of conversational dynamics, reported that gaze patterns have a fundamental influence on communication. In particular, they noted that the literature on adult conversation suggests that gaze coordination is causally related to mutual understanding within the context of communication. This conclusion is corroborated by several other strands of research.

Richardson and Dale (2005) reported that the tendency of listeners to couple their eye movements with those of speakers was correlated with their comprehension of the speakers. These authors also reported that experimental manipulation of the listeners' ability to couple eye movements with the speakers influenced the listeners' comprehension. Hanna and Brennan (2007) reported experimental evidence that adults readily use gaze following to disambiguate linguistic references in collaborative or joint action activities. Emmorey, Thompson, and Colvin (2008) have further reported that deaf native users of American Sign Language tend to engage in frequent gaze monitoring of a "speaking" signer while comprehending a spatial description. Finally, the results of a unique study have indicated that increasing the amount of information available to two strangers about an object increases their tendency to engage in joint attention while in a dialogue about the nature of the object (Richardson, Dale, & Kirkham, 2007).

Computational science also recognizes the importance of modeling gaze direction and mutual gaze in virtual collaboration and machine–human interfaces. For example, studies indicate that integrating information on human eye gaze direction into machine algorithms improves automated language processing (Qu & Chai, 2007) and improves the referential accuracy of automated speech production (Staudte, Koller, Garoufi, & Crocker, 2012). These results indicated that information on a conversationalist eye gaze substantially improved the automated processing of adult language in human–machine interaction.

The foregoing studies illustrate that the influence of joint attention on language development and social communication is not limited to the early preschool period. Rather, it is a fundamental social-cognitive mental facility involved in language learning and the support of mutual understanding in the context of conversation ambiguities across the lifespan (e.g., Diessel, 2006; Blanc, Dodane, & Dominey, 2003; Moore, 2012). It is reasonable to expect that vulnerability to difficulty with joint attention may have impacts on the learning, language, and social communication abilities of people with ASD well beyond the first years of life. Nowhere may this be more apparent than in research on reading development in school-age children with ASD.

Autism and Reading Comprehension Disabilty

As noted in earlier chapters, the CDC (2014) has recently estimated the occurrence of ASD at 1 in 68 children. The rates vary by gender, with 1 child with ASD per 42 boys, and 1 in 189 girls. The Autism and

Developmental Disabilities Monitoring Network of the CDC further reports (*www.cdc.gov/ncbddd/autism/states/comm_report_autism_2014*) that 31% of the last national sample of second-grade children that provided the data on the 1:68 prevalence ratio also indicates that 32% of the children with ASD were affected by a significant level of IDD (IQs below 70); that an additional 23% have significant intellectual vulnerabilities, with IQs in what is referred to as the "borderline range" of intelligence (75–85); and that a third group of about 46% of all children affected by ASD have average to above-average intellectual ability (IQs above 85).

This is a remarkable change in the estimates of the rates of intellectual vulnerability in children with ASD. Fifteen to twenty years ago, the estimate was that about 80% of children with ASD were also affected by intellectual vulnerability (e.g., Fombonne, 1999). It is one of the most important yet least well-recognized changes in the epidemiology of ASD over the last few decades. Although it is well known that the estimated rate of identification of ASD has increased about 25-fold since the 1990s, it is less well recognized that the estimated rate of ASD without intellectual vulnerability has tripled in that time as well. Understanding why this has occurred has deep implications for our models of the metabolic, neurodevelopmental, environmental, and/or measurement factors that contribute to the observations of many more cases of children affected by autism today than in years past. For example, I often grapple with the paradox of how increased exposures to teratogens in our environment may have led both to more cases of ASD and to a threefold increase in the proportion of children with better intellectual outcomes. The most plausible answer that comes to mind is that advances in early intervention have been so substantial and powerful that they act as a very significant counterbalance to the possible pernicious processes proposed in teratogenic models of the changes in the epidemiology of ASD.

Regardless of the possible causes of the epidemiological changes, the fact is that a substantial proportion of children with ASD today develop in such a way that they are not affected by intellectual vulnerability by school age. Consequently, many affected children receive much of their education in regular classrooms. In order to meet the needs of these children, as well as those with intellectual vulnerability, it is of paramount importance to understand how ASD affects learning from and with other people in childhood and adolescence (Mundy, Mastergeorge, & McIntyre, 2012).

One hypothesis about how ASD may affect school-based learning is that the cognitive impairments that characterize ASD interfere with the typical development of reading comprehension. Thus a vulnerability to specific reading comprehension disability is a significant part of the expression of the social learning phenotype in many elementary and secondary students affected by ASD (Nation, Clark, Wright, & Williams, 2006; O'Connor & Klein, 2004; Randi, Newman, & Grigorenko, 2010; Ricketts, 2011). Many students with ASD are at risk for impairments in the tendency to spontaneously adopt a common frame of reference between the reader (the self) as a receiver of information and the person who wrote the text as a sender of information. They also are prone to impairments in using inferential thinking in order to go beyond details to perceive larger meanings, impairments in mentally representing causal relations based on text, and the use of strategic thinking to organize behaviors and ideas in problem-solving situations (Nation et al., 2006; O'Connor & Klein, 2004; Randi et al., 2010; Ricketts, 2011). All of these cognitive characteristics place children with ASD at risk for specific reading comprehension disability.

Consistent with this hypothesis, studies of academic achievement indicate that the development of reading comprehension is among the domains of learning in which students with ASD and average IQs most frequently display impairment (Estes, Rivera, Bryan, Cali, & Dawson, 2011; Jones et al., 2009; McIntyre et al., 2015). Children with ASD often present with appropriate or above-average word-decoding skills (Jones et al., 2009; Huemer & Mann, 2010), even though they exhibit text-level reading comprehension impairments. Furthermore, the text-reading skills of affected children may fail to display the level of development across elementary and secondary school observed in children with other clinical syndromes or with typical development (McIntyre et al., 2015). This is consistent with the idea that children with ASD display developmental vulnerabilities in childhood development that are not observed in the preschool period. At least one study also raises the possibility that children with ASD not only fail to keep pace with age-appropriate text level reading development; their word-level reading skills may even decline with age (Norbury & Nation, 2011).

Evidence that reading impairment is specifically related to the social phenotype of ASD is provided by several studies. Higher scores on the Social Affect (SA) factor of the ADOS, which are indicative of greater ASD social symptom intensity, are significantly related to poorer reading ability in elementary school (Estes et al., 2011) as well as secondary school (Jones et al., 2009) in young people with ASD. Both of these studies also reported that other types of learning problems, such as math disabilities, were not related to ASD symptom presentation. In an important follow-up of the Jones et al. (2009) paper, Ricketts, Jones, Happé, and Charman (2013) reported data indicating that individual differences in language social cognition (inferring the intentions of other people), as well as revised ADOS SA scores, were associated with the intensity of reading comprehension disturbance in school-age children with ASD.

These studies provide evidence of a specific relation between reading comprehension disability and specific domains of communicative, social, and social-cognitive symptom presentation in children with ASD. My interpretation is that they provide evidence that reading comprehension impairment is part of the social learning disability strand of the social phenotype of ASD. It is possible, though, that some non-ASD-specific factor related to both reading and social symptom presentation accounts for the association between social symptoms and reading. One relevant possibility is that the presence of symptoms of comorbid ADHD symptoms in children with ASD may account for this association. This hypothesis is suggested by three observations. First, many children with ASD have been observed to display symptoms associated with ADHD (e.g., Sinzig, Morsch, Bruning, Schmidt, & Lehmkuhl, 2008). In addition, many children with ADHD have been observed to show clinical elevations of ASD symptoms on the ADOS (Reiersen, Constantino, Volk, & Todd, 2007). Finally, reading impairment is common to many children affected by ADHD (e.g., Hart et al., 2010).

A recent study has directly examined the hypothesis that reading disability is associated with ADHD symptoms rather than with the social phenotype of ASD. McIntyre et al. (2015) reported that school-age children with ASD displayed significantly lower reading comprehension development scores than age-, gender-, and IQ-matched samples of children with ADHD, as well as children with typical development. In addition, individual differences in ADHD symptoms within a sample of 80 children with ASD were not significantly associated with reading comprehension difficulties in this study. Instead, like Ricketts et al. (2013), McIntyre et al. (2015) observed that measures of oral language skills and individual differences in ADOS-2 SA scores had unique and significant associations with reading comprehension disability in children with ASD. This research group used causal modeling analyses to show that higher order language skills that involve inferential thinking explained the connection between ADOS symptom scores and reading comprehension scores in higher functioning children with ASD. The McIntyre et al. (2015) study thus presents especially compelling evidence of the link between the cognitive-communication phenotype of ASD and vulnerability for specific reading comprehension disability in school-age children with ASD.

To be sure, none of the research just described provides experimental evidence of a link among joint attention, social learning, and the expression of reading comprehension disability as part of the developmental phenotype of ASD. Nevertheless, a compelling network of data has linked joint attention to autism, and especially to the SA factor of the revised ADOS. Joint attention is also linked to language development and social-cognitive development, both of which appear to be related to reading development in ASD. All that is missing is evidence of a link between joint attention and reading development. Several studies provide such evidence.

Research on reading development has long held that joint attention in mother–infant dyads and later in teacher–child or peer–peer dyads is an essential medium of reading development (e.g., Farrant & Zubrick, 2011; Ninio, 1983). For example, a report on 2,369 children followed longitudinally from 9 to 58 months of age indicated that children who had low joint attention at 9 months and low levels of parent–child book reading across early development had lower receptive vocabularies at 58 months (Farrant & Zubrick, 2011). The authors interpreted their data as indicative of the pivotal role played by joint attention and parent–child book reading in school readiness.

In an experimental study, the eye movements of parents and children were simultaneously tracked while parent–child dyads were engaged in shared book reading (Guo & Feng, 2013). The eye-tracking data were presented to one group on video screens during the reading, and parents were instructed to on how to use this "online" information to improve joint attention in shared reading. The real-time attention feedback significantly increased both the joint attention and children's print-related learning (Guo & Feng, 2013).

I believe that the longitudinal network of indirect (i.e., nonexperimental) evidence of connections across the domains of joint attention, language, social cognition, and reading may be important to our understanding of the social learning phenotype of ASD in older children and adults. I also believe that it constitutes one example of the networks of developmental connections that potentially best distinguish the vital role of joint attention in ASD from the roles played by the dimensions of social attention, imitation, and face processing. Of course, there are other important connections to consider.

Joint Attention, Cooperation, and Collaboration

The ability to coordinate our actions with those of others to engage in cooperative joint action is crucial for individual, as well as group and societal, development and success. Studies suggest that joint attention provides an essential common perceptual and cognitive framework for cooperative behavior (e.g., Sebanz, Bekkering, & Knoblich, 2006). For example, Brownell, Ramani, and Zerwas (2006) published an informative study that examined cooperative play among dyads of 19-, 23-, and 27-month-old toddlers. The cooperative task was a toy that could be activated by pulling two handles. In one condition the handles needed to be pulled simultaneously, and in another condition the handles needed to be pulled sequentially. An adult tester modeled correct task performance for each condition for each dyad. The toddlers' IJA and RJA skills were also assessed by an independent tester with the ESCS. The results indicated that toddlers' RJA ability was significantly and positively related to their tendency to engage in simultaneous cooperative behavior, but negatively related to their tendency toward sequential cooperative behavior. IJA measurement was limited to observations of relatively low-frequency pointing and showing behavior, and was not associated with cooperative behavior in this study.

Wu, Pan, Su, and Gros-Louis (2013) reported a cross-cultural replication and extension of the Sebanz et al. (2006) study with Chinese toddlers. This study also used the ESCS to measure joint attention, but focused on 17-, 21-, and 25-month-olds who were presented with two types of *child–adult* cooperative tasks. The first task, called the "double-tube task," involved complementary (sequential) roles. One person sent a ball down a transparent tube, and the other person caught the ball at the other end of the tube with a can. The second task was called the "music-box task," and it involved parallel (simultaneous) roles. Three buttons were available on a box, and the task was to press two buttons on opposite sides of the box to turn on music and colorful lights. However, the distance between the buttons was great enough that one person could not press buttons on both sides of the box. Therefore, the two task participants needed to engage in simultaneous collaborative action.

Wu et al. (2013) utilized a more complete measure of IJA than did Sebanz et al. (2006). In addition to pointing and showing, Wu et al. included the ESCS IJA measure of alternating gaze shifts between an active toy and a social partner. Wu et al. observed that both IJA and RJA scores were significantly correlated with task cooperation in their sample, after they statistically controlled for the possible impact of language development differences among the toddlers. IJA displayed a significant association with successful cooperation in the task that involved complementary roles (different actions), and RJA was significantly associated with cooperation in the task that involved simultaneous but identical actions. These data align with the idea that IJA and RJA tap different as well as common processes. However, differences in correlations within any one study must be interpreted with caution.

These two studies provide evidence that processes involved in joint attention are involved in the development of cooperative behavior in the second year of life, in a manner that is consistent across cultures. This should not be surprising. At its core, cooperation or collaboration requires one or more partners to engage in coordinated (joint) action relative to a common object or event of reference. So mental engagement in joint attention processes is fundamental to cooperative action at any age in any context. This provides a telling example of how joint attention continues to play a fundamental role in social interaction and learning with other people after the first years of life. It also exemplifies how joint attention is involved in social cognition throughout life. Social cognition does not only involve the conceptual development of understanding the intentions of others; it also involves cognition as applied to the coordinated processing of information and action among people with regard to common points of reference. Both are vital aspects of social-cognitive development in in human nature. However, to focus on one (understanding of others' intentions) without the other (socially coordinated information processing) leads to an unnecessarily thin view of social cognition (cf. Skarratt, Cole, & Kuhn, 2012).

The distinction between social cognition as understanding of others' intentions and as socially coordinated information processing is illustrated in a study of cooperation in ASD (Colombi et al., 2009). This study examined cooperation in developmentally matched samples of 3- to 5-year-old children with ASD or other developmental disabilities. The aim of the study was to examine the hypotheses that impairments in cooperative behavior among children with ASD would be associated with their problems in imitation and understanding other people's intentions regarding action on objects, as well as joint attention.

In the first step of this study, children observed two adults modeling cooperative behaviors in one of four tasks similar to the double-tube task described by Wu et al. (2013). Children were then encouraged to play and cooperate with one of the adults on each of the four tasks. As expected, the results indicated that the children affected by ASD displayed worse performance on the intentionality, imitation, cooperation, and joint attention (but only RJA) tasks than the control sample with other developmental delays. All three dimensions of cooperation (intention understanding, RJA, and imitation) were significantly correlated in the sample with ASD, but not in the control sample.[3] Finally, an analysis indicated that the variables of diagnostic group, imitation, and joint attention explained 67% of individual differences displayed in collaborative behavior in the entire sample of 31 children. Alternatively, neither understanding of intentions nor verbal developmental age was significantly associated with differ-

---

[3]The samples of children with ASD and with other developmental delays were both small (N = 14 and 15, respectively). So negative findings need to be interpreted with caution. The correlations between RJA and imitation (r = .51) and between RJA and intention understanding (r = .38) were indicative of moderate associations that were not significant in this study, possibly because of Type 2 error. Only the magnitude of the correlation between imitation and intention understanding could be described as relatively weak (r = .18).

ences in collaborative behavior when variance in diagnostic group, imitation, and joint attention was also considered.

Finally, Dykstra-Steinbrenner and Watson (2015) have provided a very significant advance in research on the validity of childhood joint attention measurement with a report of school-based observations of student classroom engagement. Engagement here refers to participation in classroom learning opportunities. As is the case with the Early Social Communication Scales, they developed classroom observation scales of social interaction, behavior regulation, and joint attention. The primary measure of engagement comprised observations of attention during learning activities rated from passive onlooking to supported and coordinated joint attention. Their results indicated that joint engagement/joint attention was related to symptom severity scores and expressive communication scores in 25 elementary and middle school children with ASD.

Thus there is convergent evidence that joint attention is related to the development of cooperative behavior in typical toddlers. There is also some evidence that joint attention and imitation may play especially important roles in individual differences in the development of cooperative behavior within samples of children with ASD, as well as in differences in cooperative behavior observed between children with ASD and children with other developmental disorders. This last observation awaits corroboration and expansion with larger-scale and more detailed studies of this interesting topic. Perhaps most important recent research has provided evidence of the validity of joint attention as vital dimension of classroom engagement in children and adolescents with ASD.

Joint Attention, Information Processing, and Encoding

To this point, the evidence for an ongoing role of joint attention in typical and atypical child development has been drawn from studies on the relations of joint attention to childhood language and reading development, the development of cooperation, classroom engagement, and social cognition.

With regard to social cognition, three hypotheses have been raised. One is that learning in the context of joint attention contributes information that supports conceptual social-cognitive development. Second, the role of joint attention in human cognitive development is not replaced by conceptual social cognition. Instead, joint attention remains an active form of social information processing that enables us to align and maintain coordination of our thoughts, language, and behaviors relative to common reference points with other people. Third, the information-processing form of social cognition that is joint attention begins to develop in the first months of life. Just because early joint attention may not be the same as conceptual social cognition, this does not mean that early joint attention is not a true and vital aspect of lifespan social-cognitive development. The final section of this chapter looks more closely at the assumption that joint attention reflects an information-processing form in addition to a conceptual form of social cognition.

Böckler et al. (2011) reported an innovative study indicating that the experience of joint attention with another person enhanced pairs of participants' problem solving in a mental spatial rotation task. Böckler, Knoblish, and Sebanz (2012), as leaders in this field of inquiry, have since provided another illuminating study. Pairs of research participants were seated together and presented with tasks that required them to focus their attention in similar or different ways. In the former types of tasks, both participants were asked to focus their attention either on stimulus details or on the global stimulus features. In the latter types, one participant was asked to focus attention on stimulus details and the other on global features of the stimuli. The results revealed that individuals' information processing of either stimulus details or global features was significantly slower when participants were asked to engage in attention to different components of the stimulus rather than the same components.

Böckler et al. (2012) interpreted this study to indicate that participants mentally co-represented their partners' focus of attention. In the different-attention-focus condition, this induced a conflict or cognitive load that decreased participants' own task-related selective attention and information processing. Conversely, *their task performance benefited from co-representation of a common focus of attention*. According to Böckler et al. (2012), this study provides relatively strong evidence that adults tend to internally represent the visual attention of a social partner. To my way of thinking, this is tantamount to engaging in internal mental joint attention. Moreover, co-representation of convergent or divergent attention foci (or internal joint attention) may influence participants' processing of stimulus information.

Frischen and Tipper (2004) also published a seminal observation of the possible effects of joint attention on information processing. Their observations indicated that information provided by the spatial cueing of gaze direction had a longer impact on orienting and attention that did nonsocial spatial cues for visual orienting. Not surprisingly, if a nonsocial direction cue such as an arrow ($\rightarrow$) was presented, an individual would turn faster to a stimulus appearing in the area indicated by the arrow than in a noncued condition. However, this priming effect only lasted for a brief period of time (about 300 msec, or about one-third of a second) for nonsocial stimuli. By contrast, this priming effect lasted much longer (800 msec) when eyes looking left or right provided the direction cues. These findings suggest that gaze direction, or social cues for joint attention, are associated with greater saliency than are nonsocial cues, and that they have a stronger (longer) biasing impact on attention. Böckler et al. (2011) corroborated this finding in a study showing that social attention cues via hand gestures also led to a stronger, longer biasing impact on attention than nonsocial cues did.

Lachat, Hugueville, Lemaréchal, Conty, and George (2012) noted that all the previous studies of gaze-cueing effects had been conducted with analogue eye gaze stimuli. These authors conducted a gaze-cueing study with live interactive partners, and also observed evidence for faster information processing of gaze versus nonsocial spatial cues in live social interactions. Like other investigators, they also observed a small advantage for females over males in the attention-directing effects of gaze versus nonsocial cues.

The foregoing studies provide some evidence that observing gaze as a spatial cue affects information processing in adults, in terms of both latency to respond to a spatial cue, and the duration of the bias to a particular spatial location elicited by gaze versus nonsocial stimuli. Age-related decreases in response latency also constitute one measure of the development of RJA in infancy (Gredebäck et al., 2010; Vaughan Van Hecke et al., 2012). In my opinion, both shorter response latencies and longer durations of gaze cue bias are *social-cognitive information-processing phenomena* associated with joint attention across the lifespan.

More evidence of the lifespan development of joint attention has been provided by Slessor et al. (2008), who studied decline of gaze following in older age. This study compared 45 younger adults (36 women) ranging in age from 17 to 34, and 41 older adults (31 women) ranging in age from 65 to 79. The task here was simply to indicate the direction of gaze (right vs. left) in pictures of faces. However, as illustrated in Figure 4.6, the degrees of averted gaze displayed in the stimuli were either subtle (0.13 degrees from direct gaze), moderate (0.25 degrees), or clear (0.38 degrees). As expected, the older sample was significantly slower in identifying the direction of gaze (e.g., 1.4 seconds vs. 0.75 seconds on trials of clearly averted gaze). In addition, the older sample was significantly less accurate in identifying the *direction* of subtle and moderate gaze aversion in the stimuli than the younger sample was. These group differences could not be explained completely in terms of visual perception/impairment differences across the groups.

Related to the observations by Slessor et al. (2008), a recent study reported that middle-aged and elderly chimpanzees performed more poorly on an RJA task than young adult chimpanzees did (Lacreuse, Russell, Hopkins, & Herndon, 2014). Another study has reported that RJA performance was associated with grey matter in the right posterior anterior temporal sulcus (Hopkins, Misiura, et al., 2014). These authors also

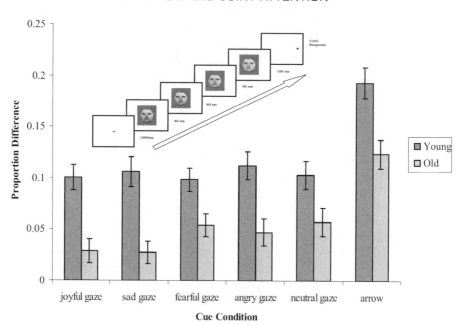

FIGURE 4.6. Graph depicting the strength of the congruity effect (proportion difference score between reaction time on congruent and incongruent trials) for younger and older adults on the gaze-cueing task (broken down by emotion condition) and the arrows task. Bars represent standard errors of the mean. From Slessor, Phillips, and Bull (2008). Copyright 2008 by the American Psychological Association. Reprinted by permission.

reported that older chimpanzees displayed poorer RJA performance than younger conspecifics, as well as significantly smaller grey matter volume in the posterior superior temporal sulcus. This area of the brain has previously been associated with joint attention and especially RJA (see Chapter 7).

Of course, all of the research described to this point concerns research related to RJA; relatively little research has been conducted on IJA. This is because RJA is a less volitional responsive behavior that is relatively easy to elicit in experimental paradigms. IJA, on the other hand, is more volitional. Therefore, it is more difficult to set up an experimental context in which examine IJA processes can be validly examined, just as it is more difficult to set up intervention conditions to advance the development of IJA (see Chapter 6). As is the case in early intervention, though, progress is being made in the experimental study of information processing associated with IJA across the lifespan.

Bayliss et al. (2013) developed a paradigm that allowed them to examine the impact of face stimuli that appeared to follow the gaze shifts of research participants (IJA emulation) or to look in the opposite direction from the participants' gaze shifts. The results indicated that the IJA condition led research participants to pay more attention to the face stimuli. The research participants also reported more positive emotional responses to the pictures they examined in conjunction with face stimuli that followed their attention.

Kim and Mundy (2012) have reported a related set of observations. This study employed a virtual reality paradigm in which college students were asked to study pictures under one of two conditions. In the IJA condition, students chose to look at and study a picture that appeared to the left or right of the central avatar, and the avatar appeared to follow the gaze of the participants. In a second (RJA) condition, students were informed to follow the gaze of the avatar and to study the picture that the avatar selected. The students were then presented with the picture they had studied, along with a picture they had not studied, and were asked to identify the familiar pictures. Students in the IJA condition correctly recognized more pictures and displayed fewer false-positive responses than students in the RJA condition. These results suggested that the analogue experience of IJA was associated with greater depth of information processing and encoding than the experience of RJA in this sample of college students.

Several other social and information-processing phenomena associated with joint attention in later development have been identified. One interesting issue is the effect of social anxiety on eye contact effects and joint attention. This is important, because it is possible that something akin to social anxiety could have an impact both on eye contact effects and on joint attention in individuals with ASD. All too little research has addressed this issue. Nevertheless, Gamer, Hecht, Seipp, and Hiller (2011) have reported data to suggest that individuals affected by social anxiety are *more* sensitive to gaze and interpret a broader cone of partner gaze averted from the midline as mutual gaze than do comparison individuals without symptoms of social anxiety. This is contrary to predictions on how social anxiety might affect social attention in ASD, because the anxiety hypothesis in ASD is often associated with aversion and decreased attention to social stimuli (e.g., Chevallier et al., 2012).

In what may be a study of a related psychological process, Wilkowski, Robinson, and Friesen (2009) examined the effects of low sense of belonging and relatedness with other people on responding to gaze cueing. In one study, belonging/relatedness was measured in terms of low trait self-esteem in research participants. In a second, more experimental study, sense of belonging/relatedness was manipulated by priming participants' self-rejection-related thoughts. Evidence from both studies indicated that lower sense of belonging/relatedness was associated with *faster* responses on gaze-cueing trials. However, a similar effect was not observed on non-social cueing trials. These results are very consistent with theory and evidence that joint attention processes are both affected by and indicative of a sense of relatedness or intersubjectivity with other people (Mundy et al., 1992; Mundy & Sigman, 2006). They add depth to this idea by demonstrating that state or trait deprivation of a sense of relatedness can affect the speed with which joint attention cues are processed.

Finally, to the degree that joint attention does involve intersubjectivity, we may be well advised to consider measures of the tendency toward spontaneously sharing experiences with others in joint attention in adults. One possibility here is to consider the social-psychological phenomenon of *capitalization* as part of the expression of joint attention (Mundy & Newell, 2007). Capitalization occurs when a marital partner initiates joint attention to share a positive experience of the day, and the other partner manifestly attends to the report of the experience and provides a positive or supportive response (e.g., Gable, Reis, Impett, & Asher, 2004). Gable et al. (2004) have provided evidence that, beyond the positive impact of the event itself, the spontaneous sharing of a positive daily experience has a unique impact on the positive affect of the reporting marital partner. Moreover, the degree to which the listening marital partner is perceived as actively attentive and supportive of the shared experience is associated with greater reported sense of intimacy and daily marital satisfaction by marital dyads.

In addition to evidence of the impact of joint attention on information processing and emotional well-being in typical development, there are studies of the effects of mutual gaze and joint attention on information processing in older individuals with ASD. Böckler, Timmermans, Sebanz, Vogeley, and Schilbach (2014) recently reported a study of 20- to 60-year-old adults with ASD, compared to a sample of typical adults matched for age, gender, and years of education. A variation of a gaze-cueing task was presented. After experiencing mutual gaze, the typical group displayed significantly faster gaze-cueing responses on congruent trials, and much longer latencies on incongruent trials. That is, mutual gaze appeared to facilitate cue processing on congruent trials and to interfere with processing on incongruent trials. However, *no such effect of mutual gaze* on speed and efficiency of information processing was observed in the sample with ASD.

Vivanti and Dissanayake (2014) examined visual attention and imitation more precisely in preschool children with and without ASD. The children in this study were between 3 and 5 years of age. The samples were matched for intellectual development, such that the control sample included 8 children with typical development and 17 children with developmental delays. Children were presented with imitation demonstrations in two conditions. In one condition, the adults only looked at the actions they were engaged with, such as the movement of their hands. In a second condition, the adults looked forward at the beginning of a trial for 2.5 seconds to allow for mutual gaze with the research participants, and then averted their line of regard to focus on their actions.

The results indicated that the control group displayed greater imitation than the group with ASD, *but only in the mutual gaze condition.* The mutual gaze condition had a beneficial effect on imitation performance in the control sample, which was not in evidence in the sample with ASD as a group. However, within the sample with ASD, individual differences in visual attention to a demonstrator's face in the mutual gaze condition were significantly and positively correlated with better imitation performance in this condition. Hence this study provided evidence of a reduced impact of mutual gaze on task processing and response in the sample with ASD, but also evidence of meaningful differences among young children with ASD in the possible impact of mutual gaze on information processing.

Lastly, Mundy, Kim, et al. (2015) used the virtual reality paradigm described by Kim and Mundy (2012) to determine whether 8- to 16-year-old IQ-matched children with typical development, ASD, or ADHD would respond to the experience of IJA with enhanced information processing. The results of this study indicated that the two control samples, but not the sample with ASD, displayed significantly better memory for pictures in the IJA than in the RJA condition. However, there were no diagnostic group differences in memory for pictures in the RJA condition. Furthermore, the diagnostic group difference in IJA-related information processing remained significant after controls for possible mediating differences in working memory across the samples. Finally, differences in IJA memory performance correctly identified 70% of the sample with ASD and 66% of the combined control samples (typical development and ADHD) in a discriminant function analysis. Thus this study provides initial evidence that the experience of joint attention with other people may not enhance information processing in some children with ASD to the degree that it does in children with typical development or with other clinical disorders. The importance of this phenomenon is emphasized in additional recent observations. Edward, Stephenson, Dalmaso, and Bayliss (2015) have reported evidence of a social cognitive system that is active in adults that detects when one is the object of others' gazes. These authors also report that differences in the responses to others' attention is related to self-reported symptoms of the broad autism phenotype.

Summary and Conclusions

Only in its most expansive or grandiose interpretation can the PDPM be viewed as an explanatory model of joint attention, or of autism. Nevertheless, the PDPM does serve a purpose: It expands the current perspective on joint attention and describes how and why its impairment in autism is more than an epiphenomenon of other processes, such as imitation, social cognition, face processing, or dyadic social orienting. This alternative perspective can be summed up in terms of several related principles and hypotheses.

First, ASD is as much about differences in self-generated activity as it is about problems in perceiving or responding to the behavior of others. Hence we need to consider the neurodevelopmental processes and networks involved in initiating behavior and attention control, as well as those involved in perceiving and responding to the behaviors of others, to understand this disorder (Mundy, 2003). Joint attention involves both reflexive/responsive functions (RJA) and volitional/self-generated functions (IJA). Other dimensions of social behavior are currently measured only in terms of reflexive/responsive behaviors. The two-dimensional nature of the functions of joint attention allow the child to engage in information processing and the social sharing of experience about a referent from two perspectives, analogous to those of a receiver/listener and a sender/speaker (Tomasello, Carpenter, Call, et al., 2005). The interaction of the experience of these two reciprocal perspectives on information processing related to shared reference points hypothetically contributes to a unique synthesis of self- and other-references—information that propels social-cognitive development. Other aspects of social behavior may play important roles in social cognition, but none supplant or mediate the role of joint attention.

Second, the interactive cognition of joint attention constitutes a form of parallel processing, because it involves the conjoint perception and analysis of information about self-attention and the attention of other people, in conjunction with spatial, temporal, or symbolic processing of information about a third entity. This conjoint or parallel analysis of information involves distributed processing across an anterior cortical system that supports self-monitoring of internal information about goal-directed attention, and a posterior cortical system for processing external information about attention related to the behavior of other people.

Third, social cognition is often thought of only in terms of the knowledge about other people that children appear to use in anticipating others' intentions, beliefs, or emotions. However, social cognition can also usefully be viewed as a form of online information processing that individuals engage in *in order to conceptualize* the mental status of other people. Accordingly, joint attention is hypothesized to be a primary type of mental information processing that is involved whenever individuals appraise what others know and feel, or don't know and feel. This is as true when the appraisal occurs through reading, listening, or watching a narrative unfold as it is in real-time processing of interactions with others. It is also a fundamental type of processing in joint action and cooperative behavior. Finally, the experience of joint attention also appears to affect the encoding of information about a common referent. So social cognition is not just about knowing other people's minds. It is also about the causes and effects of human information processing that occurs when minds try to know a common referent.

The principle of social cognition as information processing may, in part, be described as a form of executive functioning (cf. Perner & Lang, 1999). In this regard, joint attention is a social executive process supporting all forms of cognition that involve coordinating attention and the knowledge of self and others (Humphreys & Bedford, 2011; Mundy, 2003). Thus neural network activation associated with joint attention is an enduring substrate that plays a role in the unique characteristics of human cognition throughout the lifespan (Mundy & Newell, 2007). Indeed, it may be one example of the so-called "hot" executive functions that Zelazo, Qu, Müller, and Schneider (2005) theorize are central to social cognition. "Hot" executive functions are those that entail motivation processes and affect regulation specific to the support of successful goal-directed behavior in social engagements.

Following from this notion, a fourth principle of the PDPM is that individual differences in the operation of the social executive function of joint attention occur because of differences in factors involved in the flow and integration across self- and other-referenced processing networks. Understanding the nature of these processes, such as the degree to which they are mediated by learning processes, endogenous neural maturation, and motivation processes, is a vital goal for future multidisciplinary developmental research on social cognition and autism.

The principles of the PDPM encourage a multidisciplinary approach in which constructivist, connectionist neuroscience will be linked with the study of parallel and distributed processing impairments in future research on autism. Exemplary multidisciplinary efforts of this kind have already been published (e.g., Cohen, 2007; Lewis & Elman, 2008). However, the PDPM suggests that such efforts may be better informed with the appreciation of the following hypotheses. A disturbance of a distributed cortical system specifically involved in self–other representational mapping may be at the heart of human social cognition (Decety

& Sommerville, 2003). Moreover, joint attention development may be at the heart of the development of this type of representational mapping in human nature, as well as its variation in the human nature of autism.

I return to this idea in Chapter 7 with a consideration of the neurocognitive research on the development of joint attention in infancy, childhood, and adulthood in people with typical development and autism spectrum development. However, to complete the discussion of alternative interpretations of the role of joint attention in the nature of autism, I next examine the social orienting and social motivation hypotheses in Chapter 5.

Social Orienting, Joint Attention, and Social Motivation

C hapter 4 has discussed an alternative to the classic *social-cognitive hypothesis* of joint attention. According to that hypothesis, joint attention is viewed as a forerunner, but not necessarily a central component, of a later-emerging social-cognitive disturbance of knowledge about self and about others in ASD. From this point of view, joint attention is a milestone in, or something important to, the development of the central dimension of social cognition—but not necessarily important to the childhood and adult functioning of social cognition. This may be a misperception of the richness of role of joint attention in social-cognitive development in human nature and in ASD. An alternative hypothesis discussed in Chapter 4 suggests that months of practice with joint attention in the first 2 years of life provide necessary though not sufficient experience with social information processing to sculpt the development of social neurocognition. Chapter 4 also presented the premise that joint attention begins to be internalized as *mental joint attention* in the preschool years, and that mental joint attention is integral to the mechanisms involved in social cognitive mentalizing. Finally, the chapter suggested that this role of joint attention in mentalizing continues through the lifespan.

Another set of hypotheses inherent to the social orienting and social motivation models of autism have also impacted the apparent significance of joint attention in ASD. These hypotheses suggest that joint attention disturbance is an *outcome* of more primary, earlier developmental perturbations of ASD. This set of hypotheses suggests that neonatal problems in the development of social orienting, social motivation, or face processing give rise to a cascade of later-emerging disturbances in social development in ASD, one of which is atypical joint attention. Hence joint attention differences in ASD may constitute an epiphenomenon of these earlier dimensions of development effects. Scientific community buy-in to this model circa 2012 may have provided the basis for installing joint attention as a measure of face processing in the first iteration of the NIMH RDoC.

Three Questions about the Development of Joint Attention

This chapter considers this alternative view of joint attention by considering three questions: (1) When does joint attention develop in infancy? (2) What distinguishes joint attention from face processing and social orienting? (3) What motivation processes may influence the development of joint attention in typical and autism spectrum development?

Addressing the first question is important, because joint attention has often been described as a facility of mind that does not clearly manifest itself until the second year of life (e.g., Tomasello, Carpenter, Call, et al., 2005). It follows, then, that some earlier-developing behavior dimensions (e.g., face processing) may be primary and lead in a linear causal path to the impairment of joint attention in ASD. However, data obtained in the last few years have challenged the assumption that joint attention is a second-year developmental milestone. Some of these data have been considered in Chapter 4, in the form of research reports that the dimension of joint attention was useful in identifying risk for ASD by 8 months of age. This chapter provides a more detailed examination of the data on the development of joint attention in the first year of life.

The second question is also important. Some of the confusion about joint attention stems from the view that the social phenotype of ASD may be comprehensively defined in terms of differences in *social-affective engagement*. However, the phenotype is complex and may not be easily captured from one perspective. As may be clear at this point, a goal of this book is to suggest that it may useful to think about the social phenotype of ASD in terms of a social learning disability axis, as well as a social-affective engagement axis. Others have begun to reconceptualize ASD as a form of learning disability (Butterworth & Kovas, 2013).

When viewed from a learning perspective, the unique nature and role of the dimension of joint attention in ASD relative to social orienting and face processing may become more apparent. Social orienting, face processing, imitation, and other dimensions may play significant roles in social learning in autism spectrum development. The only argument here is that *they do not play the same role as joint attention*. Specifically, joint attention is an essential and distinct part of human cognition that enables partners in an interaction to share experience and information about a common referent that goes beyond the partners. Face processing, social orienting, and imitation are essentially *dyadic* forms of social engagement and social learning. On the other hand, joint attention, by definition, is critical for *triadic* social engagement and learning. This characteristic of joint attention makes it a part of social-cognitive development that enables infants and children to benefit from instruction, regardless of whether the instruction is planned or incidental. No other dimension of social-cognitive development supplants the role of joint attention in our human capacity to benefit from instructional learning.

To my mind, the two axes of the social phenotype of autism—social affect/engagement, as well as social learning—can be recognized clearly in higher-functioning elementary and secondary school students with ASD. These children vary distinctly in their social engagement tendencies according to the aloof, passive, or active but odd patterns long described by Wing and Gould (1979), as well as others (e.g., Burnette et al., 2011; Schwartz et al., 2009; Sutton et al., 2005). Moreover, it is also clear that these children vary in their social learning abilities in the classroom. For example, many but not all higher-functioning elementary and secondary students with ASD display significant difficulty with age-appropriate reading comprehension, which cannot be explained in terms of their differences in verbal IQ, attention deficits, or working memory (Estes et al., 2011; Jones et al., 2009; McIntyre et al., 2015). Several studies have also reported that differences in reading comprehension are significantly related to differences in the social phenotype of ASD, measured on the revised ADOS, in school-age children (Estes et al., 2011; McIntyre et al., 2015; Ricketts et al., 2013). The difficulty with learning to read text appears to be directly associated with a difference in how easily children can track the referential (deictic) information in the passages they are reading (Randi et al., 2010; O'Connor & Klein, 2004). It is currently difficult to understand the nature of the school-aged learning problems of children with ASD in terms of only a "social-affect" dimension in terms of problems in face processing and the like.

The validity of the dichotomy between the social engagement axis and the social learning axis of the social phenotype of ASD is also highlighted in intervention research. Modern early interventions implicitly recognize the significance of this distinction. Early intervention theory recognizes that cultivating positive social engagement is a *prepotent* context for improving social learning abilities in children with ASD. However, these interventions also recognize that improving social engagement is not sufficient to advancing social learning and development in children with ASD (e.g., Dawson et al., 2010; Kasari et al., 2008). Methods must also be used to directly advance the development of these children's capacity and motivation to engage spontaneously and actively in social learning with and from another person. In this regard, it would be hard to understand how any intervention could lead to comprehensive and cascading advances in the learning of children without ASD without advancing their joint attention skills (see Chapter 6 for details).

Finally, the third question—that is, which types of motivation processes influence the development of joint attention—may be critical to distinguishing social orienting, face processing, and joint attention in typical and autism spectrum development. In theory on autism, the role of motivation is most often conceptualized in terms of the reward value of orienting to people or their faces. However, recently a new hypothesis has emerged in the literature: In addition to considering the reward system that motivates infants and children to look at other people, it may be important for research on autism to consider the possible reward value of being the object of other people's attention. The latter may be pivotal to the nature of human social-cognitive development and autism spectrum development. This new point of view is described in subsequent sections of this chapter.

The Many Dimensions of the Social Phenotype of ASD

To the best of my knowledge, the evidence-based identification of dimensions of the social phenotype of ASD began with early reports of preschool imitation differences (DeMyer et al., 1972), followed by observations of differences in school-age face processing (Langdell, 1978), preschool joint attention (Curcio, 1978), and preschool functional and symbolic play behaviors[1] (Ungerer & Sigman, 1981; Wing & Gould, 1979). Some time later, the first report that children with ASD had difficulty appreciating that other people could hold a false belief was published (Baron-Cohen et al., 1985). This led to the idea that the social-developmental difference of ASD could be explained in terms of an alteration in *theory of mind*, or

---

[1] *Functional play* refers to the tendency of infants to use social conventions with objects in play, such as placing the receiver of a toy phone to the ear. This reflects the children's ability to recognize (mentally represent) the (social) function of the object. Subsequently, children begin to play with objects (e.g., dolls) as if they were animate, such as pretending that a doll is eating food or driving a car. This type of play act is less routinized and guided by the perceptual characteristics of an object. Play is guided by more generative and varied mental representations that eventually reach the level of symbolic actions, such as playing with a block as if it is a person. Thus functional play and symbolic play measure the development of how well children can mentally generate social action scenarios to guide their play with objects.

the capacity to identify the mental processes of other people, such as their intentions, beliefs, or emotions (Baron-Cohen, 1995).

Following the description of the theory-of-mind hypothesis, Ami Klin (1991) published his influential observation that school-age children with ASD did not display a typical pattern of preference for orienting to social sounds (parents' voices) relative to white noise. Klin's observation set the stage for the development of the social orienting model of ASD. Klin's work was followed by a similarly influential study by Geraldine Dawson and her colleagues; this study indicated that children with ASD also did not orient to social sounds such as hand clapping, versus comparable but nonsocial sounds, to the degree that comparison children did (Dawson, Meltzoff, Osterling, Rinaidi, & Brown, 1998). Indeed, Dawson et al. (1998) coined the term *social orienting deficit* in this study to raise awareness of the idea that an impairment in orienting and attending to social stimuli may be primary in the course of autism spectrum development.

Subsequently, the Yale research group of Klin, Jones, Schultz, Volkmar, and Cohen (2002b) famously showed that older individuals with ASD did not visually track the faces, and especially the eyes, of actors and an actress in scenes from a movie the way comparison research participants did. This study provided a precise means of measuring social orienting, as well as evidence that spontaneous social orienting was atypical in these individuals with ASD.

Ultimately, the Yale research group offered a variation of the social orienting/social attention hypothesis. They followed up on earlier studies (e.g., Hobson et al., 1988; Langdell, 1978) to show that atypical face processing is a measurable and significant characteristic of ASD (Klin et al., 1999; Schultz et al., 2000, 2003). This led to the proposal that face-processing disturbance could be a foundation of the atypical development of many social behaviors in both younger and older people with ASD (Schultz, 2005). In the same year, Dawson, Webb, and McPartland (2005) made an equally compelling case for the face-processing hypothesis. More recently, this hypothesis was bolstered by the observation that an EEG marker of cortical activity associated with face processing appears to becomes more like that of typical children in response to early intervention in children with ASD (Dawson, Jones, et al., 2012; see Chapter 6 for details).

In the context of these varied observations, the preeminence of social orienting/face processing in models of ASD has been reasonable. For example, if a child has a significantly robust and chronic deficit in attention to people, especially faces, the resulting attenuation of social information processing could inhibit the child's development of imitation and joint attention, and even his or her social-cognitive neurodevelopment (Mundy & Crowson, 1997; Mundy & Neal, 2000). This hypothesis has been well considered in research and theory on the genesis and meaning of joint attention disturbance in ASD.

Senju (2013) has offered a persuasive update of the social orienting hypothesis of ASD. He notes that higher-functioning people with ASD can engage in social behaviors that involve social orienting (e.g., imitation or gaze following) or social cognition when explicitly instructed to do so. However, in contrast to comparison peers, they do not consistently or uniformly attend *spontaneously* to the socially relevant information in social-cognitive, imitation, or gaze-following tasks without instruction (also see Sato, Uono, Okada, & Toichi, 2010). According to these observations, people affected by ASD do not display a disturbance of the *ability* to engage in social orienting. Such a disturbance of ability to engage in a type of cognitive-behavioral process has been called a *mediation deficit* (Dunlosky, Hertzog, & Powell-Moman, 2005). Instead, Senju (2013) argues that people with ASD display a difference in top-down (executive) cognitive control of social orienting and social cognition. This is called a *production deficit* (Dunlosky et al. 2005). This is an important distinction. It suggests that differences in ASD may stem from issues related to the development of frontal executive control of social orienting and face processing, rather than from neural networks directly associated with the ability to engage in social orienting or face processing. It also suggests that individuals with ASD may be variable or heterogeneous in the degree to which they display their social orienting or face-processing abilities.

With this review in mind, let us now consider a critical assumption that differences in social orienting and face processing may emerge very early in the development of children with ASD and lead to differences in the later emergence of joint attention,

When Does Joint Attention Develop?

Recent behavioral and imaging studies suggest that joint attention development, rather than emerging late in the first year or early in the second year of life, is well underway in the first 6 months of life. Theory also suggests that in early infancy joint attention development involves a dynamic interplay between behavior and the onset of a frontal–temporal–parietal social-cognitive control network (e.g., Mundy & Jarrold, 2010; also see Chapter 7).

Evidence of the very early neurodevelopment of joint attention was provided in an optical imaging study (Grossmann & Johnson, 2010). Observations in this study indicated that activity in left middle upper frontal cortex appeared to be specifically activated in 15 five-month-olds during an RJA task. The right dorsal frontal cortex did not display this pattern of activation. Optical imaging in this study involved passing light harmlessly through the skull to measure oxygen utilization in the surface layers of the brain during infants' task performance. Just like functional magnetic resonance imaging (fMRI), optical imaging measures changes in oxygen uptake in the brain, with the assumption that greater oxygen utilization in areas of the cortex reflects greater task-related activity in those areas. One limit of optical imaging, however, is that it does not lend itself to examining the activation patterns of deeper cortical structures.

A more recent study, though, has been able to do just that. Elison et al. (2013) used a method called *diffusion tensor imaging* (DTI), which examines the functional integrity of white matter connections between cortical areas. White matter consists mostly of myelinated bundles of axons and glial cells. The bundles of axons transmit signals from one region of the brain to another (see the illustrations in the middle of Figure 5.1). Hence

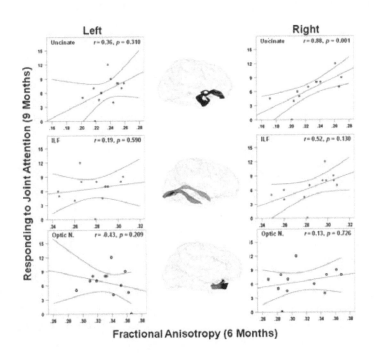

FIGURE 5.1. Scatterplots representing the associations between responding to joint attention at 9 months and an index of neural connectivity at 6 months (fractional anisotropy) within the uncinate fasciculi (top panels, left and right), the inferior longitudinal fasciculi (ILF; middle panels, left and right), and the optic nerves (bottom panels, left and right). The illustrations in the middle depict diffusion tensor imaging of the respective areas. From Elison et al. (2013). Copyright 2013 by John Wiley & Sons, Inc. Reprinted by permission.

white matter is essential to cortical connectivity, and to the flow of information across brain networks.

Elison et al. (2013) examined the degree to which evidence of fronto-temporal connectivity in 6-month-olds, via a white matter pathway called the uncinate fasciculi, predicted RJA development at 9–10 months. They also examined the degree to which occipitotemporal connectivity, via a white matter pathway called the inferior longitudinal fasciculi (ILF), predicted RJA development. The results (see Figure 5.1) indicated that functional integrity of the uncinate fasciculi pathway at 6 months significantly predicted RJA development at 9 months. No evidence was provided for the role of ILF pathway connectivity in joint attention development in this study. The uncinate fasciculi pathway connects a cortical network that involves the inferior medial temporal lobe, the rostral temporal pole (including the amygdala), the frontoinsular cortex, and the orbital and ventral medial prefrontal cortex. This network has previously been hypothesized to be part of a broader frontoparietal neural network involved in mature joint attention (e.g., Mundy, 2003; Mundy & Jarrold, 2010; also see Chapter 7).

This evidence, scant though it may be, is important for several reasons. First, the two imaging studies described above are consistent with behavioral evidence that joint attention emerges in the first 6 months of life (e.g., Farroni, Massaccesi, Pividori, & Johnson, 2004; Gredebäck et al., 2010). Recall that behavioral research suggests that responding to joint attention begins to develop in the second to sixth months of life. This is the *same period of development* that a recent longitudinal growth study of at-risk infants identified for the onset of social orienting differences in ASD (Jones & Klin, 2013).

Second, the neural systems associated with joint attention identified in these studies are not the same as the systems most prominently identified in studies of social orienting and face processing. This is especially true for face processing, which is most often attributed to functions of the fusiform gyrus (Schultz et al., 2003). The fusiform gyrus runs along the posterior ventral temporal cortex. Problems in face processing have been associated with disturbances of this gyrus, as well as the ILF, which connects the fusiform gyrus to more anterior other brain areas (Thomas et al., 2009). However, ILF was not associated with RJA in the Elison et al. (2013) study.

The latter finding is consistent with early observations published by Hooker et al. (2003). This research team specifically examined the involvement of fusiform networks in processing gaze direction (a component of joint attention), and reported that selectivity for gaze processing *was not observed in face-responsive fusiform regions*. Instead, activation of different brain networks in superior temporal sulcus and inferior parietal cortex was associated with processing directional information from gaze (also see Calder et al., 2007). Interestingly, these latter two regions of the brain, not the fusiform gyrus, are what appear to be involved in differences in gaze processing in ASD (e.g., Pelphrey, Morris, & McCarthy, 2005).

The evidence at hand thus suggests that both social orienting disturbance in ASD (Jones & Klin, 2013) and the typical development of joint attention (e.g., Grossmann & Johnson, 2010) occur during the same phase of development—that is, in the first 6 months of life. It also seems to be the case that the change in relatively fixed social orienting in the first 2 months of life to increasingly flexible social and object orienting occurs in conjunction with increasing frontal control over attention (e.g., Johnson, 1990, 1995). So, too, the emergence of joint attention in this period appears to be related to the development of frontal connectivity and functions (Elison et al., 2013). A parsimonious interpretation of the pattern of these findings is that early social orienting and joint attention development reflect many similar, if not the same, neurodevelopmental processes in early infancy. To explain one in terms of the other may be difficult at best. It may also be that the top-down processes that lead us to organize and regulate our orienting to enter into joint attention with others are similar to those processes that prioritize our looking to faces and eyes when we watch actors and actresses in a movie.

Let's begin to think a bit more deeply about the types of control and organization that are required in joint attention. In RJA, children must first socially orient to a person, but then then engage in inhibition of social orienting to the person's face, and perhaps to their names' being called, in order to redirect attention away from the person to a new spatial locale. IJA involves a similar type of executive regulation of attention. Children (or adults) must inhibit their immediate attention and information processing of an object or event that is of interest, then shift their attention to look to another person to share that person's interest, and then shift again to return attention to the object/event. The ability to shift and inhibit attention is central to so called frontal "cognitive control and executive functions." Consequently, both IJA and RJA development have repeatedly been observed to be associated with measures of executive function development in young children (e.g., Dawson, Munson, et al., 2002; Griffith et al., 1999; McEvoy, Rogers, & Pennington, 1993; Nichols et al., 2005).

Given this basic task analysis, it would not be surprising to observe that infants' initial engagement in joint attention appears to be inefficient and effortful. With months of maturation and practice, the efficiency of execution of joint attention behaviors would be expected to increase as it becomes imbedded in a routinized executive function for social attention (Mundy et al., 2009). Exactly this pattern of development has been reported in two independent studies of the development of RJA. Gredebäck et al. (2010) examined the development of RJA with caregivers and unfamiliar testers at 2, 4, 6, and 8 months of age in 36 infants. Their study indicated that RJA emerged in the 2- to 4-month period and become more consistent from 6 to 8 months. Their results are depicted in the upper left panel (A) of Figure 5.2, which illustrates three important observations.

First, the longitudinal growth of RJA accuracy was steady and measurable between 2 and 8 months of age in typical development. Second, and perhaps surprisingly, RJA behavior might be more powerfully elicited in infants by an unfamiliar tester than by the infants' caregivers. Last but not least, the reaction time required to respond to the gaze and head shift of an adult partner was initially rather long. After an adult's gaze and head shift, it took over 3 seconds for infants to respond at two months. Then across the subsequent 6 months, the reaction times on RJA trials became significantly faster. By 8 months, infants followed gaze and head turns after a delay of about 1.5 seconds. It is plausible that this increase in reaction time might be associated with advances in the integrity of white matter connectivity in the joint attention neural network.

Vaughan Van Hecke et al. (2012) reported two studies that extend our understanding of the development of joint attention in terms of increasing efficiencies of behavioral execution. Data in the first study provided information on the change in reaction time on RJA trials across a longitudinal study of infant development between 9 and 18 months of age. The 9- to 18-month data corroborated and extended Gredebäck et al.'s (2010) observations: Over this age range, the average reaction time on RJA trials for infants decreased significantly from an average of 1.77 seconds per trial to an average of 0.86 second (see Figure 5.2, upper right panel [B] and lower panel). Note that RJA reaction time observed by Vaughan Van Hecke et al. for 9-month-olds were very similar to those observed by Gredebäck at al. (2010) for 8-month-olds. This suggests that the observation of the latency to respond on RJA trials marks a replicable phenomenon in infant development. Together, the data from these two studies provide an outline of the continuous course of development of RJA in the first 18 months of life, measured not in terms of whether or not an infant has the ability to execute RJA behavior, but rather in evidence of the increasing efficiency of such behavior.

The second study more directly tested the social executive function hypothesis of joint attention (Mundy et al., 2009) by examining the degree to which differences in RJA at 12 months predicted differences in cognitive control of behavior in a delay-of-gratification task at 36 months. As noted in the previous task analysis, RJA may be regulated by an executive attention system that plays a fundamental role in the capacity to

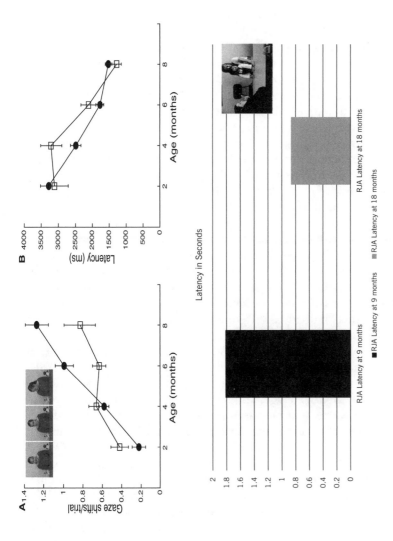

FIGURE 5.2. The average number of gaze shifts per trial (upper left, A) and latency of first gaze shifts (upper right, B) for infants in a structured interactions with a stranger (filled circles) or their mothers (open squares) from 2 to 8 months of age. The lower panel illustrates the latency of first gaze shifts in 9- and 18-month-olds by trials and direction of gaze shifts. A and B are from Gredebäck, Fikke, and Melinder (2010). Copyright 2010 by John Wiley & Sons, Inc. Reprinted by permission. The data illustrated in the lower half of the figure are from Vaughan Van Hecke et al. (2012). This graph was created by the author for this book.

disengage attention from a central stimulus in order to allocate attention to a new spatial location in a goal-directed manner (Kingstone, Friesen, & Gazzaniga, 2000; Mundy, Card, & Fox, 2000; Redcay et al., 2010; Clohessy, Rothbart, & Posner, 2001; Vaughan Van Hecke et al., 2007). Individual differences in infants' tendencies to attend to or look away from a rewarding or negative stimulus reflect differences in one of the first and most important means by which infants learn to self-regulate their affective states and goal-related intentional behaviors directed toward people and objects (Posner & Rothbart, 2000). Hence, Vaughan Van Hecke et al. (2012) examined the hypothesis that RJA development at 12 months would be related to individual differences in self-regulation in 3-year-olds.

To measure self-regulation, the researchers used a delay-of-gratification paradigm. In this paradigm, a tester examined the children's ability to delay reaching for a reward, such as a fruit snack, for up to 30 seconds. RJA at 12 months was significantly associated with individual differences in children's capacity to self-regulate by inhibiting reaching for the reward, as well as directing their attention away from the snack. The results were consistent with a previous report of a relation between 6-month RJA and 24-month delay of gratification in typical development (Morales et al., 2005). These studies provide evidence of a link between joint attention and self-regulation, both of which play pivotal roles in the development of social competence (Mundy & Sigman, 2006). They may help to explain the recent observation that preschool joint attention assessment predicts individual differences in social competence in adults with ASD (Gillespie-Lynch et al., 2012).

The foregoing studies highlight several features of joint attention development that are not always well recognized in research on ASD. Evidence indicates that the behavioral development of joint attention is underway by 2–4 months of age, and it is possible to observe the development of neural systems that support joint attention by 5–6 months of age. Moreover, important facets of the development of this dimension involve increasing efficiency in execution of joint attention behaviors. This presumably reflects the growth of a top-down executive (cognitive) control component of joint attention. In light of this observation, it is reasonable to expect that risk for joint attention disturbance in children and adults with ASD may be expressed along a continuum. In some individuals, joint attention disturbance may be displayed in terms of differences in the speed and effort involved in the execution of joint attention. In more severe cases of ASD, a near-absolute inability to engage in joint attention may be observed. In the former instance, joint attention differences in ASD seem to take the form of mediation rather than production problems (see Senju, 2013); the latter situation reflects a production problem.

The Neonatal Phase of Joint Attention

The evidence that joint attention development is underway in the first 2–6 months of postnatal life presents a challenge to the assumption that social orienting development is a foundational precursor of joint attention. Still, the developmental literature maintains that neonates and infants prioritize social orienting and face processing *in the first 3 months of life*. Even though there is little evidence of a robust difference in social orienting prioritization in infants at risk for ASD (e.g., Ozonoff et al., 2010; Jones & Klin, 2013), it remains plausible that neonatal dyadic social orienting involves precursor processes that contribute to joint attention in differences in ASD beginning at 2 months. However, Teresa Farroni and colleagues at the University of London have published a sequence of studies that raise questions about even this developmental assumption.

In one of their first reports, Farroni, Csibra, Simion, and Johnson (2002) provided evidence that 2- to 5-day-old newborns could discriminate between a face that appeared to be looking directly at them (mutual gaze) and one that appeared to be looking away from them. In an even more revealing study, Farroni et al. (2004) reported that under carefully controlled conditions, the tendency of 2- to 5-day-old neonates to orient quickly to a peripherally presented cue was significantly improved if they watched eyes shift in the congruent direction before the cue appeared. These data suggest that some aspects of joint attention may be under development in the first days of postnatal life. Moreover, these behaviors do not involve fixed orienting to the face, but rather responding to directional cues of the gaze shifts (i.e., RJA). The data reported in these two studies add to the observations of early neurodevelopment of RJA, which challenge the view that the onset of joint attention occurs after a separate and foundational period of development in social orienting and face processing.

Rather than being separate, therefore, joint attention and social orienting may share common primary processes in early development. One possibility in this regard has recently been raised by Senju and Johnson (2009) in their discussion of the *eye contact effect*, which I consider next.

Alternative Perspectives: Social Orienting, Social Motivation, and ASD

In a very interesting set of studies, Farroni and her colleagues explored the effect of adults' gaze and attention *on infants*. In one study, Farroni, Mansfeld, Lai, and Johnson (2003) investigated the degree to which observations of pupil motion were key to gaze following. They reported that

4-month-olds could consistently follow gaze when indicated by only pupil motion without head turn cues, but *only* if this was preceded by the opportunity to experience a period of mutual gaze, or adult attention directed to the infants. Senju, Csibra, and Johnson (2008) also observed that the experience of mutual gaze, or attention to the self, also facilitated more advanced RJA abilities in 9-month-olds. In addition, Farroni, Massaccesci, Menon, and Johnson (2007) have examined the impact of mutual gaze or social attention on children's face processing. Four-month-olds displayed better recognition when they studied faces that appeared to look directly at them than when they studied faces with averted gaze. Moreover, if they *first* studied faces with mutual gaze, this enhanced their processing and recognition for subsequently studied faces with averted gaze.

The observations of Ferroni and others bring to mind an idea that slightly, though fundamentally, turns the typical social orienting model in a new direction. The current social orienting model suggests that choosing to look at faces and social stimuli is insufficiently rewarding for children with ASD (Chevallier et al., 2012; Kim et al., 2014; Mundy, 1995). Senju and Johnson (2009) raise a different possibility to consider: *Infants may find social attention directed to them rewarding or arousing in a way that organizes and promotes their ability to engage in information processing.* This raises the possibility that differences in responsiveness to being the object of attention of another person play a role in autism spectrum development. More specifically, being the object of another person's attention may not organize early social orienting and joint attention development in the same way or to the same extent in autism spectrum development as it does in typical development.

Indeed, there is already one study that supports this possibility. Grice et al. (2005) have observed that neural correlates of social attention (mutual gaze) in 4- to 7-year-old children with ASD may be delayed in their development and more comparable to those of infants. However, at least 50% of the sample of children with ASD in this study also appeared to be affected by moderate to severe IDD. Control for this factor was not part of the research design. Therefore, it is difficult to know whether the results reflect effects associated with ASD, IDD, or both.

Nevertheless, the idea that infants respond to mutual gaze, and the experience of being the object of social attention, with enhanced information processing of stimuli is consistent with numerous observations of similar phenomenon in adults and children (e.g., Bayliss, Paul, Cannon, & Tipper, 2006; Becchio, Bertone, & Castiello, 2008; Hood, Macrae, Cole-Davies, & Dias, 2003; Kim & Mundy, 2012). This has been called the *eye contact effect* by Senju and Johnson (2009), who proposed three causal explanations for this phenomenon.

The *arousal model* stipulates that eye contact during mutual gaze directly activates brain arousal systems and/or an emotional response. Hence this model posits an affect-based reward mechanism for preferential social orienting early in life (Senju & Johnson, 2009). The increased reward arousal then influences subsequent perceptual and cognitive processing. This model holds that a subcortical system including the amygdala is responsible for cortical and cognitive activity that can lead to enhanced information processing subsequent to eye contact.

Alternatively, the *communicative intent model* suggests that eye contact directly triggers a higher-order cognitive awareness of the communicative intent of another person's mutual gaze. This stems from the activation of social-cognitive/theory-of-mind brain modules thought to guide the development of joint attention and referential information processing (Baron-Cohen, 1995; Becchio et al., 2008; Wicker et al., 2003; Pelphrey, Viola, & McCarthy, 2004; Schilbach et al., 2006). It is this incipient social-cognitive awareness that leads to social orienting prioritization, and the social-cognitive network activation leads to enhanced information processing in response to eye contact.

Third, Senju and Johnson (2009) propose a *fast-track modulator model,* which they believe provides a better account of the development of the eye contact effect than either of the other two models does. According to this third model, a very fast subcortical visual processing network that involves interactions of superior colliculus, pulvinar, and amygdala is triggered by mutual eye contact. This system does not involve activation of cortical face-processing systems (e.g., the fusiform gyrus) and is much faster than cortical face processing. It is responsible for a *bias* in responding to eye gaze and faces in young infants, even before cortical face processing fully develops (Johnson, 2005).

Accordingly, the fast-track modulator is responsible for infants' preference for attention to faces and people (Senju & Johnson, 2009; Johnson, 2005). However, rather than an affect-based/emotional reward mechanism, or a cognitive awareness mechanism, this model posits that the subcortical fast-track network also leads to the rapid activation of the orbital and medial frontal cortex (150–170 msec after gaze fixation). This frontal activation is equated with cognitive arousal, or an interest-driven tendency to attend to (spotlight) faces and eyes. Moreover, fast-track modulator activation is thought to kindle incipient frontal top-down modulation of attention and attention-related information processing, which spurs on the development of a social-cognitive network (Senju & Johnson, 2009, p. 6). The nature of the early social-cognitive network is not yet fully specified. Yet Senju and Johnson (2009) describe a fast-track modulator network in which subcortical, amygdala, and frontal nodes would conceivably be interconnected by the uncinate fasciculi, which research suggests plays a role in RJA development at 5 months (Elison et al., 2013).

Senju and Johnson's (2009) hypothesis *may* take us a few steps closer to understanding some of the primary neurodevelopmental systems and functions that are involved in social attention, face processing, and joint attention impairments in young children affected by ASD. They have described an innate effect of mutual gaze that triggers an enhanced attention spotlight and associated greater cognitive processing during and subsequent to mutual gaze. In dyadic interactions, this could lead to enhanced processing of information from and about a social partner. In triadic social interactions involving joint attention, this could contribute to enhanced information processing about concrete or abstract things in the world (points of reference) that are the common object of attention of two or more people. In adults this processing may not even require eye contact. Boothby et al. (2014) reported that information processing was amplified when individuals tasted the same type of sweet or bitter chocolate in the presence of others (but without eye contact), compared to isolated conditions.

A precedent for such a bias toward enhanced information processing may be provided by the literature on the effects of novel stimuli on recognition memory in infants.

From the 1950s to the 1980s, Robert Fantz and then Joseph Fagan at Case Western Reserve University conducted a sequence of observations indicating that neonates often display an inherent visual preference to attend to novel stimuli. This came to be known as the infant *novelty preference effect*. Given a choice between looking at a novel stimulus or a familiar stimulus, infants from the first weeks will often spontaneously look to and engage in active information processing/memory encoding of the former (Bornstein & Sigman, 1986). It seems to me that Senju and Johnson (2009) have described a similarly automatic early attention and information-processing bias with their fast-track modulator explanation of the eye contact effect. Like the novelty preference effect, the eye contact effect appears to triggers not so much liking or disliking of a stimulus, but rather interest, exploration, and processing of stimulus information.

I return to additional details and thoughts related to Senju and Johnson (2009) fast-track modulator model in Chapters 7 and 8. For now, the important ideas are these: Both evidence and theory indicate that mutual gaze or social attention to the self facilitates information processing in people. Moreover, the eye contact effect, and the neurocognitive systems believed to support it, emerge early in typical infant human development. Remarkably, these ideas are consistent with two strands of joint attention theory.

Attention to Self and Joint Attention

Back in the 1970s, Elizabeth Bates thought about the possible role of motivation in infants' initiations of joint attention, or what she and her colleague called *protodeclaratives*. Bates et al.(1975) suggested that the joint attention bids of infants and toddlers involved the "use of an object (through pointing, showing, giving, etc.) as a means to gain adult attention [to the child]" (p. 115). Thus Bates et al. hypothesized that early joint attention development may be influenced by children's intrinsic positive response to social attention directed toward one's self.

While Bates proposed the kernel of this idea, it has been more completely articulated by Vasudevi Reddy (2003) in her discussion of the emotional and cognitive impact of *being the object of others' attention* in early child development. Reddy suggests that an intrinsic discriminant response to social attention, or mutual gaze to self, begins to serve a critical organizational function in the dynamic process of human development by no later than 2 months of age. Accordingly, perception of attention to self stimulates infants in a way that triggers a cascade of developmental cognitive and affective processes involved in differentiating self and other. Reddy's hypothesis carries with it the inference that differentiation and identification of a sense of self and others may be an important part of joint attention. Equally, differences in joint attention in autism spectrum development may involve differences in processes associated with self-identification, or the discrimination but integration of self-referenced and other-referenced information processing (Hobson & Hobson, 2007; Mizuno et al., 2011; Mundy et al., 2010). It is also consistent with the suggestion by Bates et al. (1979) that sharing experience through IJA may become motivated by the goal of eliciting attention to self. According to Reddy (2003), the expressed human motivation to elicit attention to self becomes even clearer in the second and third years of life, with increased frequency in the display of four types of related behaviors by children.

These four behaviors are (1) *showing off*, or the performance of exaggerated or unusual actions to gain attention when it is absent or to retain it when a child is the center of attention; (2) *clever actions*, which are repeated acts to elicit further praise, or checking on others' attention with pleasure after the completion of difficult actions; (3) *clowning*, or the repetition of odd actions that have previously led to laughter to elicit more laughter; and (4) *teasing*, or deliberate provocation through the performance of actions contrary to existing expectations or routines. All of these behaviors are less frequently displayed by many children with ASD than by groups of comparison children (e.g., Reddy, Williams, & Vaughan, 2002)

This line of theory proposes that atypical early intrinsic responsiveness to being the object of others' attention may make contributions to the differences in development of joint attention in ASD. Again, this formulation deemphasizes the role of a lack of social orienting in ASD, in favor of the possible role of differences in the effect of mutual gaze as an attractor and organizer in development. Indeed, Schietecatte et al. (2012) have reported that 6-month preference for looking at social stimuli was not related to later joint attention development in typically developing infants. However, the tendency of 6-month-olds to look more at pictures or videos that offered the opportunity to experience mutual gaze did predict later RJA and IJA in the course of typical development.

The small difference in conceptualization between directing attention to others and receiving attention from others as the operative process in social orienting phenomena may have significant ramifications. It suggests that we may need to go beyond current approaches to the measurement of social attention effects in the study of early markers of ASD. Measuring only the frequency or duration of looks to people or faces may not capture all the critical phenomena associated with social attention. Behavioral or physiological measures of children's responsiveness to social attention (mutual gaze) in the first months of life may be also useful. Combining measures of tendencies to deploy attention to other people and of reactions to the social attention of other people may be better than using either type of measure alone in the search for early markers of ASD.

Second, the current social orienting hypothesis suggests that children with ASD do not look to people and faces because social stimuli are not rewarding enough to attract typical levels of attention. However, the basis of the attraction to social attention is not well defined. The fresh hypothesis here is that at least one component of the *attractor of attention* may operationally be defined as the stimulating effect of mutual gaze on the cognitive processing of an infant.

Accordingly, a lack of typical response to social attention to self may play a critical role in impairments of cognitive activity that contribute to impairments not only in joint attention, but also in imitation and social-cognitive development, for children with ASD. Recent studies have provided some evidence that atypical responses to the social attention of others do play a role in joint attention, imitation, and social-cognitive development in children with ASD (Schilbach, Eickoff, Cieslik, Kuzmanovic, & Vogeley, 2012; Stagg, Davis, & Heaton, 2013; Vivanti & Dissanayake, 2014).

The work of Stagg et al. (2013) is illustrative in this regard. This Cambridge- and London-based research group worked with three groups of 10-year-old children. One group of 14 higher-functioning children with

ASD (average verbal mental age, 10.8 years) did not display delayed language onset. Another group of 18 children with ASD did display delayed language onset (average verbal mental age, 10.0 years). A comparison group of 18 children with typical development also participated (average verbal mental age, 11.0 years). All the groups were matched on nonverbal cognitive ability.

The children with ASD but without early language delays reportedly began to acquire phrase speech by 17 months, whereas the children with ASD and language delays reportedly did not acquire phrase speech until about 37 months of age. All children were presented with a series of computer-generated but realistic faces with gaze directed straight ahead (social attention toward participants), gaze directed left or right, or eyes closed. Stagg et al. (2013) used a measure of galvanic skin response (GSR) to examine subtle differences in the autonomic nervous system markers of arousal during exposure to the face stimuli across the groups of children.

The results of this study indicated that the group with ASD and later onset of language displayed evidence of hypoarousal to all face stimuli, regardless of eye gaze or eyes-closed conditions, compared to the typical control group (see Figure 5.3). The group with ASD but without early language delays displayed an intermediate response pattern (see Figure 5.3): They displayed the same pattern of GSR response to faces with mutual

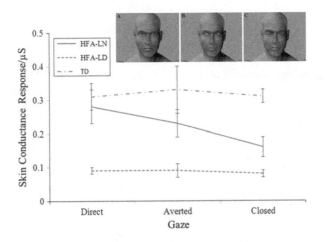

FIGURE 5.3. Illustration of the virtual avatar gaze stimuli and skin conductance responses to eye gaze for typically developing children (TD in the figure), children with normal language and higher-functioning ASD (HFA-LN in the figure), and children with language delays and higher-functioning ASD (HFA-LD in the figure). From Stagg, Davis, and Heaton (2013). Copyright 2013 by Springer Science+Business Media. Reprinted by permission.

gaze as their language-delayed peers. However, these children with ASD displayed more evidence of arousal to faces with averted gaze, or eyes closed, than did the children with ASD and language delays. The two groups with ASD significantly differed on GSR collapsed across all face stimuli (total average GSR). However, the children with ASD but without language delays did not significantly differ from the typically developing sample on the total average GSR measure.

Retrospective parent report of eye contact in the first year of life was also examined. These data indicated that parental reports of amount of their children's eye contact in the first year of life were significantly correlated with greater arousal to faces across the groups at age 10. This observation in conjunction with the group comparison data prompted the authors to suggest: "For infants with ASD, early over- or under-arousal [to gaze] may be reflected in upstream difficulties in joint-attention and language acquisition" (Stagg et al., 2013, p. 2309).

It may be apparent that the fast-track modulator model brings us back to the notion that a lack of responsiveness to others plays a critical role in the development of ASD. However, it is not a pervasive lack of responsiveness. Rather, we are talking about a rather specific early developmental vulnerability. This vulnerability could be expressed as a transient delay in the timing and intensity of the eye contact effect, and could degrade a vital organizer of social and cognitive development early in the development of children affected by ASD. This could contribute to a dynamic cascade of developmental disturbance in children; alternatively, this could be a more chronic condition that continues to have an impact on social-cognitive development well into adulthood. That is, it could have variable timing, intensity, and/or duration across children. Regardless, one vital impact may be that a lack of responsiveness to mutual gaze may impede the organization of early joint attention development in some children with ASD in the first 6 months of life. This in turn may lead to a cascade of problems in social learning—problems that play a significant role in the subsequent development of the cognitive and social-behavioral phenotype of ASD. It is useful to delve deeper into the pivotal role of joint attention in learning before we examine the effect of targeted interventions for joint attention in the next chapter.

Joint Attention, Language Development, and Social Orienting

The chapter to this point has reviewed evidence that social orienting, face processing, and joint attention emerge more or less concurrently in the first 6 months of life. Moreover, they may share one or more sources of initial disturbance; it may not be the case that impairment in one dimension causes impairment in the other. However, subsequent developmental differentiation is likely to yield distinct functional identities for these dimensions that have different roles in the social, communicative, and cognitive development of people with ASD.

Social orienting serves security, threat, attachment, and affiliative goal-related needs for tracking the locations and actions of other people. Face processing serves many functions, such as identifying familiar and unfamiliar social agents and processing nonverbal emotional cues in social interactions. Alternatively, joint attention begins to enable infants to adopt a common point of reference with others in order to begin to share information and meaning with others about objects and events in the world. The referential function is a defining utility of the social-cognitive neurodevelopmental dimension of joint attention. The referential function is also pivotal to the role that joint attention plays in social learning for all of us throughout all our lives. This role is perhaps best illustrated by research on the strong connection between joint attention and language development.

Joint Attention and Typical Language Development

From the beginning of its study, theory and research suggested that joint attention is vital to sharing information and human learning (Bruner, 1995). Some of the first empirical evidence of this was provided by the observation that joint attention and functional language development were significantly correlated in 8- to 13-month-olds (Bates, 1976; Bates et al., 1979).

More recently, computational cognitive scientists have increasingly recognized the need to include parameters that reflect joint attention, in order to effectively model the development of language, sharing meaning, and social cognition (e.g., Scassellati, 1999; Steels, 2003; Kwisthout, Vogt, Haselager, & Dijkstra, 2008). For example, Kwisthout et al. (2008) reported a computer simulation study in which adding parameters reflecting three types of joint attention (checking attention, following attention, and directing attention) substantially improved the performance of models in successfully simulating functional discourse between agents in virtual interactions. To my knowledge, computational approaches do not make a comparable case for the need for parameters reflecting dyadic social orienting or face processing in accurate computational models of social and language development. One of these models, though, indicates that it may be important to consider the interaction between imitation and joint attention in accurately modeling human communicative development (Scassellati, 1999). Likewise, a meta-analysis of 25 studies of research on the relation between IJA pointing and language was reported by Colonnesi et al. (2010). These studies included a total of 734 children, and the meta-analysis indicated average effect sizes ($r = .52$ and $r = .35$) across concurrent and longitudinal studies, respectively, of the association between pointing and language development. The association was clear for pointing that served a declarative function (i.e., IJA pointing), but not for pointing with an imperative function (requesting). Evidence for the association between joint attention and language development, though, extends beyond research on pointing. For example, a longitudinal study provides evidence of significant relations between infant individual differences in RJA and IJA and later typical language development (Mundy et al., 2007). The IJA measures in this study did not emphasize pointing. Moreover, comparable relations between joint attention and language development were observed regardless of infants' language backgrounds, maternal education, or rate of cognitive development.

Dare Baldwin (1995) encapsulated a pivotal aspect of the contribution of joint attention to language development by describing its role in referential mapping. Early language learning often takes place in unstructured, incidental situations where parents spontaneously refer to a new object (see Figure 5.4 for an example). How do infants know how to link their parents' vocal labels to the correct parts of the environment, amidst

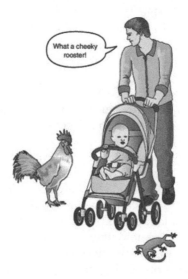

FIGURE 5.4. Illustration of the incidental context of language learning and the utility of infant joint attention (e.g., gaze following) in self-organizing information to reduce referential mapping errors in interactions with adults. Based on Baldwin (1995).

a myriad of potential referents? Baldwin (1995) suggested that infants use RJA, or their parents' direction of gaze, to cue them to search a more limited part of the environment, where they are more likely to map the label to the correct object or event.

Wu, Gopnik, Richardson, and Kirkham (2011) have recently provided an elegant study of this model. Their research indicates that in relatively simple or constant environments, such as rooms in their homes, infants can use statistical learning to detect repeated consistencies (invariant associations) between labels and objects or event. However, as the environment becomes less consistent or more complicated with distractors across learning opportunities, infants also use social cues (RJA) in order to improve accurate referential mapping. So joint attention is not necessary for all early vocabulary development, but it does have an impact on individual differences in the breadth of vocabulary development.

Infants also use IJA to reduce the chance of referential mapping errors. IJA serves to denote something of immediate interest to a child. This allows parents to follow their child's attention better, and to provide new information in the context of the child's interest and attention, which is optimal for language learning (Tomasello & Farrar, 1986). Hence joint attention may be conceived as a self-organizing faculty of mind by which the active participation of infants in social interaction facilitates their adaptive information processing and learning in social interactions (Mundy, 2003). This self-organizing element of the social "learning function" is fundamental to the nature of joint attention as a milestone of early development (Bruner, 1975). In turn, joint attention differences in autism syndrome development are markers of a difference in this self-organizing aspect of development, which contributes directly to subsequent problems in language and communication development. The latter are also defining features of the syndrome.

Joint Attention and Language Learning in ASD

A study by Bono et al. (2004) exemplifies how differences in the self-organizing nature of joint attention play a role in language development and its impairment in children with ASD. This study was conducted with a small sample of 29 three- to five-year-olds with ASD, to examine how differences in intensity of community-based intervention affected their language development. Children were assessed for language, cognitive, and joint attention development at the beginning and end of 12 months of community-based preschool education. In those 12 months, intervention intensity ranged from 6 to 53 hours a week, and averaged 28 hours a week for the group. Bono et al. (2004) hypothesized that higher-intensity intervention would lead to better language outcomes for the children with ASD. To their surprise, they observed no relation between intervention intensity and language development in their sample. Additional data analysis showed that infants who displayed mastery of RJA at the beginning of the study did display greater language gains with greater intervention intensity; however, children without RJA mastery at the beginning of the study showed little effect of intervention at any intensity on language development. This small study suggested that children who displayed more mastery of RJA were better able to learn in the context of intervention than were children with less well-developed joint attention.

This observation is consistent with the notion that development of RJA may be an important developmental foundation for learning from instruction during early development in children with ASD. Moreover, the results of this study belied an earlier observation that children with ASD display a joint attention production deficit and cannot use social gaze cues for referential mapping (Baron-Cohen, Baldwin, & Crowson, 1997). Instead, RJA difficulty in children with ASD displays a pattern more in keeping with a mediation disturbance. Whereas some children with ASD display very little RJA, many display a range of RJA development that may be more effortful but approaches levels observed in typical development (Mundy et al., 1994; Nation & Penny, 2008). Indeed, recent experimental research indicates that some children with ASD clearly use RJA to resolve referential ambiguity in word learning (Luyster & Lord, 2009; Norbury, Griffiths, & Nation, 2010). Moreover, Hani, Gonzalez-Barrero, and Nadig (2013) observed that performance on an experimental measure of the use of gaze cues in referential mapping was related to individual differences in the language development of children with ASD. Hani et al. also reported that many of these children with ASD were comparable in their level of RJA use to language-level-matched typically developing children, *albeit less consistent in its use*. The latter is the hallmark of a top-down mediation deficit.

Several studies have provided data on the concurrent or predictive relations of joint attention with language development in ASD. However, as often as not, these studies also indicate that other behaviors (such as imitation and symbolic play development) are associated with language in children with autism syndrome development.

One study examined the association between language development in 59 children with ASD from ages 2 to 5 years, and joint attention measures from the Prelinguistic version of the original ADOS (Thurm, Lord, Lee, & Newschaffer, 2007). This study also included parental reports of children's tendency to imitate sounds and simple movements. Observations from this study indicated that IJA and RJA measures predicted expressive language development, but that RJA and imitation predicted receptive language development, in children with ASD. In a study of 164 toddlers with ASD, Luyster, Kadlec, Carter, and Tager-Flusberg (2008) also reported that a measure of RJA was associated with receptive language, even after the investigators controlled for age, gesture use, and cognitive ability. Smith, Mirenda, and Zaidman-Zait (2007) observed that verbal imitation, symbolic play, and IJA predicted vocabulary growth in 35 children with ASD from 20 to 70 months of age.

Maljaars, Noens, Scholte, and van Berckelaer-Onnes (2012) observed that the combined scores on IJA and RJA items from Modules 1 and 2 of the ADOS were associated with expressive and receptive language development in young children affected by ASD and IDD, even after the researchers controlled for symbolic play ability.

In research aimed at longer-term prediction, Sigman and McGovern (2005) observed weak but significant associations: RJA and social conventional object play in 48 children ages 3–5 years was associated with about 8% and 13%, respectively, of their variance in language assessed in adolescence after the authors controlled for initial language differences. Poon, Watson, Baranek, and Poe (2012) measured joint attention, imitation, and symbolic play from retrospective videos of 29 children with ASD at 9–12 and 15–18 months of age. They reported that these measures predicted language development measures in this sample when the children were measured at ages 3–7 years.

One of the difficulties of fully interpreting the data in the foregoing studies is that the patterns of results are variable, and we do not fully understand the possibly overlapping roles that imitation, symbolic play, and joint attention differences may play in the language development of children with ASD. The nature of this problem was well illustrated by Toth, Munson, Meltzoff, and Dawson (2006), who examined joint attention, play, and imitation in relation to language development in 60 children with ASD from 34 to 52 months of age. They reported that children's levels of performance on the measures of joint attention, imitation, and symbolic play were significantly correlated (i.e., they shared about 8–40% of their variance), and that these measures were all concurrently associated with a measure of language. If all the measures were correlated, it would be very difficult to understand whether each dimension made a distinct contribution to language development. It could be that all three dimensions reflect a common process or set of processes explaining their roles in language learning among children with autism spectrum development.

One way to approach to examining this possibility is called *mediation analysis*. A mediation analysis is a statistical (regression) method that can be used to answer the question of whether one variable (e.g., joint attention) explains the apparent correlation between another variable (e.g., language) and a third variable (e.g., imitation) or vice versa. Van der Paelt, Warreyn, and Roeyers (2014) provided such an analysis in a study of 83 children with ASD in an early intervention program. Similar to observations reported by Toth et al. (2006), Van der Paelt et al.'s data suggested that processes associated with joint attention may play a greater role in the early rather than the later stages of language development for children with ASD. More specifically, IJA and RJA measures mediated relations of play and imitation to receptive and expressive language development among children with ASD who displayed very little evidence of language development at the beginning of intervention.

The results of these studies support several broad conclusions. First, the impairment of joint attention in ASD is likely to involve some of the same processes involved in impairments in imitation and symbolic play development. However, they also suggest that each of these dimensions reflects unique facets of social-communicative development in ASD. Unfortunately, we are far from definitively understanding the common and unique processes associated with these dimensions of early development. Understanding the dynamic development of cognitive processes involved in joint attention, imitation, and representation cognition remains an elusive goal in the science of ASD (e.g., Roeyers, Van Oost, & Bothuyne, 1998). I return to research related to this issue in subsequent chapters.

Social Orienting, Face Processing, and Language Learning

Whereas there is a large literature on the role of joint attention in language development, the roles of social attention and face processing in the language learning of children with ASD are not so extensive. Nevertheless, some studies do provide some relevant information.

The study by Stagg et al. (2013) connects social orienting and face processing to language development in children with ASD. The process implicated in this linkage, though, is arousal related to the eye contact effect. Young, Merin, Rogers, and Ozonoff (2009) provided an informative study of 33 high-risk infant siblings of children diagnosed with autism, and 25 infant siblings of children with typical development. They then examined the predictive validity of data on social orienting and face processing at 6 months for ASD symptom development and language through 24 months of age. This study revealed no evidence that the 6-month measures of social orienting and face processing were associated with ASD symptoms as 24 months. The symptom index included the M-CHAT (see Chapter 3), which includes multiple joint attention items as measures of ASD symptoms.

In interpreting this finding, the research group noted that the internal consistency across the measures of social orienting and face processing was quite low, suggesting the presence of significant measurement error with respect to the latent construct of social orienting at 6 months. However, face processing—specifically, attention to mouths (but not eyes) at 6 months—was associated with more advanced language development at 18–24 months. Thus this study provided evidence of an association between attention to a component of face processing and language development. The component of face processing, however, was not of a kind (i.e., attention to eyes) that would theoretically be most directly linked to joint attention and its relations to language development.

A third elegant study provided perhaps the more direct test of the possibility that social orienting or face processing could explain joint attention relations with language development in children with ASD (Dawson et al., 2004). This study used mediation statistical analysis to investigate language development in 72 children ages 3–4 years with ASD; 33 age- and IQ-matched children with IDD but not ASD; and 39 children ages 12–46 months with typical development who were matched with the other two groups for mental age. The study examined three possible predictors of autism spectrum language development. A social orienting measure assessed children's tendency to orient and attend to social versus nonsocial stimuli. Joint attention was also assessed, via the ESCS and the RJA and IJA measures from the ADOS. Finally, a combined face-processing and empathy measure, *attention to distress*, was included. This measure assessed children's tendency to look to a tester and react with facial and vocal affective expressions of concern after the tester pretended to hurt her finger while playing with a toy.

The results indicated that the children with ASD performed more poorly than the controls on all three dimensions of social attention. Dawson et al. (2004) also reported that the multiple measures of joint attention, social orienting, and attention to distress all displayed significant levels of internal consistency, so that the three sets of measures formed three unique social attention factors or dimensions. These factors were intercorrelated, supporting the assumption that they shared a set of processes to some extent, and three dimensions were differences in language development in the sample with ASD. However, the mediation analysis revealed something very important: The relations of the Social Orienting factor and the Attention to Distress factor with language were completely explained by their associations with the Joint Attention factor (see Figure 5.5). In other words, social orienting and response to distress were only related to language through their relations with joint attention.

As I see it, the study by Dawson et al. (2004) epitomizes the differences among joint attention, social orienting, and face processing in the study of ASD. Processes associated with the dimension of joint attention are more directly related to language development and learning from

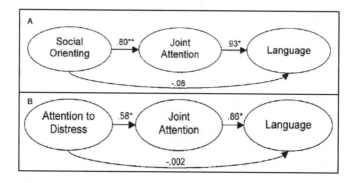

FIGURE 5.5. Illustration of structural equation model analyses indicating that joint attention mediated the association between social orienting and language development (A), as well as the relations between attention to facial/vocal distress and language development (B), in 3- to 4-year-old children with ASD. From Dawson et al. (2004). Copyright 2004 by the American Psychological Association. Reprinted by permission.

other people in ASD. Results of a very different type of research also run counter to the notion of a mediational role of social attention or face processing in joint attention disturbance in ASD. Joint attention appears to be a robust developmental domain that emerges even without typical levels of social experience and/or face processing. For example, children who are congenitally blind are delayed in acquiring joint attention, but ultimately develop joint attention abilities (Bigelow, 2003; Bruce, 2005). Their delays in joint attention and other elements of social development, however, are not as profound as the delays seen in children affected by ASD (Hobson, 2005).

Other informative studies have employed methods to test whether joint attention's role in autism spectrum development is mediated by other variables. These studies have also shown that the relations between joint attention and language, symbolic play, and symptom development in children with autism cannot easily or fully be explained by variance in measures of typical executive functions, imitation, knowledge about others' intentions, or global measures of mental development (e.g., Charman, 2003; Roeyers et al., 1998; Kasari et al., 2007; Naber et al., 2008; Rutherford, Young, Hepburn, & Rogers, 2007; Sigman et al., 1999; Smith et al., 2007; Thurm et al., 2007; Toth et al., 2006).

Accordingly, the evidence reviewed up to this point indicates that joint attention has a very early onset in development. Joint attention differences among infants may be observed no later than 8 months of age, and these contribute significantly to identification of early risk for ASD.

It's difficult to assign disturbances in social orienting or face processing to such primary roles in the differences in ASD. This is because these dimensions develop concurrently, and there is no robust evidence of the onset of differences in social orienting or face processing before joint attention differences in the development of ASD. Finally, there is evidence that joint attention plays a pivotal role in the differences in learning from and with other people that are characteristics of the ASD phenotype. However, there is little evidence that other dimensions of development mediate the relations of joint attention to learning, at least in young children with ASD.

Joint Attention and Cognitive Processing in Infancy

Recall from Chapter 4 that the potential for a deeper understanding of the role of joint attention in ASD, as well as human social-cognitive development, has emerged recently. Several studies in children and adults indicate that the experience of joint attention effects often benefits depth of information processing and encoding. However, this is not simply a joint attention phenomenon of later development. It begins early in infancy and may well be linked to the eye contact effect.

Striano and her colleagues (Striano, Chen, Cleveland, & Bradshaw, 2006; Striano, Reid, & Hoel, 2006) reported a study in which 9-month-olds looked at pictures while their mothers sat with them. In one condition, the mothers made eye contact with their infants (social attention to child) and then also looked at the pictures. In another condition, the mothers also looked at the picture but did not make eye contact with their infants. Infants in the eye contact condition displayed better information processing, measured by short-term picture recognition memory, than the infants who received no eye contact. They also displayed EEG data indicative of associated enhanced neural activation associated with encoding and information processing. It is quite possible that the phenomena described in this study and the one described below reflect the continuation of the eye contact effect observed by Ferroni et al. (2004) and discussed earlier in this chapter.

The observations of Striano and her colleagues have been replicated and extended by Kopp and Lindenberger (2011), who observed that joint attention in 9-month-olds was related to EEG evidence of depth of processing that was associated with long-term as well as short-term picture recognition memory in infancy. Wu and Kirkham (2010) have shown that 8-month-old infants learned the associations between pairings of specific sounds and visual stimuli when cued to attend to the latter by a face and eye gaze rather than by a blinking light. Similar effects have been noted even earlier in development: Kopp and Lindenberger (2011) found that 4-month-olds displayed EEG activity indicators of enhanced long-term (1-week) memory for pictures that were viewed in a condition with a tester who engaged in active joint attention (e.g., alternating gaze between an infant and the pictures) versus a condition where the tester was only looking at the pictures. Finally, a study with older toddlers has provided evidence of widespread frontal–central–parietal neural network activity and better depth of processing during a word-learning task that involved in joint attention, versus a similar task that did not involve joint attention (Hirotani, Stets, Striano, & Friederici, 2009).

These studies raise the distinct possibility that in the course of development, joint attention may serve to transfer the eye contact effect of enhanced information processing of another person in a dyadic context to enhanced information processing about a third object, event, or idea that is a point of common social reference for two or more people. More colloquially, the hypothesis here is that the awareness of joint attention with another person typically is, or becomes, a strong signal to our brains: "Pay attention! There's something important to look at, listen to, and encode information about."

It is clear that children with ASD do not engage in joint attention as readily as many other groups of children do. What is less clear is whether joint attention, when it develops more fully, takes on this type of information-processing signal value for people affected by ASD. If not, a child may appear to display a typical frequency of joint attention behaviors, but still may not reap the typical level of social learning benefits from joint attention. Fortunately, it now appears that the early course of joint attention development can be changed for the better in many young children with ASD. Moreover, experimentally changing the course of joint attention development through early intervention appears to have direct effects on the learning and symptom presentation of such children. Indeed, the spate of new research on targeted treatments for joint attention provides perhaps the strongest evidence of the fundamental causal link between joint attention and social learning in the phenotype of ASD. The evidence for these assertions is detailed in the next chapter.

Chapter 6

Early Intervention, Joint Attention, and ASD

The previous chapters have reviewed evidence indicating that differences in joint attention are fundamental to the diagnosis of ASD. Furthermore, differences in joint attention by 8 months of age appear to predict risk for ASD. The latter observation is consistent with data from several studies indicating that facets of joint attention development are underway in the first 6 months of life. This means that joint attention probably begins to develop concurrently with the onset of face processing and social orienting. Their concurrent onset makes it difficult to ascribe developmental primacy to any one of these three dimensions. Rather, all three may be expressions of common factors in the first 6 months of life. After that, though, they become functionally differentiated. In particular, a distinguishing feature of the dimension of joint attention is the role it plays in learning from and with other people. In short, joint attention is necessary for children to benefit from systematic or incidental instructional opportunities provided by other people.

Research on language development has been reviewed in Chapter 5 to illustrate the role joint attention plays in learning. However, the evidence stemming from that review is entirely correlational in nature. Theory on the development of deictic or referential cognition predicts that joint attention should be related to learning and especially to language development. So when individual differences among children with typical or autism spectrum development have repeatedly been observed to correlate with language acquisition, the studies provide evidence consistent with this theory. However, observations of correlations cannot be interpreted as evidence that joint attention plays a causal role in differences in learning language—or learning anything, for that matter. Evidence for the causal role of joint attention in learning can only come from experimental rather than correlational studies.

The controlled manipulation of a dimension, such as joint attention, is the most powerful means by which to examine the developmental significance of a dimension in the study of ASD (Jones et al., 2014). In clinical research, experimental studies often take the form of intervention trials. The most rigorous type of intervention trial is a *randomized controlled trial* (RCT), where great care is taken to ensure that groups receiving different types of interventions are as comparable as possible.

To better evaluate the legitimacy of the claim that joint attention is a primary dimension of ASD, this chapter scrutinizes intervention studies that target joint attention development. Studies of interventions that more broadly target the social learning disability of ASD are also considered. It is no exaggeration to say that the development of effective early interventions for children with autism has been one of the greatest achievements in the science of ASD and other neurodevelopmental disorders over the last 50 years (e.g., Dawson et al., 2010; Rogers & Dawson, 2010; Kasari et al., 2006; Kasari, Gulsrud, Wong, Kwon, & Locke, 2010; Kasari, Gulsrud, Freeman, Paparella, & Hellemann, 2012; Lovaas, 1987; Smith, Eikeseth, Klevstrand, & Lovaas, 1997; Smith, Groen, & Wynn, 2000; Reichow & Wolery, 2009). The recognition of the efficacy of early intervention for children with ASD parallels our emerging understanding of the role played by impaired social learning in the developmental etiology and phenotype of ASD.

Models of Early Intervention

When research on autism first began, operant theory (Skinner, 1957) was the preeminent influence on thoughts and beliefs about the mechanisms of learning. Accordingly, many if not all types of learning-related changes in behaviors and thinking were thought to be dependent on contingent reinforcement. Children would learn to increase behaviors (e.g., using words) that led to a reward, or would learn to decrease behaviors that led to loss or lack of reward. One fundamental feature of the operant perspective is that it is based on what has been called a "black box" theory of learning. Operant theory explains learning singularly in terms of the causal relations of input (stimulus) with behavior and its outcomes (reinforcement contingencies). It makes no reference to the effects that the internal workings of the mind, such as cognitive mechanisms, may have on human learning or its variations across people.

Because of operant theory's preeminence in the 1950s and 1960s, it is not surprising then that first reports of successful attempts to treat ASD were based on operant, stimulus–response reinforcement learning principles (e.g., Lovaas, 1987). This approach was also consistent with the notion that children with ASD displayed a pervasive lack of responsiveness to others. Operant methods were well designed to increase responsive to external contingencies, or to decrease behaviors that interfered with responsiveness to instruction, in young children with ASD. It was very reasonable, then, to think that external reward-based methods could slowly increase successive approximations of adaptive social and communication responsiveness in children with ASD. This turned out to be true to a significant extent.

The Operant Learning Model and Early Intervention

Operant-based intervention methods are now known collectively as *applied behavior analysis* (ABA) approaches to early intervention. The operant principles of ABA have become more sophisticated with time, and numerous studies have documented their efficacy (see Reichow & Wolery, 2009, for a review). ABA may be described as a rehabilitation approach to intervention for children with ASD. The goal is to rebuild the children's adaptive behaviors, one behavior at a time. The development of each behavior is encouraged by using discrete, adult-directed trials that present rewards to increase specific adaptive task-related behaviors. These methods can be very effective in increasing language development and some adaptive social behaviors in preschool children with autism. They can also reduce the risk for IDD in children with ASD. The work of Cohen, Amarine-Dickens, and Smith (2006) provides an illustration of the effectiveness of ABA intervention with young children with ASD.

Cohen et al. (2006) examined the outcomes of 21 two- to three-year-old children with ASD who received 2 years of ABA discrete-trial intervention in preschools, versus 21 peers with ASD who received community preschool intervention that did not use systematic ABA discrete-trial methods. Although this research was not an RCT, it was designed to examine the effectiveness of ABA when used in a community setting. Earlier studies had demonstrated the efficacy of ABA in highly resourced university-based implementation.

The results indicated that both the ABA and non-ABA treatment groups of preschool children improved in IQ performance. However, at the end of the study, fewer children in the ABA group than in the non-ABA group qualified for a designation of IDD (then defined as IQ > 75; see Figure 6.1, left panel). In addition, the children's parents reported that the children in the ABA group made more gains on the Vineland

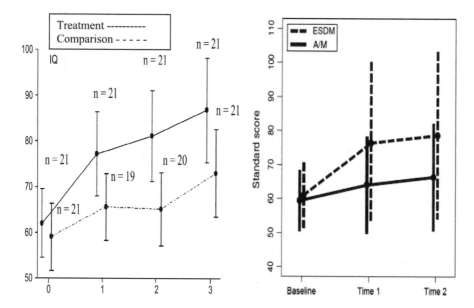

FIGURE 6.1. The effects of early intensive behavioral treatment (EIBT, left panel) and the Early Start Denver Model intervention (ESDM, right panel) on IQ outcomes, compared to those of treatment-as-usual control groups. The study of EIBT was a community-based preschool effectiveness study of 2- to 4-year-olds with ASD. The study of ESDM was a randomized controlled trial (RCT) efficacy study of 2- to 3-year-olds with ASD. A/M, assessment/monitoring. Left panel from Cohen, Amerine-Dickens, and Smith (2006). Copyright 2006 by Wolters Kluwer Health, Inc. Reprinted by permission. Right panel from Dawson et al. (2010). Copyright 2010 by the American Academy of Pediatrics. Reprinted by permission.

Adaptive Behavior Scales than did children in the non-ABA treatment group.

The ABA approach provides a very important and effective foundation for interventions for many children with autism. However, it does have some drawbacks. Because it seeks to rehabilitate the impairments of children one behavior at a time, it is labor-intensive and costly. It often requires 30–50 hours per week of one-to-one implementation with a child, for 1 or more years, to have substantial effects. Moreover, it is primarily designed to improve children's *responses* to adult directives in instructional settings. This is necessary for development and learning. However, recall that ASD is characterized as much by impairments in the ability to initiate behaviors spontaneously and engage in self-organized learning activities as by deficits in the tendency to respond to the directives of others. Therefore, the best practitioners recognize that ABA approaches may need to be augmented by methods designed to increase the children's spontaneous initiation of learning opportunities with other people (Cohen et al., 2006).

In response to this perceived need, *developmental interventions* have been fashioned that attempt to balance the adult-directed, child-responsive, discrete-trial methods of ABA with increased use of child-directed, incidental learning formats. For example, interventionists and/or parents are trained to pay attention to what a child's interests are, such as by following the child's direction of gaze. Interventionists then frequently present *structured* learning opportunities in the context of joint attention to the child's focus of interest. These learning trials are designed to take advantage of the child's manifest interests when the child may be most amenable to learning new information about and object or event. To use incidental learning methods, though, means that an adult does not fully control the focus of learning opportunities or when and how these are presented. Incidental learning trials are included, but are not necessarily the singular focus of developmental approaches to intervention. They are used to promote greater child engagement and self-initiated, active learning. However, more traditional ABA learning trials may also be used.

Developmental Models of Early Intervention

The developmental approach to early intervention in ASD grew out of several lines of research. One of these was the early recognition of Koegel, Dyer, and Bell (1987) of the fundamental importance of using a child's preferred activities and interests as a *pivot* around which engagement, social interaction, and learning could be best be promoted. One of the difficulties in instruction with young children is that they may not be interested in a topic or referent chosen by an adult. The very nature of ASD can make this a frequent impediment to effective instruction or scaffolding. However, if a child is already interested in something in the environment, a *teachable moment* presents itself. Helping interventionist and parents identify and capitalize on teachable moments with young children with ASD is a mainstay of what has become known as *pivotal response intervention* or *pivotal response training* for ASD (Koegel, Carter, & Koegel, 2003).

Child-directed teachable moments are often indicated by the child's focus of visual attention. Following the child's focus allows interventionists to imbed a learning trial more easily within an episode of joint attention. ABA approaches also often use adult-selected external reinforcements to motivate behavior change. Koegel et al. (1987) recognized that it was possible, if not preferable, also to recognize a child's intrinsic (internal) motivation and capitalize on that in the delivery of learning trials.

The developmental approach to ASD intervention was also spurred on by related developmental research. Studies of parents differed in the ways in which they presented learning opportunities to their infants with typical development. Some parents more frequently followed their children's line of regard to establish joint attention, and offered instruction in accordance with child-directed joint attention to and object or event. Other parents often tried to redirect their infants' line of visual regard to establish joint attention to provide instruction. A sequence of seminal studies by Michael Tomasello and his collaborators indicated that infants of parents in the former group tended to acquire vocabulary faster than infants of parents in the latter group (e.g., Tomasello, 1988; Tomasello & Farrar, 1986; Tomasello & Todd, 1983).

These observations on typical development were consistent with, if not a foundation for, the development of pivotal response intervention. Moreover, the same processes occurring in parent–child interaction in typical development appeared to hold true for the development of children with ASD. Siller and Sigman (2002) observed that language development in children with ASD is predicted not only by their joint attention ability, but also by the tendency of parents to follow the attention of their children to establish joint attention and deliver instruction related to the children's own activities and interests.

The Early Start Denver Model (ESDM; Rogers & Dawson, 2010) provides an outstanding example of how these and other elements of research can be molded, with considerable clinical acumen and innovation, to produce a contemporary developmental approach to early intervention. Developed by Sally Rogers over many years, the ESDM does not eschew adult-directed behavioral methods, but rather integrates them with plenty of child-directed incidental learning opportunities, to create a new hybrid approach to early intervention. This hybrid early form of treatment has also been described under the rubric of *naturalistic behavioral interventions* (Ingersoll & Schreibman, 2006).

A recent study of the ESDM shows just how effective this hybrid approach can be. Dawson et al. (2010) randomly assigned 48 young children (ages 18–36 months) to either a group that received an ESDM intervention or a group that received comprehensive assessment, referral to community intervention, and monitoring (the assessment/monitoring or A/M group). The ESDM group received about 15 hours of therapist-delivered intervention per week, and parents reported spending another 16 hours per week using ESDM strategies with their children, for an average total of 31 hours. The A/M group received an average of 18 hours a week of individual and group community-based intervention.

The ESDM treatment resulted in an increase in cognitive IQ performance over the 2 years of the study that was greater than the increase for the A/M group, and comparable to the ABA treatment effects observed by Cohen et al. (2006) (see Figure 6.1, right panel). Thus evidence indicates that both the ESDM and ABA approaches can have a very significant impact on reducing risk for IDD in samples of young children with ASD. Both interventions also led to significant and comparable increases in parents' reports of the social and/or communication behaviors of their children. However, neither the ABA nor the ESDM intervention led to observations of reduced observations of *social symptoms* on standardized diagnostic assessments used with the children with ASD in these studies. Nevertheless, a recent study raised the prospect that ESDM early intervention may lead to positive neurodevelopmental changes in face processing among young children with ASD.

Dawson, Jones, et al. (2012) have reported EEG data on cortical activation to face versus object pictures in 15 of the 24 children who received the ESDM (63%) and 14 of the 24 children in the A/M condition (58%) in the Dawson et al. (2010) study. Loss of children from the samples was primarily due to some children's inability to comply with the EEG procedure, or to excessive movement, which degrades the clarity of EEG data (Dawson, Jones, et al., 2012, p. 1153).

The results of the study indicated that the group of children who received ESDM displayed a more typical pattern of cortical activation (i.e., greater activation to pictures of faces than to pictures of objects) than was observed in the A/M treatment control group. This pattern of cortical activation was thought to correspond to greater attention and cognitive processing of the face pictures in the ESDM group. Seventy-one percent (12 of 17) children in a typical control sample displayed this EEG pattern of cortical activation to faces versus objects, and 11 of 15 children in the ESDM group (73%) displayed this pattern. Alternatively, only 5 of 14 children (36%) in the A/M group displayed this pattern of cortical activation to faces or pictures.

This study, and others (Voos et al., 2013; Vaughan Van Hecke, Stevens, Carson, Karst, et al., 2013), are very important because they provide evidence that behavior-focused interventions, not just medical intervention, have the power to affect the course of neural development in children with ASD. This is consistent with the tenets of a dynamic systems theory approach to human development, which emphasizes that engaging in behavior over time influences nervous system structure and function (Fausto-Sterling et al., 2012b; Spreng & Grady, 2010). However, not unexpectedly for the first study of its kind, the Dawson, Jones, et al. (2012) study has limitations that are important to keep in mind.

Dawson, Jones, et al. (2012) acknowledged that a central limitation of the study was that sample selection may have affected the results and their interpretation. Only 60% of the children in the ESDM and A/M treatment groups participated in the EEG paradigm. This subset of children with ASD had significantly higher verbal IQs and lower ADOS Social Affect scores prior to intervention than did those children with ASD who could not sit for the EEG procedure (Dawson, Jones, et al., 2012, p. 1152). So the results may be limited to children who were brighter and less symptomatic when they began ESDM treatment.

The children receiving ESDM treatment were also trained in face recognition during the intervention with individualized booklets of color photographs of the faces of four *familiar* people, such as a child's mother, father, sibling, and therapist (Dawson, Jones, et al., 2012, p. 1152). Whether or not the face recognition training trials are a standard part of the ESDM was not clear. Nevertheless, the inclusion of specific face-processing training trials makes it difficult to know whether the results of the study reflected general ESDM effects, or specific effects of the face recognition training protocol. In addition, it might have been useful to include training on unfamiliar as well as familiar faces. This is because research suggests that the processing of familiar faces is more likely to elicit activation of "typical" face-processing neural networks among children with ASD than is the processing of unfamiliar faces (Pierce & Redcay, 2008).

Perhaps more importantly, there is little evidence to link changes in face processing to changes in early learning, language, and cognitive development in young children with ASD. It is not yet clear, then, that an EEG measure of face processing is an optimal biomarker of behavioral intervention effects in research on ASD. Consistent with these observations, Dawson, Jones, et al. (2012) reported that no significant correlations among the event-related potential latency or EEG spectral power indicators, and measurements of autism symptoms, IQ, language, and adaptive behavior development, were observed in this study (p. 1156). It was the case, however, that higher cortical activation to faces than to objects was associated with parental reports of social communication development. Therefore, face processing may be associated with some effects on sociability or social engagement, which could have had an impact on learning in the subsequent development of the children with ASD who participated in this study.

Beyond face-processing measures, it will be useful to consider other aspects of behavioral development and neurodevelopment that have theoretical and empirical links to early learning and language development in future research on intervention biomarkers. One alternative approach is to examine biomarkers of the development mechanisms that research suggests are most closely tied to learning and intervention response in children with ASD, such as the biomarkers of joint attention (Elison et al., 2013). Of course, that assertion may only be valid with experimental evidence that changes in joint attention may be causally related to changes in learning in children with ASD. Such evidence has begun to be reported in studies of targeted interventions for joint attention development. Just as ABA emerged from theory on the operant nature of learning, targeted interventions for joint attention have emerged from the cognitive revolution, which presented an alternative to the operant theory of learning.

The Cognitive Revolution and Targeted Joint Attention Treatments

Recall that ABA interventions and, to a lesser extent, naturalistic behavioral interventions are based on operant learning theory. These models are steeped in the notion that utilizing or manipulating the links between behaviors and environmental reinforcement in adult- or child-directed learning trials is primary to early intervention. Their focus on the systematic study and manipulation of environmental contingencies in learning trials is both a great strength and a weakness of these approaches. The strength has allowed interventionists to develop systematic and detailed sequences of learning trials (curricula) that both theory and evidence indicate are beneficial in early intervention (Cohen et al., 2006; Rogers & Dawson, 2010). The development of these curriculums also greatly facilitates the transfer of effective intervention methods across research groups, clinics, or community- and home-based intervention milieus.

One drawback, though, may be that implementation of behavioral approaches within a typical curriculum moves interventionists into a very goal-directed role in interaction with young children. Whether in discrete trials or incidental learning/naturalistic learning trials, the interventionists are often responsible for recognizing and/or eliciting critical behaviors from children, and then delivering external rewarding responses contingent on these behaviors. It may be, though, that manipulation of contingencies and delivery of reward are not effective for all important dimensions of human social, cognitive, and communicative development.

Another related potential drawback of behavioral approaches, whether they involve discrete or naturalistic trials, is that they implicitly adopt a "black box" perspective on the mind. Therefore, they do not specifically target the development of cognitive dimensions that are fundamental to learning in human nature. Another way to say this is that few current approaches to early intervention with children are based on the wave of research on human learning that came after the development of operant theory. This wave of research was called the *cognitive revolution* of the 1950s and 1960s (e.g., Miller, 2003).

The cognitive revolution provided an alternative to the operant conceptualization of human learning. The operant model stipulated that human learning could be understood in terms of stimulus–response effects. The cognitive revolution suggested that stimulus–response links could explain some but not all aspects of human learning. Instead, to explain many quintessential elements of *human* learning, such as language learning, it was important to understand the role that the *human mind* played in learning.

One famous example was Noam Chomsky's (1959) argument that children learn language through inherent cognitive mechanisms, not just, or even mainly, in response to external rewards. In place of the operant model, Chomsky suggested that early infant development is typically characterized by the maturation of a cognitive module he referred to as the *language acquisition device*. A *module* refers to a dedicated neural system that develops to support advanced types of learning, such as language learning. Chomsky described a component function of the language acquisition device as *innate generative grammar*, or a facility of the human mind that enables the direct perception of the correct ordering of morphemes and words in any language to which a human infant is exposed.

There were many other important contributions to the cognitive revolution. One involved the recognition of the role that human memory and its limits play in human learning (Miller, 1956). Another was the prescient observation that human learning involves information processing in problem solving that goes beyond reward processing, and that this information processing could be modeled with software in early computers (Newell & Shaw, 1957).

Most relevant to the topic at hand was the publication of a book called *A Study of Thinking*, in which Bruner, Goodnow, and Austin (1956) argued that stimulus–response models of learning could not explain how or why people developed the ability and motivation to share meaning with others. For Bruner and colleagues, and for many other cognitive scientists (e.g., Steels, 2003; Tomasello, 2008), the ability to share meaning (e.g., communicate) is a major outcome of evolution that is common to many animals, from insects to mammals to primates and whales (Cavalli-Sforza & Feldman, 1983). However, it reaches its epitome in human development. Much of Bruner's career was focused on understanding the development of this pivotal aspect of human cognition (Bruner & Sherwood, 1983).

Relative to Chomsky's modular approach to language development, Bruner envisioned that *less modular and more general prelinguistic cognitive foundations* emerge in human development; as he saw it, these are necessary for language learning, but not specific to language development. His search for these prelinguistic cognitive processes that help infants and toddlers crack the linguistic code led him to the idea of shared reference and joint attention. Bruner often referred to joint attention in terms of a *deictic function* (e.g., Bruner, 1975). He borrowed this term from the study of linguistics and grammar, where *the* deictic function serves to specify identity, or spatial or temporal location, from the perspective of one (or more) persons to another person or people. Bruner understood that the development of the deictic function is an essential cognitive dimension of the human mind—one that begins to emerge early and is necessary for the human capacity to share meaning, whether in language or in social cognition.

Caregivers do not need to actively sculpt the development of joint attention in infants through stimulus–response caregiving. However, once joint attention begins to become apparent, caregivers can increasingly capitalize on it to engage more effectively in scaffolding and instruction to advance the socialization, language, and cognitive development of their infants (Bruner, 1995; Bruner & Sherwood, 1983). Moreover, the same inherent constructivist activity that enables joint attention to development continues as infants use joint attention to self-organize their own social information processing to the benefit of learning from other people (Baldwin, 1995; Mundy et al., 2009; Tomasello, Carpenter, Call, et al., 2005).

The idea that caregivers do not need to actively foster the development of joint attention in typical development finds support in the literature on attachment (Mundy & Sigman, 2006). If caregiver responses play a primary role in the initial phases of joint attention, one might expect joint attention to be moderately if not strongly associated with caregiver–child attachment in development. This is because variation in attachment is thought to go along with differences in the quality and consistency of caregiver responses to their infants. However, there is little evidence of this in the research to date. Indeed, initiating joint attention bids may be maintained in the face of a primary caregiver's *unresponsiveness* early in development, in order to decrease developmental vulnerability by maintaining an infant's capacity to elicit positive nurturance from secondary caregivers (Mundy & Sigman, 2006, p. 300).

A recent study supports this assertion. Higher rather than lower levels of initiating joint attention with *an unfamiliar experimenter* in 15-month-olds were associated with insecure-avoidant attachment (Meins et al., 2011). However, insecure-avoidant attachment at 15 months *was* associated with lower levels of initiating joint attention in *mother–child* interactions. Meins et al. concluded that although insecure–avoidant infants presumably experience less frequent or less positive caregiver responsiveness, they may compensate for reduced social contact with their caregivers by initiating more interaction with other social partners. This emphasizes the possibility that IJA development is inherent in the child, rather than primarily a consequence of child–caregiver interaction.

The idea that decreased parental responsiveness to children may have a negative impact on social development, including joint attention, has also been considered in the literature on ASD (e.g., Naber et al., 2007). Recall from Chapter 1 that there is little evidence of syndrome-specific attachment problems in the interactions of caregivers and their children with ASD (Rutgers et al., 2004; Sigman & Mundy, 1989). Equally important, studies directly examining this issue have found no evidence of significant relations between individual differences in the dyadic attachment status of caregivers and their children with ASD, and joint attention development in the children with ASD (Capps, Sigman, & Mundy, 1994; Naber et al., 2007).

If joint attention is a pivotal cognitive function for early learning in children, but it develops from internally motivated, child-based developmental processes, how do we intervene in the joint attention development of children with ASD? The conundrum here is that interventions based on stimulus–response methods may increase external behaviors that look like joint attention, but may not foster the underlying cognitive and motivation foundations children need to share meaning spontaneously with others. Worse, stimulus–response methods may actually be contraindicated as intervention approaches, because they may disturb the naturalistic constructivist engagement that could be necessary to the functional development of this cognitive domain in children and adults! When I left UCLA, I had doubts about the possibility of interventions for IJA. However, because of the deeply insightful methods that have since been developed at UCLA (Kasari et al., 2006, 2008) and elsewhere, it has become clear that targeted approaches to joint attention, including IJA, are possible and effective for children with ASD.

Approaches to Joint Attention Intervention

Much of the literature reviewed up to this point leads to the following proposition: *If* joint attention differences are fundamental to social learning difficulties in ASD, *then* early intervention targeting joint attention may be an important treatment approach to ASD. A consensus is beginning to emerge across countries and disciplines with regard to this logic (e.g., Cheng & Huang, 2012; Patten & Watson, 2011; White et al., 2011). It may not be surprising, then, that there have been many recent experimental tests of methods designed to advance joint attention in children with ASD. Table 6.1 provides a nonexhaustive list of some of the more prominent and relevant research reports. One observation that can be drawn from Table 6.1 is that there have been numerous, albeit, relatively unheralded, RCTs of the efficacy and effectiveness of targeted interventions for joint attention.

The development of targeted intervention methods for joint attention is challenging. It is one thing to design methods to increase the frequency of joint attention behaviors in young children. It is something altogether different to design methods for effectively advancing the intrinsic motivation and cognitive constructivism that enable joint attention to become an enduring, self-organizing, and generalized means of facilitating learning for young children.

Several different approaches to joint attention intervention have been reported. ABA approaches have been used in studies to train children with ASD to display both RJA and IJA behaviors (e.g., Meindl & Cannella-Malone, 2011). Most of these studies have employed single-subject research designs, and many provide evidence of improved RJA behavior. Perhaps not surprisingly, though, their effectiveness with spontaneous IJA is less consistent. In addition, behavioral approaches to targeted joint attention interventions have rarely reported evidence of generalizability of effects over time and context. Moreover, the single-case design studies provide limited information about individual differences in treatment response across a diverse array of children.

With regard to generalizability, though, there are a few noteworthy exceptions in the single-case design intervention literature on joint attention. At least three such studies have reported that behavioral interventions specific to joint attention are associated with collateral advances in language development, imitation, and other social behaviors (Jones, Carr, & Feeley, 2006; Whalen & Schreibman, 2003; Whalen, Schreibmann, & Ingersoll, 2006). This cascade of treatment effects is what one might expect if the intervention allows children to increase their self-organizing use of joint attention in many subsequent learning opportunities. However, alternative explanations for these effects cannot be rejected. In particular, it may be that some form of nonsystematic intervention effects in these studies had direct influence on children's language or imitation development.

Other studies, using pivotal response training, suggest that systematic interaction involving children's favorite objects may provide an effective means to elicit and respond to joint attention bids in children with ASD (e.g., Naoi, Tsuchiya, Yamamoto, & Nakamura, 2008; Vismara & Lyons, 2007). Suggestive evidence that the ESDM may influence joint attention development in very young children has also been provided in a case study (Vismara, Colombi, & Rogers, 2009).

TABLE 6.1. Intervention Studies with Effects on Joint Attention in Children with ASD

Study	Intervention	Design	Participants in experimental treatment group: Number (ages)	Joint attention outcomes
		Small-*n* studies (<15 participants in experimental treatment group)		
Aldred, Green, & Adams (2004)	Developmental communication intervention (Aldred, Phillips, Pollard, & Adams, 2001)	RCT (vs. routine community care control)	14 (2–5 yrs.)	No change in CJA
Baker (2000)	Thematic ritualistic play intervention	MBL by participants	3 (5–6 yrs.)	Increase in CJA
Cheng & Huang (2012)	Joint Attention Skills Learning (virtual reality system/tool)	MBL by participants	3 (9–12 yrs.)	Increase in IJA
Ezell et al. (2012)	Imitation	RCT (vs. contingently responsive play control)	10 (4–6 yrs.)	Increase in IJA and RJA
Field et al. (1997)	Touch therapy	RCT (vs. nontherapeutic touch control)	11 (mean 4 yrs., 6 mos.)	Increase in RJA and IJA
Hwang & Hughes (2000)	Social interactive training: Following child, imitation, natural reinforcement	MBL by participants	3 (2–3 yrs.)	Increase in IJA
Ingersoll & Schreibman (2006)	Reciprocal imitation training	MBL by participants	5 (2–3 yrs.)	Increase in RJA; mixed results for IJA
Ingersoll (2012)	Reciprocal imitation training	RCT (vs. community treatment control)	14 (2–4 yrs.)	Increase in IJA

Study	Intervention	Design	Participants	Outcome
Isaksen & Holth (2009)	Reinforcement, prompting, modeling	MBL by participants	4 (3–5 yrs.)	Increase in IJA and RJA
Jones, Carr, & Feeley (2006)	Pivotal response training (discrete trials)	MBL by behaviors and participants	5 (2–3 yrs.)	Increase in IJA and RJA
Jones & Feeley (2007)	Pivotal response training (discrete trials), parent training	MBL by behaviors and participants	3 (3–4 yrs.)	Increase in IJA and RJA
Jones (2009)	Pivotal response training: Modeling, prompting	MBL by behavior	2 (3–5 yrs.)	Increase in IJA
Klein, MacDonald, Vaillancourt, Ahearn, & Dube (2009)	Reinforcement	MBL by participants	3 (4–6 yrs.)	Increase in RJA
Krstovska-Guerrero & Jones (2013)	Direct instruction in smiling and eye contact, prompting, reinforcement	MBL by participants and behaviors	3 (2–4 yrs.)	Increase in IJA and RJA
Lawton & Kasari (2012)	JASPER (see chapter text; teacher-implemented)	RCT (wait-list control)	9 (3–5 yrs.)	Increase in IJA
MacDuff, Ledo, McClannahan, & Krantz (2007)	Auditory scripts, reinforcement	MBL by participants	3 (3–5 yrs.)	Increase in IJA
Martins & Harris (2006)	Reinforcement	MBL by participants	3 (3–4 yrs.)	Increase in RJA; no change in IJA

(continued)

TABLE 6.1. *[continued]*

Study	Intervention	Design	Participants in experimental treatment group: Number (ages)	Joint attention outcomes
Naoi, Tsuchiya, Yamamoto, & Nakamura (2008)	Joint attention reinforcement, modeling, preferred objects	MBL by participants	3 (5–8 yrs.)	Increase in IJA
Pierce & Schreibman (1995)	Pivotal response training (peer-implemented)	MBL by participants	2 (10 yrs.)	Increase in CJA
Rocha, Schreibman, & Stahmer (2007)	Parent training (discrete trials), pivotal response training	MBL by participants	3 (2–4 yrs.)	Mixed results for IJA and RJA
Rogers et al. (2006)	Early Start Denver Model (ESDM)	RCT (vs. Prompts for Restructuring Oral Muscular Phonetic Targets [PROMPT] control); MBL for participants and behaviors	5 (2–5 yrs.)	Mixed results for IJA and RJA for both interventions
Salt et al. (2002)	Scottish Center for Autism Treatment Programme: Social-developmental naturalistic intervention	Treatment (vs. wait-list control, not randomized)	14 (3–4 yrs.)	Increase in IJA and RJA (collapsed)
Schertz & Odom (2007)	Joint attention mediated learning (JAML) intervention (Schertz & Odom, 2007)	MBL by behaviors	3 (1–2 yrs.)	Mixed results for IJA and RJA

Study	Intervention	Design	N (age)	Outcome
Schertz, Odom, Baggett, & Sideris (2013)	JAML intervention	RCT (vs. community treatment control group)	11 (1–2 yrs.)	Increase in RJA; no change in IJA
Goods, Ishijima, Chang, & Kasari (2013)	JASPER	RCT (vs. community-based intensive applied behavior analysis treatment control)	7 (3–5 yrs.)	No change in IJA
Taylor & Hoch (2008)	Behavioral: Prompting, reinforcement	MBL by participants	3 (3–8 yrs.)	Increase in IJA and RJA
Tsao & Odom (2006)	Sibling-mediated: Stay, Play, Talk	MBL by participants	4 (3–6 yrs.)	Increase in CJA
Vismara & Lyons (2007)	Parent training, pivotal response training, following child's lead	Reversal; MBL by participants and behaviors	3 (2–3 yrs.)	Increase in IJA
Vismara & Rogers (2008)	ESDM (Rogers & Dawson, 2010)	Case study	1 (1 yr.)	Increase in IJA
Whalen & Schreibman (2003)	Pivotal response training (discrete trials)	MBL by participants	5 (4 yrs.)	Increase in RJA; mixed results for IJA
Zercher, Hunt, Schuler, & Webster (2001)	Peer-supported play, modeling	MBL by participants	2 (6 yrs.)	Increase in RJA; mixed results for IJA

(continued)

TABLE 6.1. *(continued)*

Study	Intervention	Design	Participants in experimental treatment group: Number (ages)	Joint attention outcomes
	Large-*n* studies (≥15 participants in experimental treatment group)			
Green et al. (2010)	Preschool Autism Communication Trial (PACT)	RCT (vs. community treatment as usual)	77 (2–4 yrs.)	Increase in CJA
Gulsrud, Kasari, Freeman, & Paparella (2007)	Targeted joint attention intervention (based on Kasari et al., 2006)	RCT (vs. symbolic play intervention control)	17 (2–4 yrs.)	Increase in CJA
Kaale, Smith, & Sponheim (2012)	Targeted joint attention intervention (based on Kasari et al., 2006)	RCT (vs. community preschool program control)	34 (2–5 yrs.)	Increase in IJA
Kasari, Freeman, & Paparella (2006)	Targeted joint attention intervention	RCT (vs. symbolic play intervention vs. control in existing early intervention program)	20 (3–4 yrs.)	Increase in IJA, CJA, and RJA
Kasari, Paparella, Freeman, & Jahromi (2008)	JASPER (6-and 12-month follow-up to sample in Kasari et al., 2006)	RCT (vs. symbolic play intervention vs. control in existing early intervention program)	20 (3–4 yrs.)	Increase in IJA and CJA

Study	Intervention	Design	N (age)	Outcome
Kasari, Gulsrud, Wong, Kwon, & Locke (2010)	Focused joint attention intervention; parent training (based on Kasari et al., 2006)	RCT (vs. wait-list control)	19 (2–3 yrs.)	Increase in RJA; no change in IJA
Landa, Holman, O'Neill, & Stuart (2011)	Interpersonal synchrony intervention	RCT (vs. non-interpersonal-synchrony intervention)	24 (1–2 yrs.)	No change in IJA in either intervention
Wong, Kasari, Freeman, & Paparella (2007)	Behavioral interventions (prompting, social/natural reinforcement, imitation); joint attention intervention	RCT (vs. symbolic play intervention in existing early intervention program)	20 (3–4 yrs.)	Increase in IJA
Yoder & Stone (2006)	Responsive education and prelinguistic milieu teaching (RPMT)	RCT (vs. Picture Exchange Communication System [PECS; Bondy & Frost, 1994] vs. control)	16 (1–3 yrs.)	Increase in IJA in both treatments; children with >10 IJA acts at pretest had greater gains from RPMT; children showing <2 IJA acts at pretest had greater gains from PECS

Note. IJA, initiating joint attention; RJA, responding to joint attention; CJA, coordinated joint attention; RCT, randomized controlled trial; MBL, multiple-baseline design. Studies were included in this table if (1) a behavioral treatment, with or without a specific focus on joint attention, was employed with children with autism, ASD, or pervasive developmental disorder not otherwise specified; and (2) either RJA, IJA, or CJA was assessed before and after the employed treatment. Typical measurement for RJA and IJA included various paradigms, such as gaze-following tasks, individual IJA or RJA scores from the original Autism Diagnostic Observation Schedule (ADOS; Lord, Rutter, DiLavore, & Risi, 1999), or the Early Social Communication Scales (ESCS; Mundy, Delgado, et al., 2003), among others. CJA was typically measured as a proportion of time children were engaged in focused, cooperative, free play with an adult or peer, wherein gaze alternating and eye contact occurred.

Treatments designed to increase interventionists' awareness and responsiveness to joint attention and other nonverbal communication bids have also been developed. Yoder and Stone (2006) reported an RCT of this intervention approach. The intervention successfully increased the tendency of children with ASD to initiate joint attention, but only for those children who displayed some IJA behaviors prior to the intervention. In two related studies, Schertz and Odom (2007; Schertz, Odom, Baggett, & Sideris, 2013) have described an approach called *joint attention mediated learning* (JAML). Based on earlier work (Klein, 2003), JAML provides methods to increase parental responsiveness to their children's RJA and IJA bids, as well as to turn-taking opportunities with their children, and to occasions when the children look to faces. In an RCT, a group of 2- to 4-year-olds who received parent-implemented JAML displayed significant improvement on RJA but not IJA, relative to children in a control comparison intervention.

Another interesting and instructive approach involves imitation-based intervention. Recall that some of the first studies to raise questions about the model of a pervasive lack of responsiveness in autism involved reports that *affected children responded to imitation.* That is, when adults imitated the actions of children with autism, the children soon started to pay more attention to the adults (Dawson & Adams, 1984; Tiegerman & Primavera, 1984)!

Many years later, three studies now suggest that imitating children with ASD may be a valid tool for cultivating joint attention in young children with ASD (Ezell et al., 2012; Ingersoll, 2012; Ingersoll & Lalonde, 2010; Ingersoll & Schreibman, 2006). The report by Ingersoll (2012) is especially illuminating. This study reported an RCT of *reciprocal imitation training* (RIT). RIT involved targeting imitating children's gestures and object play for 1 hour per day, 3 days per week, for 10 weeks. To promote reciprocity, the therapist contingently also imitated each child's verbal and nonverbal behavior, described the child's actions in simplified language, and expanded the child's utterances. To teach imitation, the therapist modeled an action, either with an object or a gesture, once a minute on average.

The sample consisted of 27 children with ASD (ages 2–4), who were randomly assigned to the RIT group or a control intervention group. The results indicated that the RIT group made significantly greater gains than the control sample on IJA (measured with the ESCS), as well as on social-emotional regulation (measured during a cognitive-developmental assessment). Ingersoll (2012) also provided a mediation analysis to examine whether change in children's own imitation ability explained the gains in outcomes in the intervention versus control sample.

The results of the mediation analysis indicated that growth in imitation was associated with intervention effects on social-emotional functioning, or the ability to regulate behavior and attend to task performance on items of a cognitive assessment. Surprisingly, though, growth in imitation ability did *not* mediate the effect of RIT on growth in IJA. To explain this finding, Ingersol raised the post hoc hypothesis that it may have been the impact of RIT on children's *awareness of being imitated* by others that influenced IJA development in this study. She noted that previous observations of the positive impact of adult imitation on the social behavior of children with ASD in older studies (Dawson & Adams, 1984; Tiegerman & Primavera, 1984), as well as more recent efforts (Escalona, Field, Nadel, & Lundy, 2002; Lewy & Dawson, 1992), were consistent with this hypothesis.

Ingersoll's hypothesis is also consistent with joint attention theory (Bates et al., 1975; Bates, 1976; Reddy, 2003), which suggests that methods that increase a child's awareness of being the object of others' social attention may be important components of targeted interventions for joint attention development in ASD. The recent observations of Edwards et al. (2015) noted in Chapter 5 also speak to this aspect of joint attention theory. These authors note that in a sense of when our direction of gaze is followed "another individual has imitated our attentional state" (p. 1). They then went on to present experimental evidence that lower awareness of gaze following by others was related to higher self-reports of autism-related symptoms in typical adults. This awareness of the attention-to-self feature of joint attention theory is central to an innovative approach to targeted joint attention intervention—a program called Joint Attention, Symbolic Play Engagement and Regulation (JASPER), developed by Connie Kasari at UCLA.

The JASPER Intervention

JASPER is a theory- and evidence-based targeted approach to early developmental–behavioral intervention for children with ASD. The development of JASPER began in 1997, with one of the first intervention studies funded in the National Institutes of Health CPEA/STAART/Autism Centers of Excellence (ACE) national network of autism research centers, and research on JASPER has been continuously funded since that time. The efficacy and community effectiveness of JASPER are supported by one of the most substantial and programmatic bodies of evidence available, including multiple RCTs.

JASPER Methods and Theory

JASPER is a targeted treatment rather than a comprehensive intervention, such as ESDM or many ABA approaches. It is not an attempt to advance a child's development across many domains. Rather, it is designed to advance development in two dimensions that will allow children to become more engaged and active in learning with and from others. These dimensions are joint attention and symbolic play. JASPER is a focused, brief intervention approach that can contribute to longer-term, more comprehensive interventions by helping children learn to learn. It is based on the idea that fostering joint attention and especially IJA development in children with ASD will improve their capacity for taking a more constructivist and engaged orientation to sharing information with other people in social learning opportunities across contexts (Kasari et al., 2000; Mundy & Crowson, 1997; Sigman & Kasari, 1995).

Chapter 5's discussion of the eye contact effect and the impact of being the object of other people's attention helps us to understand the methods of JASPER that seem to foster IJA. A fundamental aspect of JASPER is repeatedly presenting children with social interaction contexts designed to increase the likelihood of the children's discovery and enjoyment of being the objects of others' attention. Although this awareness is likely to be fostered in other intervention approaches, the methods of JASPER have been designed to address this target more concertedly, systematically, and consistently in children with ASD. This requires interventionists to adopt a relatively nondirective, supportive style of scaffolding activity around the children's interests and actions. Indeed, this type of scaffolding is prioritized, so that stimulating a child's latent joint engagement capacities is the primary goal. Some interventions may eschew this approach as not sufficiently directed to the goal of helping the child learn *about* something (e.g., language expression or reception, imitation). Other approaches may emphasize attending to children without the use of sufficiently evidence-based methods to cultivate the initiation of joint attention and joint engagement in social learning with others. JASPER, though, has been shown to provide evidence-based methods that increase learning in children in many studies.

Training begins with preparing clinicians, teachers, or parents to continually follow children's attentional focus in JASPER sessions. In these sessions, children have the opportunity to play with a variety of toys matched to their cognitive level. Interventionists follow the children's attention and make their presence known by judiciously imitating the children's play acts. Interventionists also often talk to the children and narrate events as they occur.

In learning to implement JASPER, adults are encouraged to recognize the utility of rearranging and adjusting each child's environment to provide the optimal engagement opportunities when the need arises. However, adults are also sensitized to the difference between optimizing engagement opportunities and *directing or recruiting* a child's attention to an adult-generated task or goal. Instead, the adults learn to watch the interaction with the child carefully, and to present novel opportunities for object play within the context of the child's manifest interest in play. In this way, JASPER therapists present many structured but incidental learning "trials" in an intervention session, without interrupting the child-focused nature of the intervention by recruiting or redirecting the child's attention. For example, adults are shown how to slow the pace of their language to match a child's and to avoid directive language (e.g., commands, demands, and test questions). Alternatively, they comment on objects of interest, imitate actions, model elaborations of actions, and model functional language in a manner that the child can learn from, without redirecting or recruiting the child's attention.

The goal here is to encourage the development of each child's latent capacity for initiation of joint attention, engagement, and a more self-organized, constructivist role in social learning. However, the only way this can develop is through the child's own slow but consistent self-discovery and practice. We assume that this domain of development has significant latent potential in all children with ASD, but that their vulnerabilities obscure this potential for affected children. Therefore, they need many experiences with adults who are attentive and creative with respect to offering stimulating novel activities, but far less directive than in many intervention approaches for children with ASD. The latter can feel counterintuitive at first. It can be very difficult for adults to recognize and pull back from a natural inclination to try to intervene with children by directing them to accomplish goals the adults envision as helpful and educational. So a significant part of JASPER training involves understanding and adopting this seemingly "counterintuitive" approach. In other interventions, children with ASD may experience a lot of time and opportunities with goal-directed learning trials. In learning JASPER, a task for adults is to decrease investment in getting a child to display Behavior *X* or *Y*, while systematically investing effort in a type of interaction designed to encourage the child to share experiences actively with others.

The idea that many children with ASD are ready to advance when provided with enough experience with social contexts that trigger their internal constructivist development of joint attention may seem to belie the idea that joint attention disturbance is central to ASD. However, as first noted in Chapter 1, joint attention differences are not a primary *cause* of autism. It may be useful to think of joint attention as an engine of human social-cognitive development. Autism causes this joint attention engine to stall in its development in affected children. Recall from Chapter 5 that boys may be especially vulnerable to this type of stalled development (Fausto-Sterling et al., 2012b). Without intervention, it becomes a primary dimension of cognitive etiology that impedes subsequent social and communicative development (e.g., Mundy & Crowson, 1997). Joint attention differences moderate the development of children with ASD (e.g., Bono et al., 2004). However, symptomatic impairment and the complete absence of the potential for joint attention are two very different things. Many children with ASD have a significant capacity for joint attention development, and the degree to which joint attention develops is associated with how socially related the children appear to be to other people (e.g., Mundy et al., 1994). The trick is to figure out how to kindle the stalled internal engine of joint attention development in many young children with ASD. Several potentially worthwhile methods for joint attention-based interventions have been developed that may be useful in this regard (e.g., Gutstein, Burgess, & Montfort, 2007; Schertz et al., 2013). To date, though, evidence suggests that the theory and methods of JASPER are best suited to this task.

Within this emphasis on repeatedly exposing children to nondirective interactive sessions, JASPER systematically shows adults how to target joint attention developmental milestones. Modeling and direct teaching of behaviors are employed once children begin to demonstrate increased and consistent joint attention and engagement with adults across session.

Another primary target domain of JASPER is to increase the diversity of children's play skills. Appropriate play acts are modeled; joint attention is facilitated within play routines; and greater diversity in types of play is encouraged. The overall goal is to help the children increase their diversity and flexibility in play and to reach higher levels of play. Although reaching levels of symbolic play (use of objects "as if" they represent something else) is an ultimate goal, functional play (social-conventional use of objects) is also targeted, depending on a child's developmental level.

JASPER scaffolds engagement in the child from being unengaged or solely focused on objects to higher states of joint engagement with others. This is done initially through following the child's attentional lead and mirroring (imitating) the child's behaviors to promote both awareness and acceptance of another person as a partner in joint engagement.

Finally, the JASPER approach stresses the importance of emotion and behavior regulation. Adults are provided with a series of strategies to handle self-stimulatory behaviors that interfere with engagement and learning. Since these are often associated with dysregulation, many of these strategies emphasize the (early) recognition of onset of dysregulation, and provide steps to promote a child's development of the capacity to recover from dysregulation in social interaction. In the initial stages of intervention and/or with developmentally very young children, this requires more adult scaffolding to enable children to experience and practice regulation of their own behaviors within an interaction.

JASPER intervention begins with a series of assessments to measure a child's joint attention, play, and engagement, so that appropriate targets for intervention can be chosen. Next, the adult (teacher, paraprofessional, therapist, or parent) and child meet with a trained professional for a series of sessions. Depending on the context (home, school, clinic), these sessions for learning the JASPER strategies vary from twice a week to 5 days a week. The adult learns to adjust the environmental arrangement, balance modeling with imitation, and expand on language and play routines as needed to promote joint attention and engagement during play.

The decidedly targeted nature of JASPER distinguishes it from many other intervention approaches. Comprehensive ABA or naturalistic behavioral interventions are presented for 20 or more hours a week, for 1 or more years (e.g., Cohen et al., 2006; Dawson et al., 2010). In contrast, JASPER is designed to be presented in brief sessions (20–60 minutes) daily or consistently over a moderate interval (e.g., 5–12 weeks). In one of the initial RCTs of the efficacy of JASPER, for example, Kasari et al. (2006) implemented this intervention for 30 minutes a day over 5–6 weeks with 3- to 4-year-olds with ASD. This characteristic of JASPER allows it to be incorporated as a module to be used in conjunction with other intervention approaches. Indeed, JASPER may be considered a targeted intervention specifically designed to enhance young children's ability to engage with and benefit from learning opportunities presented in the home and more structured comprehensive interventions such as ABA (Kasari et al., 2006).

It is also important to recognize that the focus of JASPER is not the only important target for early intervention with ASD. Far from it: JASPER may be best conceived as a targeted approach to intervention that can be used most optimally in conjunction with more comprehensive approaches. JASPER provides a useful balance to interventions designed with more specific teaching goals in mind, which rely more (though not exclusively) on recruiting and directing child attention. JASPER methods cultivate joint attention in order to help children learn to learn in all social interactions that are vital to their longer-term development and education (Mundy et al., 2009). Of course, theory demands evidence—and evidence in support of JASPER abounds.

Evidence for Efficacy and Effectiveness

Kasari and her colleagues at UCLA have worked to specify the effectiveness of different components of JASPER. For example, recall that JASPER focuses on developing both joint attention and symbolic play skills. In one of the initial JASPER studies, Kasari et al. (2006) conducted an RCT to examine the separate effects of joint attention and play intervention methods on 2- to 4-year-olds with ASD. All children in this study were receiving 20 hours or more of ABA intervention. Children were randomly assigned to intervention groups to determine whether the addition of 30 hours of joint attention or symbolic play intervention in a 5- to 6-week period would improve outcomes above and beyond the effects of ABA alone.

The results of this study showed that joint attention methods led to developmental advances in RJA and IJA on the ESCS, and in observations of children's IJA in interaction with their parents. The symbolic play methods also led to very clear increases in the frequency and diversity of play acts displayed by children with adult testers and parents. Moreover, the symbolic play methods also led to advances in showing on the ESCS, and in IJA alternating looking with caregivers. Hence both the joint attention methods *and* the symbolic play methods of JASPER benefited joint attention development. The joint attention condition, though, did not lead to advances in symbolic play (Kasari et al., 2006).

Kasari et al. (2008) subsequently reported follow-up outcome data on the efficacy of these JASPER treatment components for improving language learning. Expressive and receptive language development in children receiving joint attention, symbolic play, or control (ABA-only) treatment were compared at four time points: pre- and postintervention, and 6 and 12 months after intervention. The results of this study revealed three main observations.

First, both the joint attention and symbolic play intervention groups displayed greater growth on IJA across the four assessment intervals than did the ABA-alone control group. A similar treatment effect was not observed for RJA growth. Second, all three intervention groups displayed improved language growth across the 6–12 months after intervention. However, the joint attention and symbolic play groups displayed significantly better expressive language development across the four assessments than did the ABA-alone control group (see Figure 6.2, upper panel). This pattern of data is consistent with the idea that the targeted joint attention intervention in JASPER improves the intrinsic social learning ability of children with ASD, and that this adds to or boosts the benefits they receive from other, more comprehensive interventions.

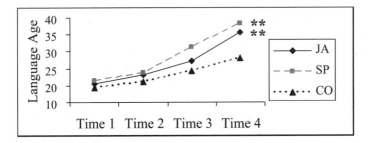

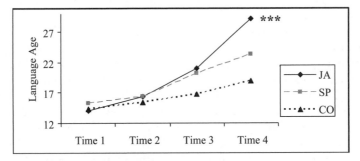

FIGURE 6.2. The results of an RCT efficacy study of joint attention and symbolic play targeted interventions for children with ASD. Children randomly assigned to all groups received the same applied behavior analysis (ABA)-based early intervention for 30 hours per week. Children in the control (CO) group received only the ABA treatment, but children in the joint attention (JA) group received targeted joint attention intervention plus ABA treatment and children in the symbolic play (SP) group received targeted symbolic play intervention plus ABA treatment. The upper panel illustrates the significant boost to language development exhibited by children in the JA and SP groups. The bottom panel illustrates the relatively stronger effects of the JA intervention on language development in a comparison of the subset of children who displayed lower expressive language achievement at the beginning of the interventions. From Kasari, Paparella, Freeman, and Jahromi (2008). Copyright 2008 by the American Psychological Association. Reprinted by permission.

The third observation was that the joint attention component of JASPER was more effective than the symbolic play component for the subgroup of children who began the intervention with the lowest levels of language development (see Figure 6.2, lower panel). This is consistent with theory (e.g., Baldwin, 1995) and previous observations from longitudinal studies that joint attention development may be an especially important "bootstrap" for early language development in children with ASD (Toth et al., 2006; Van der Paelt et al., 2014).

Kasari et al. (2012) then went on to gather rare long-term follow-up data at ages 8–10 years from 40 of the children who had experienced the preschool JASPER joint attention and symbolic play interventions or ABA alone. Thirty-two of these children had displayed spoken language at outcome, and the other 8 children had had minimally verbal outcomes. The elementary school-age children who had received preschool JASPER joint attention treatment scored 12.5 points higher than the ABA-only controls on a standardized language measure. The JASPER symbolic play treatment group scored an average of 10.6 points higher than the ABA-only controls on the language measure. The difference between the two JASPER treatment groups was not significant.

Gulsrud, Hellemann, Freeman, and Kasari (2014) have subsequently reported a growth curve analysis of the same data set described in Kasari et al. (2012). This report was designed to examine the expectations that (1) JASPER has a direct impact on the growth of joint attention in children, and (2) the growth of joint attention in children with ASD has a direct impact on their long-term developmental and/or symptom outcomes. Individual differences in rate of growth in IJA was measured across five points: pretreatment, immediate posttreatment, 6 months posttreatment, 12 months posttreatment, and 5 years posttreatment.

The results of this study revealed that children in the group that had received the joint attention component of JASPER displayed greater positive growth in the IJA skills of coordinated joint looking and showing than did children in the ABA-alone control group or the group that had received the symbolic play component of JASPER. The control group and the symbolic play group were not significantly different from each other with respect to the growth trajectories of these two skills.

Most importantly, the data indicated that different patterns of children's IJA growth were associated with different symptom intensities on the original ADOS 5 years after treatment. One group of 8 children received subclinical ADOS scores at 5 years posttreatment. They displayed greater growth in coordinated joint looking than the 27 children who continued to meet criteria for autism, as well as 5 children who met criteria for ASD. The least symptomatic group also displayed positive growth for showing that was greater than observed for either of the other two groups. Finally, the group with autism symptoms displayed a greater decline in IJA pointing across time than did the group with ASD, but not the least symptomatic group.

This study provided some of the first longitudinal evidence that IJA intervention and growth may be associated with declines in categorical ratings of the intensity of autism symptoms in school-age children. One might expect joint attention intervention to have an impact on symptom presentation, simply because joint attention measurements play such a central role in ASD diagnostic assessments (see Chapter 3). However, 27 of the children in this study were assessed with Module 3 of the ADOS, which does not include a Joint Attention factor.

The analyses of the growth trajectory data in Gulsrud et al. (2014) also documented that more positive growth in expressive language development was apparent in the data for children who received either the joint attention or symbolic play component of JASPER and the ABA intervention, compared to children who received ABA alone. Moreover, this report provided evidence that IJA pointing behavior was causally related to language growth outcomes in this study.

Together, these studies of JASPER provide relatively detailed appraisals of the short- and long-term efficacy of this early intervention approach. In addition to efficacy research, the UCLA group has also engaged in several avenues of research to explore the effectiveness of JASPER when implemented in homes by caregivers, and in preschools by teachers. Finally, Kasari and her colleagues have begun to examine the effectiveness of JASPER for meeting the very substantial intervention needs of older, minimally verbal, school-age children with ASD.

Preschool Intervention Effectiveness

One way to make effective treatments available to more children with ASD is to implement them in public preschools. The need for this type of effectiveness research with JASPER is clear. Recent observations of 27 children with autism and 28 children with other forms of developmental delay in community-based preschools indicated that the children with ASD spent more time unengaged in structured activity and less time engaged in joint attention and symbolic play. Moreover, lacking training, teachers rarely focused on teaching joint attention or symbolic play (Wong & Kasari, 2012).

To begin to examine teacher training and the teacher-implemented JASPER intervention, Lawton and Kasari (2012) reported a small study of 16 children with ASD. The children and their primary preschool teachers were randomly assigned to 6 weeks of JASPER plus the regular preschool curriculum, or a control condition of only the regular curriculum. At the end of the intervention, the children receiving JASPER intervention used more joint attention behaviors in their classrooms than did the children receiving the control condition. The children receiving JASPER also spent more time engaged with an unfamiliar tester in a play interaction than did the control children.

An independent research group has replicated these observations in a larger study of 61 preschool children in Norway (Kaale, Smith, & Sponheim, 2012). In this study, 34 children with ASD between the ages of

29 and 60 months were randomly assigned to 8 weeks of joint attention intervention using JASPER strategies and methods. Twenty-seven children with ASD were randomly assigned to a condition involving a regular preschool curriculum only. At the end of the intervention, children in the JASPER treatment group engaged in more joint attention with teachers than did children in the control group. In addition, some evidence of treatment generalization was observed: Children in the JASPER treatment group engaged in significantly longer bouts of joint attention with their caregivers, compared to children in the control condition. A second report from this group indicates that these intervention effects on joint attention were maintained and became more generalized over a 12-month follow-up period (Kaale, Fagerland, Martinsen, & Smith, 2014).

These studies suggest that JASPER methods can be implemented by preschool teachers, and that this implementation has the expected effects of improving the joint attention and joint engagement of young children with ASD. These studies do not address the question of whether or not teacher-implemented JASPER improves longer-term social, cognitive, and communicative outcomes for preschool children with ASD. However, they do establish the feasibility of examining this critical hypothesis in future research.

Parent Intervention Effectiveness

Teacher implementation is vital to the effective dissemination and community implementation of an effective intervention approach like JASPER. Equally important, though, is the implementation of parent-mediated JASPER intervention for toddlers. The potential for parent-mediated joint attention intervention was made clear by the observation that parental following of child attention is correlated with better language development in children with ASD. Siller and Sigman (2008) reported a longitudinal study of growth in the language abilities of 28 children with ASD (ages 30–60 months). Children's responsiveness to caregivers' bids for joint attention (i.e., RJA) predicted language development. In addition, Siller and Sigman reported that the *relative* frequency with which parents were aware of and responsive to their children's attention and activities was a unique predictor of language development in this sample of children. Subsequently, Bottema-Beutel, Yoder, Hochman, and Watson (2014) have replicated and extended this observation.

It is important to be clear about the meaning of these observations. They do not mean that recruiting and directing children's attention is bad, or that parents should minimize this type of behavior in interacting with their children with ASD. If so, the children's responsiveness to parent or adult attention directing (RJA) would be unlikely to show a positive association with language development. What these results do suggest, though, is that balance is needed. Directing the attention of a child with ASD is important. However, it is important to balance this with ample opportunities for the child to lead and initiate the topic of interaction. JASPER is a systematic method for enabling parents and teachers to achieve this balance.

Another informative study was conducted by Patterson, Elder, Gulsrud, and Kasari (2014). This study observed 85 toddlers in interaction with their caregivers. Parents' interactive style was characterized as relatively responsive or directive. The degree to which parent–child joint engagement episodes were initiated by parents or children was also rated. Observations from this study indicated that the children initiated more joint engagement with parents who displayed a *relatively* responsive rather than a *relatively* directive style. In addition, the tendency of children to initiate joint engagement more frequently was observed to be associated with their tendency to initiate joint attention bids, display positive affect, and imitate during the interactions. Of course, these results do not establish a causal link between parent and child behavior. At a minimum, though, these data are consistent with the hypothesis that JASPER may provide an effective parent-mediated approach to targeted intervention for improving joint attention and joint engagement in young children with ASD.

To test this hypothesis more directly, Kasari, Gulsrud, Hellemann, and Berry (2015) worked with 86 children with ASD (ages 30–36 months) and their parents. All the children participated in an outpatient early intervention (OEI) program for 10 weeks, 30 hours a week. This OEI provided children with speech, occupational, and behavioral therapy sessions each day. Forty-three children and their caregivers were also randomly assigned to receive parent training and implementation of JASPER. This involved 10 weeks of two 30-minute sessions per week of actively coaching parents in JASPER strategies during interactions with their children. The other 43 parent–child dyads were assigned to a stress reduction intervention, which presented parents with information about early child development and autism, as well as strategies for managing parent stress.

The results indicated that parents were able to learn the JASPER methods, and that their use had positive impacts children that were observed in the home and by teachers in OEI classrooms. Across the 10-week intervention interval, children's duration of joint engagement in interactions with parents more than doubled in the JASPER intervention group, but did not change in the control group. This advantage for the JASPER group was again observed in an assessment 6 months after the end of the intervention. In addition, the amount of time that children in the JASPER group spent jointly engaged with a play partner in the OEI classroom increased significantly across the 10-week intervention protocol (from 5.7 minutes to 8.9 minutes within repeated 15-minute observations). The control sample did not display evidence of a comparable increase (from 6.9 to 7.4 minutes). This brief intervention, however, did not lead to evidence for treatment effects on children's IJA, play, language, or cognitive development.

More evidence of the impact of parent-mediated JASPER on child joint attention and play skills was reported in a second RCT (Kasari, Lawton, et al., 2014). This was a multisite study involving five universities across the country and 112 toddlers. To begin to determine how applicable JASPER methods would be to all families, this study included 60% or more low-income families in all treatment groups.

The caregivers and children were randomly assigned to either a caregiver-mediated JASPER (CMJ) group or a caregiver education intervention (CEI) group. The former condition involved two 1-hour sessions of JASPER coaching in the homes of parents with their children each week for 12 weeks. The CEI control condition involved two 1-hour small-group meetings for parents, conducted in homes, community centers, or schools each week for 12 weeks. These meetings focused on providing parents with information about ways to teach communication skills to their children, behavior management methods, and the value of developing routines with their children. Children were not present at these sessions, so direct coaching and modeling of intervention strategies were not provided.

Children of parents in both types of interventions displayed a pre–post improvement in the total duration of joint engagement in interaction with caregivers. However, the children in the CMJ group displayed a significantly stronger 47% increase in duration of joint engagement during caregiver interactions, compared to a 3% increase in the CEI control group. The advantage for the children in the CMJ group was maintained through a 3-month follow-up. The children in the CMJ group also displayed a significantly greater improvement on IJA in interactions with an unfamiliar tester, which was also maintained through the 3-month follow-up. This suggests that the parent-mediated JASPER not only affected joint engagement in interaction with the caregivers, but also generalized to improve the children with ASD's capacity of the children with ASD for spontaneous IJA. In addition, the JASPER intervention improved the symbolic play skills of children with ASD, but only if the children displayed measurable amounts of symbolic play at the beginning of treatment. Significantly, parents in the two intervention conditions did not report differences in how frequently they used strategies with their children that they learned in either the CMJ or CEI group.

As the research with teachers has done for implementation of JASPER in preschools, these studies provide evidence strongly suggesting that parent-implemented JASPER may be a feasible and efficacious component of treatment plans for families of young children with ASD. Additional information is now needed on the impact of parent-implemented JASPER on language, social, and cognitive development later in childhood. The current data suggest it is reasonable to expect that this type of research will yield evidence of the efficacy of JASPER as a means to facilitate learning in young children with ASD. However, only time will tell if this important possibility is true.

JASPER and Minimally Verbal School-Age Children

One of the more edifying aspects of the programmatic nature of research on JASPER research program is the research group's willingness to challenge the efficacy of the approach by testing it in community settings with a diverse range of samples. A prime example of this is the recent report of the application of JASPER to improving the language development of school-age children with ASD who exhibit minimal verbal skills (Kasari, Kaiser, et al., 2014).

This report has been described as "a landmark paper [that] should be required reading for all clinicians and educators who work with minimally verbal children with ASD" (Tager-Flusberg, 2014, p. 613). Approximately 30% of children with ASD have not developed consistent sentence-level language use by kindergarten, even though some of these children have graduated from high-quality preschool intervention programs. The lack of optimal response to early intervention, at least with respect to language development, has serious consequences for these children and their families. Yet little evidence is available concerning the intervention methods that can meet the urgent needs of these children once they enter elementary education settings; hence the landmark nature of the Kasari, Kaiser, et al. (2014) study.

The earlier report by Kasari et al. (2008) that the joint attention component of JASPER was especially effective for young children with ASD and lower language attainment sets the stage for research applications with minimally verbal children. So does a recent report of a study of preschool children with ASD who were slower than their peers with ASD in developing language (Paul, Campbell, Gilbert, & Tsiouri, 2013). This intervention team randomly assigned 22 minimally verbal children with ASD (ages 3–6 years) to a 12-week course of either a behavioral or a naturalistic intervention designed to target their slow language development. Paul et al. (2013) reported that that both of these interventions were effective, but only with about 50% of the children. However, they also reported that individual differences in joint attention significantly moderated the responsiveness of these children to the targeted language interventions.

This observation is consistent with the possibility that targeted intervention for joint attention may improve language intervention responsiveness in minimally verbal children with ASD.

Kasari, Kaiser, et al. (2014) examined this possibility in a very sophisticated multisite RCT of JASPER and other interventions for 61 minimally verbal children with ASD (ages 5–8 years). Children were randomly assigned to two intervention groups in which JASPER was combined with one or two other types of intervention. In one condition, JASPER was combined with enhanced milieu teaching (EMT; Kaiser, Hancock, & Nietfeld, 2000). EMT is a naturalistic behavioral intervention that uses adult responsiveness, modeling, and prompting to promote children's use of functional language. The second group of children received the JASPER + EMT intervention, as well as training in the use of a speech-generating device (SGD). An SGD allows children to select an icon or symbol on a computer tablet to produce voiced words for functional communication with other people.

Children received two intervention sessions a week for 3 months. Their progress was monitored with a sophisticated design of repeated measurements at baseline and at Weeks 12, 24, and 36. Based on their response to treatment by Week 12, they either continued on their initial treatment protocol, received an increased intensity of treatment (increased number of sessions), or began to receive training in the use of an SGD. This type of "smart" intervention design anticipates that there will be significant individual differences in responsiveness to any treatment. It also examines how a response-to-intervention protocol implemented in the course of a study can optimize the power of the treatment for more, if not all, of the children involved (Kasari, Kaiser, et al., 2014).

The results of this study indicated that spoken communication improved in both groups, but that the combination of JASPER + EMT + SGD had significantly stronger positive effects on children's social-communicative utterances, use of different word roots, and total number of comments at the end of treatment and at the 3-month follow-up assessment. Equally important was the observation that adding the SGD component was singularly more useful than increasing the intensity of intervention in facilitating language development for children who were at the low end of treatment responsiveness at the 12-week assessment point.

This study indicates that it is possible to facilitate functional language development among older children with ASD who have minimal functional speech. Of course, it is not clear from this first study which components of the intervention contributed to these results. In particular, this study cannot be used to claim that JASPER or intervention for joint attention per se contributed to the language gains displayed by children in this study. However, several observations suggest that this was probably the case.

First, previous research on therapies for minimally verbal children, including the use of SGD or lower-tech picture boards to augment communication, has indicated improvements in the children's use of speech to request. However, these previous studies have rarely if ever reported significant improvement in varied speech acts and social-communicative functions, *including commenting,* as the Kasari, Kaiser, et al. (2014) study did. Recall that joint attention, especially IJA, serves a nonverbal commenting communicative function. Therefore, it seems plausible, if not likely, that JASPER had an impact on the breadth of communicative speech functions facilitated in this intervention study.

Previous research has also indicated that differences in joint attention mediate response to interventions in older preschool children with ASD (Paul et al., 2013; Yoder & Stone, 2006). These findings are also consistent with the hypothesis that JASPER was an active component of the intervention effects observed in the Kasari, Kaiser, et al. (2014) study. Further research is clearly needed, but this study provides hopeful and helpful evidence that targeted intervention for joint attention can be combined with other methods to improve effective educational practices for minimally verbal school-age children with ASD (Kasari, Kaiser, et al., 2014; Tager-Flusberg, 2014).

Joint Attention and Intervention for Older Verbal Children

Joint attention theory suggests that perturbations of joint attention may continue to play a role in ASD throughout childhood and adulthood, regardless of an affected individual's level of language. If so, then interventions directed to ameliorate these perturbations may be of use in intervention batteries for older people with ASD. However, a stumbling block here is that, beyond measures used in imaging studies (see Chapter 7), we have developed few measures of joint attention for older individuals. Therefore, we know relatively little about the strengths and weaknesses of joint attention in older individuals, and we certainly have few measures that could inform intervention development. To begin to address what may be a significant gap in the field, the following nonexhaustive description of new avenues of approach to joint attention assessment has been developed. Not only may a new generation of measures be useful in broadening the scope of joint attention intervention research; there may be revealing applications for these measures in future research on the neuroscience, as well as the genetic and genomic science, of joint attention. These areas are addressed in the final two chapters of this book.

Latency Measures in Assessment and Intervention

As noted earlier, the significant variations in the patterns of neural network activation associated with IJA and RJA in adults with and without ASD indicate that meaningful differences in joint attention can be measured across the lifespan (e.g., Mizuno et al., 2011; Pelphrey et al., 2005; Redcay, Dodell-Feder, et al., 2013). However, the clinical utility of imaging-based measures is not yet clear. Moreover, some of these studies indicate that the differences in the neural underpinnings of joint attention may coexist with evidence of intact behavioral performance on joint attention tasks in adults with ASD (e.g., Redcay, Dodell-Feder, et al., 2013). The lack of observed differences in basic competencies in joint attention behavior is a problem for the inclusion of this dimension in the clinical measurement of the phenotype (Lord & Jones, 2012).

However, recall that theory says that joint attention involves a social-cognitive control system (see Chapter 4), and that differences in its development may be measured in terms of latency of response to joint attention tasks (e.g., Gredebäck et al., 2010; Vaughan Van Hecke et al., 2012). This is a very important measurement consideration with respect to older individuals. A 16-year-old may be able to demonstrate the capacity for IJA or RJA. However, unless the teen can also employ that ability smoothly and efficiently in social situations, the joint attention dimension may not have reached an age appropriate level of adaptive development. For example, by 10 years of age, the capacity to manage rapid shifts with other people in the consensus point of reference in social learning and affiliative communication interactions is likely to be part of age-appropriate joint attention development. Hence measures that are sensitive to differences in latency as well as accuracy in real-life or virtual social attention paradigms (e.g., Jarrold et al., 2013) may be increasingly useful in assessing the development of this dimension after the preschool period. Measurement of differences in fluidity and efficiency of use of joint attention in social interactions may also help us better visualize important targets for social skills intervention for children and adults with ASD.

Information-Processing Measures and Intervention Assessment

When we conceptualize the measurement of joint attention/joint engagement in older children, especially in the context of intervention, it will

be also useful to recall that joint attention involves information processing (see Chapters 1 and 5). One important but only recently recognized
aspect of social cognition involves the positive effects of eye contact and
joint attention on human information processing (e.g., Bayliss et al., 2013;
Böckler et al., 2011; Boothby et al., 2014; Frischen & Tipper, 2004; Kim &
Mundy, 2012; Kopp & Lindenberger, 2011; Linderman et al., 2011). With
this aspect in mind, we can anticipate that children and adults affected by
ASD may display basic joint attention behaviors, but may not display the
typical levels of benefit to information processing in the context of joint
attention (Mundy et al., 2009, 2010; Mundy, Kim, et al. 2015). A recent
eye-tracking study provides an excellent example of research with children with ASD that is related to this idea.

This study examined RJA in 3-year-old children with ASD and comparison groups of children with other developmental disabilities or typical development (Falck-Ytter, Thorup, & Bölte, 2014). The results of this
study indicated that the children with ASD did not differ from the control
groups in following the gaze of a social partner to objects. However, analyses of the duration of fixation times to the objects showed that these times
were significantly shorter for the group with ASD than for the controls.
The observation prompted Falck-Ytter et al. (2014) to interpret this pattern of results as perhaps indicating that the group with ASD was more
weakly engaged in processing information about the objects in response
to RJA bids than were other groups of children. The authors went so far
as to suggest that attenuated processing bias in RJA may negatively affect
learning opportunities in ASD. I agree that this hypothesis not only is
valid, but should motivate one line of research: to improve assessment of
joint attention in older children and measurement of factors related to
variability in responsiveness to intervention among children with ASD
(Mundy, Kim, et al., 2015).

Social Engagement Measures of Joint Attention and Intervention

It may be that the engagement facet of joint attention/joint engagement
lends itself to one of the more effective approaches to measurement of
this dimension in the phenotype of ASD from infancy to adulthood.
There are varied definitions of *social engagement*, but these typically
emphasize three characteristics of a capacity for a prosocial behavior
style: (1) the capacity to monitor, relate, and integrate the behavior of self
and others; (2) the ability to regulate attention and emotional reactivity
in the dynamic flow of social interaction effectively enough to maintain
these interactions; and (3) the tendency to express positive emotions and

to be friendly and agreeable with peers as well as adults (Eisenberg et al., 1997; Masten & Coatsworth, 1998; Mundy & Acra, 2006; Rothbart & Bates, 1998).

Longitudinal studies of typically developing children as well as children with ASD indicate that early joint attention development is a predictor of difference in the childhood development of prosocial engagement (Sheinkopf et al., 2004; Vaughan Van Hecke et al., 2007; Sigman et al., 1999). A very recent study has provided further evidence of this linkage: Joint attention at age 3 years has been observed to significantly predict reports of higher sense of closeness and less conflict in friendships at ages 8–9 years in a group of higher-functioning children with ASD (Freeman, Gulsrud, & Kasari, 2015).

Research and theory (see Chapters 4 and 5) also emphasize that the joint attention/joint engagement dimension is fundamental to children's and adult's capacity to engage in joint action and cooperative behaviors that are critical to collaborative engagement in social problem solving, learning, games, and affiliation. Recall that one example here is *capitalization*, or the reciprocal initiation and response to shared positive work experiences as a means to maintain and deepen a sense of relatedness and intersubjectivity in marital relations (e.g., Gable et al. 2004). Consequently, it should be possible to develop items on both joint attention and cooperative/collaborative behavior to form valid and efficient parent or self-report measures of the lifespan development of joint attention and joint engagement.

Preliminary research provides an example of how this might be done (Mundy, Novotny, et al., 2015). Three categories of behaviors appear to elicit valid and relevant parent report data on joint attention/joint engagement in childhood. One of these categories is a child's tendency to use nonverbal behaviors to share experiences, such as "The child makes eye contact with you when something in the environment interests him or her." Another is joint or cooperative action, such as "The child works cooperatively in groups of more than one other child to achieve a common goal." The third is verbally sharing positive or interesting experiences (i.e., capitalization; Gable et al., 2004), such as "The child shares exciting events with you that happened in school."

To develop a measure of these three categories, we examined many parent and teacher report measures of ASD for use with children and adolescents to identify an item pool. However, we could find few to no measures of symptoms that concertedly reflected these elements of joint attention/joint engagement in any of the prominent measures of ASD in verbal children and adults. So a pool of 65 items was developed de novo. In a preliminary study of 80 higher-functioning 8- to 15-year-old children with ASD, 40 children with ADHD, and 40 children with typical development, 49 items in the 65-item pool constituted a scale with significant internal consistency (Mundy, Novotny, et al., 2015). The total score for this measure displayed a sensitivity of 82% for the identification of children with ASD in this sample, and a specificity of 86% for the identification of children with ADHD and typically developing children. Much work remains to be done on the measure. However, these initial observations are encouraging and suggest that it may be possible to develop a rating scale for childhood social development and joint attention.

Summary and Conclusions

There are many dimensions of the social differences involved in ASD, including but not limited to dyadic social attention, face processing, imitation, and triadic joint attention. All are important. There are likely to be some sources of disturbance that are common in the development of all these dimensions in children with ASD. However, just because dimensions share common processes, this does not mean that the nature and significance of impairments in one dimension can be explained by impairments in another dimension (Happé et al., 2006).

Atypical joint attention development is a unique dimension of ASD—one that the current science suggests begins to develop in the first months of life (see Chapter 5). Its developmental impairment occurs in conjunction with the onset of atypical dyadic social attention and face processing, but its role in autism should not be counted as an expression of either. The distinctiveness of joint attention in ASD is illustrated by its central and uniquely powerful role in the early identification and diagnosis of ASD. Moreover, starting in the second 6 months of life, the singular importance of joint attention is evident in the role it plays in mediating learning and language development in children with ASD. This mediational role in ASD is supported not only by correlational longitudinal research, but also by experimental intervention studies that provide more direct evidence of a causal relation among joint attention, language development, and learning in young children with ASD. Few if any other social dimensions of ASD currently have as much experimental intervention support for their role in mediating learning in affected children. Evidence for the central role of joint attention in the early social phenotype of ASD and in mediating learning suggests that the social phenotype of ASD may be well conceived in terms of both a social learning disability and a social engagement disability.

The nature of the social learning disability axis is not yet well described. However, it likely involves a dynamic developmental transaction among social, motivational, cognitive, neural network, and genomic factors. This chapter, as well as Chapter 5, has begun with a discussion of ideas about several possible social, motivational, and cognitive factors that may be involved in the developmental disturbance and disruption of social learning about the world in children with ASD. The final two chapters of this book elaborate on these ideas. Chapter 7 reviews newer and older theory and research on the neurodevelopment of joint attention in typical and atypical development. Finally, Chapter 8 discusses what we know—or, more precisely, what we need to know—about the genomics of joint attention and social-cognitive development in order to advance out understanding of ASD.

Before I begin those discussions, one last conjecture is in order about research on targeted interventions for joint attention. Numerous authors have recently pointed out that the identification of valid biometrics is vital to the advanced understanding, earlier and more precise identification, and more effective treatment of ASD (Dawson, Jones, et al., 2012; Vaughan Van Hecke et al., 2012; Voos et al., 2013). I believe that the increasingly clear evidence of joint attention's role in early identification, diagnosis, and treatment argues for more research on the neurodevelopment of joint attention as a biomarker of risk and intervention response in ASD. To my mind, this research could involve at least three lines of inquiry.

Pertinent research may be directed to identifying early differences in neural network organization associated with joint attention (e.g., Elison et al., 2013) and its impairment in ASD. Another approach would be to begin examining the degree to which joint attention development is associated with variations in autonomic reactivity to social attention (e.g., Stagg et al., 2013), and to begin determining which neural networks may mediate that effect (e.g., Senju & Johnson, 2009). Third, it may prove useful to begin examining the degree to which intervention facilitates joint-attention-related cognitive or affective processing of objects or events (e.g., Bayliss et al., 2013; Frischen & Tipper, 2004), and to begin identifying the neural network processes involved in amplified cognitive processing in joint attention (e.g., Hirotani et al., 2009; Kopp & Lindenberger, 2011).

By now, I hope I have made it clear that joint attention is a unique and fundamental social and social-cognitive dimension in both typical and autism spectrum development. Recall, though, that joint attention "impairment" is not an explanation of ASD. It is not a dimension that fully accounts for ASD; rather, it is a dimension that must be included in any full account of ASD. Developing a deeper appreciation of the nature and measurement of joint attention over the last several decades has advanced research on diagnosis, early identification, and targeted behavioral intervention for ASD. To qualify for dimensional status within the NIMH RDoC, however, joint attention would also need to be shown to guide advances in research on the biological basis of ASD. The degree to which understanding the biological basis of joint attention may inform the basic and clinical biological sciences of ASD is examined in the following two chapters.

Chapter 7

Neurodevelopment
of Joint Attention

U nderstanding functional neurodevelopment is a primary goal of the
science of ASD. One approach is to describe the specific neurodevelopmental systems associated with a dimension of behavior that may
be central to ASD. Indeed, the description of the neurodevelopment of
neural networks specific to its behavioral functions may be necessary to
the validation of a dimension as significant to the study of ASD (e.g.,
Cuthbert & Insel, 2013). Accordingly, this chapter discusses theory and
evidence for the development of a functional joint attention neural network. The claim is made that the neurocognitive development of joint
attention is integral to the human *social brain*. To begin this discussion, it
is important to first recognize some of the challenges and complexities of
developmental cognitive neuroscience.

The Need for Caution in the Cognitive Neuroscience of ASD

The study of cognitive neurodevelopment began with research on the
functional roles of distinct brain structures, such as the amygdala, fusiform gyrus, or regions of the cerebellum (Friston, 1994). The study of the
neurodevelopment of ASD initially adopted this *region-of-interest* approach
(Wass, 2011). Recently, however, cognitive neuroscience has begun to go
beyond the study of the function of brain structures in isolation, to the
examination of neural networks that encompass functional systems of
multiple brain structures. This shift has been motivated in part by the

idea that complex human cognitive functions do not emerge from individual brain structures, but rather from the exchange of information across multiple local and distal brain structures (e.g., Barrett & Satpute, 2013; Spreng et al., 2013; Wass, 2011).

With the shift to a network approach, however, the complexity of cognitive neuroscience is multiplied (Bassett & Gazzaniga, 2011). Estimates suggest that there are billions of neurons in the mature human brain, and trillions of connections between those neurons. Developing methods to map, identify, and understand the development of neural networks is a challenge that neuroscience is just beginning to address (e.g., Spreng et al., 2013). Nevertheless, the shift to a neural network level of analysis dovetails well with the contemporary *connectivity hypothesis* of ASD.

According to this hypothesis, the development of ASD is thought to be characterized by a pattern of significant differences in the quantity or quality of network features involved in the transfer of information within and between local or distal neural systems of the brain. In ASD, the current speculation is that differences in the development of functional connectivity within and between the frontal lobes and the posterior parietal lobes of the brain may be especially important ([see Figure 7.1]; e.g., Belmonte et al. 2004; Courchesne & Pierce, 2005; Just, Cherkassky, Keller, Kana, & Minshew, 2007; Just, Keller, Malave, Kana, & Varma, 2012; Geschwind & Levitt, 2007). Differences in neural connectivity presumably change the characteristics of the flow of signals across structures within brain networks. Following from the notion that the exchange of information across local and distal brain structures is fundamental to complex human cognitive functions (e.g., Barrett & Satpute, 2013; Wass, 2011), changes in the characteristic flow of information are thought to result in the differences in the efficiency, organization, and content of cognition that are characteristic of people affected by ASD.

Given that we are in the early years of a systems approach to cognitive neuroscience, it should not be surprising that questions abound about the particulars of the connectivity differences in autism spectrum development. Across studies, evidence of underconnectivity (e.g., Wicker et al., 2008) and evidence of overconnectivity (e.g., Supekar et al. 2013) have been reported in different neural networks. Moreover, cross-age developmental data provide evidence that the patterns of over- versus underconnectivity may change with development in groups of people with ASD (Courchesne, Campbell, & Solso, 2011; Thompson-Schill, Ramscar, & Chrysikou, 2009). ASD may also be characterized by differences in connectivity across widespread (distal) brain networks and/or local (proximal) brain networks, and these patterns may also change over age (Khan et al., 2013; Keehn, Wagner, Tager-Flusberg, & Nelson, 2013). Finally, there is debate about whether the differences in neural networks involved

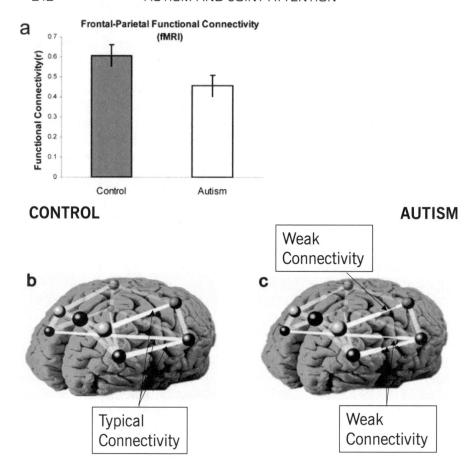

FIGURE 7.1. An illustration of evidence of lower frontal–parietal connectivity in autism on an executive function planning task (a), and a two-part schematic of white matter connectivity: (b) typical connectivity; and (c) less efficient connectivity in ASD, with narrowing of several of the white matter paths between neural networks illustrated with circles located across the parietal (upper rear) and frontal cortices. From Just, Keller, Malave, Kana, and Varma (2012). Copyright 2012 by Elsevier/Pergamon Press. Reprinted by permission.

in ASD are best characterized in terms of networks that support many different aspects of cognitive development (Barrett & Satpute, 2013; Corbetta, Patel, & Shulman, 2008; Spreng et al., 2013), or a more narrow band of neural networks that are specific to social-cognitive development (e.g., Happé & Frith, 2014; Kennedy & Adolphs, 2012; Wolf, Dziobek, & Heekeren, 2010). Complicating matters further, there is also evidence that atypical connectivity is not specific to autism, but also plays a role in other disorders, such as IDD (Chechlacz & Gleeson, 2003), ADHD (Konrad & Eickhoff, 2010), and schizophrenia (Karlsgodt et al., 2008).

Currently, connectivity can be studied by using imaging methods such as DTI (mentioned briefly in Chapter 5) to examine the structural integrity of the white matter[1] that provides connections and communication between brain regions. However, DTI does not directly measure the flow of information between or within neural networks during the execution of specific cognitive processes.

Alternatively, statistical methods can be used to detect patterns of correlations across multiple brain regions during cognitive task performance as measured with fMRI or EEG-related methods. This approach can provide another type of evidence of proximal and distal functional neural network connectivity. However, the causes of correlations are often open to different interpretations. In part, this is because correlation network analyses are not yet well linked to data on the structural characteristics of connectivity derived from DTI studies. Significant progress in resolving some of these methodological challenges may be on the horizon (e.g., Hernandez, Rudie, Green, Bookheimer, & Dapretto, 2015; Yates, 2011). Nevertheless, the cognitive neuroscience of ASD is currently as much (or more) about collecting observations that may lead to new hypotheses, as it is about conducting well-controlled tests of a priori causal hypotheses that lead to firm conclusions.

At least two other issues complicate developmental cognitive neuroscience. One is that data on the test–retest reliability of the types of imaging or EEG data used in the study of ASD have rarely been presented. At a minimum, this significantly constrains the comparative interpretation of findings across studies. Another problem is the so-called "developmental issue." The valid study of neurodevelopment demands that we examine

---

[1] *White matter* consists mostly of glial cells and the myelinated axons of neurons that connect to other neurons to transmit signals from one region of the cortex to another and between the cortex and lower brain centers. The neurons (or cell bodies) are referred to as *grey matter*. Whereas grey matter is primarily associated with processing and cognition, white matter transmits the results of information processing between networks of grey matter. For example, white matter integrates information from the networks of grey matter involved in processing external and internal sensory information (see Fields, 2008).

phenomena such as connectivity with equal precision, *on comparable tasks*, within many people at many different points in their development (Hernandez et al., 2015). This necessitates a type of programmatic, longitudinal research that requires considerable theoretical guidance, as well as considerable personal and institutional investment and support. These methodological challenges are surmountable, but remain to be addressed in the field. The rest of this chapter has been written, and should be read, with at least these caveats in mind.

Choosing Dimensions in the Developmental Cognitive Neuroscience of ASD

Some of the challenges of studying developmental connectivity in ASD may be reduced by examining the neural network development of cognitive dimensions that best discriminate ASD from other neurodevelopmental differences in in human nature. There are several dimensions to choose from. However, it should be obvious at this point that a goal of this book is to argue for the advantage of research on neurodevelopment of the dimension of joint attention. The previous chapters have provided evidence of several features of joint attention that support this assertion. First, joint attention is a dimension with extensive evidence of its validity and reliability in the diagnosis and early identification of ASD. Joint attention assessments reflect neurocognitive systems involved in responding to the social-communicative signals of others, and in the intentional, self-generated initiation of social communication to others. Its experimental manipulation in targeted treatment studies provides rare causal evidence of its role in learning and social-communicative development in young children with ASD. Joint attention reflects cognitive processes (e.g., adopting a common point of reference) that are linked conceptually and empirically to the subsequent emergence of other dimensions of behavior that are integral to the developmental phenotype of ASD. These include learning from other people; symbolic thinking; the development of language, joint action, and cooperative behavior; the development of social cognition; and enhanced information processing in social interactions. Finally, joint attention can be measured with similar types of measures from infancy to adulthood. Research indicates that the development of the neural networks involved in joint attention can be validly examined across ages, from the fifth and sixth months of life through old age (Brunetti, et al., 2014; Elison et al., 2013; Grossmann, Johnson, Farroni, & Csibra, 2007; Lachat et al., 2012), as well as comparatively across human and primate development (e.g., Hopkins, Keebaugh, et al., 2013).

Other dimensions of the social phenotype of ASD, such as social orienting, face processing, imitation, or even social cognition, may be comparable to joint attention on some of these features. It is debatable, though, whether there is evidence that other dimensions encompass all of these features. Evidence also suggests that that joint attention is characterized by a unique path of developmental continuity in ASD that may not be fully explained in terms of other social or cognitive-behavioral dimensions (e.g., Morgan, Maybery, & Durkin, 2003). Understanding the neurodevelopment of joint attention, then, may be one key to fully understanding the human nature of ASD. This hypothesis, though, is not yet well recognized in the field of social-cognitive neuroscience.

Theory on the neural network foundations of social cognition in either typical or autism spectrum development often include little discussion (e.g., Happé & Frith, 2014) or no discussion (e.g., Johnson, Grossmann, & Kadosh, 2009; Kennedy & Adolphs, 2012; Wolf et al., 2010) of the possible contributions of the neurodevelopment of joint attention. For example, research has long suggested that children process information about other people's attention in solving theory-of-mind problems (Lee et al., 1998). Consistent with this observation, Corbetta et al. (2008) have provided an insightful account of how theory-of-mind abilities may be an outgrowth of the developmental interplay between neural systems for endogenous (self) and exogenous (other) orienting and attention. The many insights in this potentially seminal argument notwithstanding, Corbetta et al. do not include any recognition of the relevance of joint attention theory or research to the argument they make in their paper. By the same token, Mahy, Moses, and Pfeifer (2014) have provided a cogent and compelling proposal that integrating knowledge from developmental psychology with that from imaging research on theory of mind may yield a more informed and veridical social-cognitive neuroscience. Yet the contribution of the developmental psychology and developmental neuroscience of joint attention to knowledge about the development of theory of mind has escaped notice in this otherwise very informed and informative paper.

The lack of recognition for joint attention research and theory in current social-cognitive neuroscience is unfortunate. Certainly, considerable support can be mustered for a neurodevelopmental model that describes joint attention as integral to social-cognitive development, and to its impairment in ASD. This chapter describes the evidence for this model. Elements of the model have been developed in a previous sequence of papers on the basic assumptions and evidence for the hypothetical sequence of the cognitive neurodevelopment joint attention and social cognition (e.g., Mundy, 2003, 2011; Mundy & Jarrold, 2010; Mundy

& Neal, 2000; Mundy et al., 2009). However, new observations in cognitive neuroscience allow for a much more detailed appraisal of neurodevelopmental joint attention theory in this chapter than has previously been possible.

Evidence for the Neural Network of Joint Attention

Similar methods and measures may be used to study joint attention across the lifespan. This continuity of method provides a foundation for mapping the growth and change of neural networks associated with the development of this cognitive dimension. Such a map, to date, is far from detailed or complete. Nevertheless, the outlines of this map can now be perceived. It is based on the burgeoning literature of infant, childhood, and adult studies of the neural substrates of joint attention.

Infant Neurocognitive Studies

Part of Chapter 5 has suggested that the neurodevelopment of joint attention begins with the transition from relatively involitional attention to more frontally regulated, intentional attention control at about 2 months of age. The first 2 months of life are marked by a bias toward looking at people and especially faces, but from 2 to 6 months of age, infants begin to pay less attention to faces and begin to attend to objects in the environment in addition to faces (Bakeman & Adamson, 1984; Johnson & Mareschal, 2001).

The development of the intentional control of visual attention between 2 and 6 months of age is expressed by infants' increased tendency to shift attention more flexibly between people and objects (Bakeman & Adamson, 1984; Farroni et al., 2003; Striano & Stahl, 2005; Striano, Stahl, Cleveland, & Hoehl, 2007; Tremblay & Rovira, 2007). At the beginning of this period, a pathway from the frontal eye fields (Brodmann's area [BA] 8/9) begins to release the superior colliculus from inhibition, which enables the development of active prospective control of saccades and visual attention (Canfield & Kirkham, 2001; Johnson, 1990; Kennedy & Adolphs, 2012; see Figure 7.2).[2] The function of this pathway may underlie 4-month-old infants' ability to suppress automatic visual saccades in order to respond to a second, more attractive stimulus (Johnson, 1995),

-----

[2]I often refer to illustrations of neuroanatomy when I try to map ideas about joint attention to information from cognitive neuroscience. Assuming that many readers may also find this useful, I provide sets of illustrations in Figure 7.2. To avoid repetition, though, this figure is not always mentioned where it may be useful.

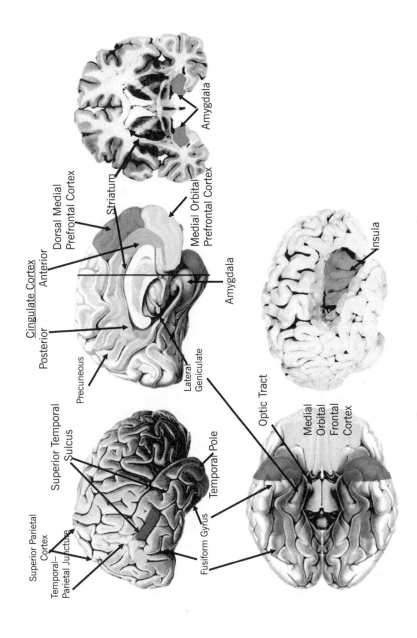

FIGURE 7.2. An illustration of brain regions most pertinent to imaging research on joint attention and social cognition. Adapted from Kennedy and Adolphs (2012). Copyright 2012 by Elsevier Ltd. Adapted by permission.

217

and 6-month-olds' ability to respond to a peripheral target when central, competing stimuli are present (Atkinson, Hood, Wattam-Bell, & Braddick, 1992). The functions of this pathway also enable intentional gaze alternation between interesting events and social partners (Mundy, 2003).

Evidence related to this hypothetical system of functions in joint attention has been provided in a study of infants 9–11 months of age. Benga (2005) showed that IJA behaviors correlate with *antisaccade performance*—the ability to suppress automatic saccades. Infants with more than 50% antisaccade responses on trials displayed significantly higher numbers of IJA behaviors than did infants with lower antisaccade response rates. Benga (2005), however, obtained no correlation between initiating behavior requests (IBR)/imperative joint attention and antisaccade performance. This suggests that the task demands of IJA may involve the frontal cognitive control of social attention more than requests or IBR, in this phase of development. The suppression of automatic saccades is a cornerstone of evidence for the onset of frontal control of attention in 4- to 6-month-olds (Johnson, 1995). It is linked to the activity of frontal eye fields (BA 8) and also the anterior cingulate cortex (ACC).

As described in Chapter 5, a new element of theory has been proposed by Senju and Johnson (2009). The tendency to engage actively in alternating gaze from an object to a person, or from a person to an object, may be influenced by a fast-track modulator that accounts for the eye contact effect. The *eye contact effect* is a name for the observation that the experience of mutual gaze is associated with increased arousal and enhanced information processing in infants, children, and adults (e.g., Bayliss et al., 2006; Becchio et al., 2008; Hood et al., 2003). The eye contact effect is hypothesized to organize behavior in young infants by motivating interest and information processing in social and especially triadic interactions with adults (again, see Chapter 5). Senju and Johnson (2009) suggest that the eye contact effect is mediated by very fast processing and responding to eye contact via a subcortical network involving the superior colliculus, pulivinar, and amygdala (see Figure 7.3). This network may be considered part of the nonconscious emotional processing network (Tamietto & de Gelder, 2010) and is connected to frontal networks via a major bundle of axons called the uncinate fasciculus. The idea that Senju and Johnson's fast-track processor may be involved in joint attention development is supported by the recent observation of the relation of early joint attention development to the uncinate fasciculus. Elison et al. (2013) conducted a DTI study of 14 infants, which examined 6-month neural network connectivity and 9-month RJA development. The results indicated that 6-month differences in the development of the uncinate fasciculus—a white fiber tract that connects the rostral temporal pole (and the cortical nuclei of the amygdala) with the frontal insular, orbital, and

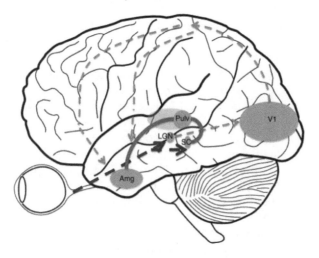

FIGURE 7.3. An illustration of components of the hypothetical fast-track subcortical neural circuit for the eye contact effect, including the superior colliculus (SC in the figure), the pulvinar (Pulv), and the amygdala (Amg). In this system, visual information processing flows rapidly from the retina to the SC, Pulv, and Amg, and interacts with frontal, parietal, and visual cortical (V1) areas to mediate the arousal of attention directed to oneself. From Garrido (2012). Copyright 2012 by Elsevier Ltd. Reprinted by permission.

ventromedial cortices (see Figure 7.4)—was a reasonably strong predictor of differences in 9-month RJA development ($r = -.88$) in this sample of infants. We need to understand that the data from this small study probably overestimate the strength of the correlation, because a correlation must appear to be very strong for it to be observed as significant in such a small sample. Nevertheless, by comparison, a tract that connects the occipital lobe, fusiform gyrus, and ventral temporal lobe (the inferior longitudinal fasciculus, or ILF), and an overlapping tract that provides a direct pathway between the occipital, posterior temporal, and orbitofrontal cortex (the fronto-occipital fasciculus), were not associated with RJA development in this small study.

According to the notion that joint attention is best subsumed under the rubric of face processing, one might have expected the tract involving connections with the fusiform gyrus to be more strongly related to joint attention development. However, the finding that the association between the left ILF and later joint attention development "approached" significance in this study indicates that the possibility of this network connection in joint attention development requires additional consideration.

The pattern of data reported by Elison et al. (2013) points to an important feature of the neural network development of joint attention that goes beyond the principal network of the fast-track modulator. Their pattern of data suggests that at a very early stage, joint attention is likely to involve the integration of regions of the frontal cortex with temporal/amygdala and subcortical network nodes. Little is currently known about the functional role of the uncinate fasciculus. However, a recent review suggests that the functions of the neural network served by this long-range white fiber tract are likely to be involved in semantic naming, learning based on individual valuations of objects and people, and related episodic memory and updating of people/object valuations based on experience (Von Der Heide, Skipper, Klobusicky, & Olson, 2013; see Figure 7.4).

The role of the frontal cortex in early joint attention development is also emphasized in a study by Grossmann and Johnson (2010). Optical imaging or near-infrared spectroscopy was used to examine the brain

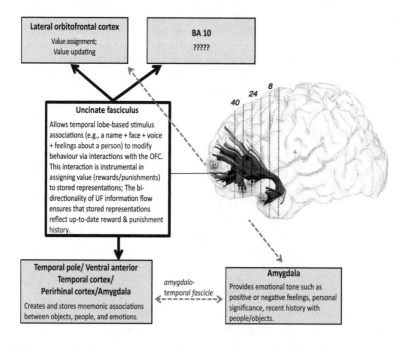

FIGURE 7.4. An illustration of the connective paths of the uncinate fasciculus across the temporal pole and frontal lobes, which a diffusion tensor imaging study (Elison et al., 2013) has implicated in the development of RJA in 6-month-old infants. The possible uncinate fasciculus branch connecting with BA 10 of the frontal cortex remains unclear. From Von Der Heide, Skipper, Klobusicky, and Olson (2013). Copyright 2013 by Oxford University Press. Reprinted by permission.

activity of 15 five-month-olds. Each infant observed videos of an adult who looked at the baby and then shifted gaze to look at a target to the adult's left or right that was also visible to the infant. Control comparison conditions were also included. Optical imaging was used because it provides a means of examining time-locked, localized metabolic cortical activity (changes in cortical oxygenation) simply by passing light through the top of the head of the infant during task performance (see Vanderwert & Nelson, 2014, for details).

The results of the Grossmann and Johnson (2010) study indicated that brain activity in the left *dorsal frontal cortex* was specifically correlated with an infant's processing of RJA events rather than control conditions (an adult's looking to no object or looking to an object without looking at the infant). This was especially true for the most dorsomedial diode site of the optical-imaging network of receptors (see Figure 7.5). I have italicized *dorsal frontal cortex* above to emphasize that when we study any aspect of social attention, we may expect frontal areas involved in self-referenced and goal-related allocation of visual attention, such as the frontal eye fields and the superior frontal gyrus, to be involved (e.g., Mundy, 2003; Sajonz et al., 2010).

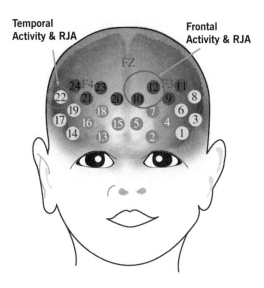

FIGURE 7.5. An illustration of optical imaging measures of dorsal frontal, ventral frontal, and possible temporoparietal cortical activation selectively associated with RJA in 5-month-old infants. From Grossmann and Johnson (2010). Copyright 2010 by The Royal Society. Reprinted by permission, through a Creative Commons License Deed.

A role of frontal functions in early joint attention development was identified in what was perhaps the first neurocognitive study of joint attention, conducted by Caplan et al. (1993) at UCLA. Caplan and colleagues used positron emission tomography (PET) imaging methods in a study of postsurgical outcomes for 13 infants and toddlers who underwent cortical surgery to treat intractable seizure disorders. IJA, IBR, and turn-taking social interaction measures from the ESCS were used as outcome measures. The severity of participants' seizure disorders prevented valid presurgical behavioral assessment. However, baseline presurgical cortical activity (glucose utilization) was measured with PET in the infants' dorsal and orbital prefrontal cortex; the superior, inferior, and middle temporal cortex; and the parietal and occipital cortex. The results indicated that baseline dorsal prefrontal cortical activity in the infants and toddlers was a significant predictor of postsurgical IJA development. However, neither other cortical regions nor other ESCS measures were observed to be involved in significant brain–behavior associations in this study. Thus this study provided the first evidence of a frontal contribution to early joint attention development.

This imaging study was followed with a succession of EEG studies of brain–joint attention relations. In the laboratory of Nathan Fox, an EEG study was conducted to assess the hypothesis that evidence of frontal cortical activity would be a specific correlate of IJA development in typical infants (Mundy, Card, & Fox, 2000). Baseline EEG and ESCS joint attention data were collected on 32 infants at 14–18 months of age. The results indicated that individual differences in 18-month IJA were predicted by a complex pattern of 14-month EEG activity that included indices of left medial frontal EEG activation and coherence between left medial frontal and left dorsal central EEG activation, as well as indices of right central deactivation, left occipital activation, and right occipital deactivation.

The location of the generators of the EEG data could not be definitively determined in this study. Nevertheless, the resting state EEG correlates of IJA reflected activity from electrodes positioned near the left medial frontal cortex (BA 8; see Figure 7.5). This area includes the frontal eye fields and supplementary motor cortex involved in attention control (Posner & Petersen, 1990). Moreover, Posner and Petersen suggested that medial frontal cortical activity associated with attention regulation probably reflected activity in the ACC (BA 24), a subcortical structure contiguous with the ventral surface of BA 8.

Neither RJA nor IBR measures were associated with a similar pattern of EEG activity. RJA at 18 months, however, was predicted by EEG indices of left parietal activation and right parietal deactivation at 14 months. This observation was consistent with research suggesting that parietal areas specialized for spatial orienting and attention, along with temporal systems specialized for processing gaze, contribute to gaze following and RJA performance in adults (Kingstone et al., 2000; Kawashima et al., 1999).

These were important observations for several reasons. The observations of Caplan et al. (1993) on the specificity of frontal correlations with IJA in infancy were replicated with different methods and samples of infants. The evidence from the Mundy et al. (2000) study of an association between RJA and parietal cortex activity in infants replicated observations of similar brain–behavior correspondence in adults. Hence this research provided evidence of reliable brain activation associations with joint attention across infant and adult samples, and across imaging and EEG methods.

It was also significant that the patterns of findings on IJA were consistent with observations from early brain–behavior studies of social cognition that theory-of-mind task performance was also consistently associated with activity in BA 8 of the dorsal medial prefrontal cortex (e.g., Frith & Frith, 1999, 2001). The observations of the brain activity of joint attention and theory of mind in similar cortical localization findings suggested that continuity in the neurodevelopment of joint attention and social-cognitive development warranted consideration (Mundy, 2003).

Several studies have meaningfully extended and improved on the methods used in these early studies. Kühn-Popp et al. (2015) have replicated the observation that proximal EEG coherence between frontal medial and central dorsal electrode sites reflect a cortical activation pattern specifically associated with joint attention in infancy. In this study, declarative pointing was the measure of joint attention observed in 32 infants. Moreover, Kühn-Popp et al. (2015) reported that joint attention and proximal left frontal central EEG at 15 months of age predicted children's use of mental state terms (e.g., *think, know, guess, believe*) at 48 months when they were describing characters' actions in a storytelling task. Consistent with other studies described in Chapter 4, this observation provides evidence of a behavioral and neurocognitive relation between infant joint attention and the childhood development of social cognition.

Grossmann et al. (2007) examined fast and slow EEG gamma band oscillations to examine local and distal neural networks associated with processing gaze direction in 12 four-month-olds. This study revealed a sequence of network activation associated with the discriminant processing of mutual gaze versus averted gaze in young infants. A large occipital network was activated at 100 msec. This was followed by frontal medial activation at 250–350 msec, and an overlapping pattern of parietal activation was identified at 250–450 msec. Thus, beyond the parietal activation associated with RJA in infant behaviors observed in the Mundy et al.

(2000) study, Grossmann et al. (2007) provided data indicative of fronto-parietal connectivity in the neural networks associated with RJA or gaze direction processing and responses in 12-month-olds.

Henderson et al. (2002) examined the 14-month resting state EEG predictors of 18-month pointing for joint attention and pointing for requesting as measured on the ESCS. To improve the specificity of the EEG data, this research group used a higher-density array (64 electrodes) than the one used in the Mundy et al. (2000) study, and they also examined data from multiple bandwidths. Their comparison of types of pointing behavior enabled a more controlled comparison of social attention coordinating behaviors that shared the same motor-behavioral topographies, but could be reliably be distinguished in the basis of ratings of their communicative functions. These functions were social attention coordination to share experience (joint attention) or social attention coordination to attain an object goal (requesting).

The Henderson et al. (2002) results indicated that activity in the bilateral left dorsal medial prefrontal cortex at 14 months of age predicted 18-month-olds infants' pointing for joint attention, but not their pointing for requesting. Moreover, joint attention pointing was also associated with activity in the orbital and dorsolateral frontal cortex, as well as in the temporal cortex. Again, however, evidence of such associations with pointing to request was lacking. These seminal data began to outline a network of cortical activation in infancy that was specific to the performance of joint attention in social communication.

Recent replications and extensions of these studies have appeared in the past few years. Brunetti et al. (2014) have extended Henderson et al.'s (2002) previous infant observations in a study of cortical correlates of pointing in adults. Brunetti et al. examined the brain activity of 14 adults during four conditions in which the participants pointed to request or pointed for joint attention. Participants were also asked to view videos of another person pointing to request, or another person pointing for joint attention. Brain activity was measured with magnetoencephalography (MEG). MEG is a functional imaging technique that can identify variations in magnetic fields associated with brain activity, which can be well localized to specific cortical as well as subcortical brain regions. The results of this MEG study indicated that activity in the dorsal medial prefrontal cortex (specifically, the ACC) and in the right posterior temporo-parietal cortex was significantly stronger in pointing for joint attention than in pointing to request.

The pattern of results reported by Brunetti et al. (2014) was very consistent with that reported by Henderson et al. (2002) in their observations of 14-month-old infants. This suggests that some level of continuity in the neural networks involved in joint attention exists across age and development. Moreover, it is very consistent with a basic hypothesis of joint attention theory: that functions of the ACC are likely to be integral to joint attention development and its impairment in ASD (Mundy, 2003). I discuss this hypothesis and its empirical support later in the chapter.

Finally, another recent and informative study compared the specifics of network activation patterns in 5-month-olds to joint visual attention behaviors versus other gestural signals. Lloyd-Fox, Blasi, Everdell, Elwell, and Johnson (2011) used optical imaging to compare the infants' cortical activation patterns in response to videos of actors who presented left and right eye movements. This was compared to how the infants responded to videos of testers opening and closing their mouths, or closing and opening their hands and pointing. Eye movements were selectively associated with inferior frontal and temporal pole activation. Hand gestures and pointing were associated with activation of the prefrontal cortex and posterior temporoparietal cortex. Mouth movements were associated with anterior temporal and motor cortex activation patterns.

In summary, there is now a small but growing literature on the neural networks associated with joint attention development in infancy. Studies provide evidence that by 4–6 months of age, neural networks of the frontal/prefrontal cortex and parietal cortex, as well as the temporal cortex (including the amygdala), probably play functional roles in gaze following and RJA development. Studies of brain–behavior relations suggest that a dorsal medial frontal and parietal cortical network may contribute to joint attention development by the beginning of the second year. Data from studies also raise the hypothesis that the relative degree of activation of the frontal network component (including the ACC) and the parietal network component may discriminate the development of IJA from RJA functions, as well as that of IJA functions from social attention coordination for requesting. Let us now turn our attention to the study of brain–behavior relations of joint attention in adults.

Adult Neurocognitive Studies

Williams et al. (2005) reported what I believe was the first fMRI study of the experience of joint attention in adults. This study was motivated by theory suggesting that RJA is a type of imitation. Twelve adult participants were asked to track a red ball that appeared and then disappeared in different regions of the perimeter of a video screen. A video image of an adult male face was visible in the middle of the screen. On some trials, the visual gaze of the video face shifted to a region of the screen just prior to the red ball's appearing there, thus predicting the correct location of the ball's appearance. On other trials, the visual gaze of the video face shifted to a region of the screen where the ball did not then appear, thus not predicting the correct location of the ball's appearance. The former (*congruent*) trials provided an analogue of RJA, and participants tracked the position of the ball more quickly. The latter (*incongruent*) trials required inhibition of gaze following, and participants consequently tracked the ball more slowly.

Contrasts of the two types of trials revealed a network of brain activation associated with the RJA analogue that included the medial frontal cortex (BA 9, 10), ACC, and parietal (precuneous) cortex, as well as the caudate nucleus (Williams et al., 2005). These observations were consistent with data from infant studies and with the hypothesis that joint attention is supported by a distributed dorsal medial prefrontal and parietal cortical network (Mundy et al., 2009). However, networks for imitation overlap with those proposed for joint attention with respect to regions of the inferior frontal gyrus and adjacent ventral premotor cortex, as well as the rostral inferior parietal lobule (e.g., Iacaboni, 2005; Shih et al., 2010).

So the data in this study may be interpreted as specific to RJA, or to imitation processes that may be part of RJA. Thus, as I have noted in Chapter 5, understanding the shared and unique neurocognitive processes of joint attention and imitation remains an important goal for developmental science and its application to ASD. I believe it is likely that the two dimensions both involve differentiated and integrated frontal and parietal self-referenced and other-referenced information processing. It may be noteworthy that a recent EEG study of preverbal infants suggests that infants' perception of being imitated by another person is associated with correlated activity across a frontoparietal network activation (Saby, Marshall, & Meltzoff, 2012). This observation may be important for autism research, because imitating young children is one initial path to stimulating joint attention in affected toddlers (e.g., Kasari et al., 2006, 2008; Ingersoll, 2012; Lewy & Dawson, 1992). Moreover, as noted in Chapters 5 and 6, this imitation effect may be linked to the eye contact effect and possible differences in the response of people with ASD to being the object of attention to others (Edwards et al., 2015; Gordon et al., 2013). These observations raise two interesting questions. First, does imitating children encourage the activation of self–other neurocognitive processing, which then potentiates joint attention behaviors? Second, are individual differences in integrated processing in the frontoparietal network predictors of intervention responsiveness in ASD, and/or biomarkers of intervention outcome in targeted joint attention interventions?

The foregoing also suggests that there may be a line of neurocognitive continuity between the dimensions of imitation and joint attention in early development and in the development of ASD. Whether or not this is so, it may not be useful to try to explain all of joint attention in terms of imitation processes or all imitation processes in terms of joint attention (see Chapter 5). Aside from a dynamic model, which suggests that these are better conceived as interacting development dimensions, another reason for this assertion stems from the observation that the Williams et al. (2005) study only involved a measure analogous to RJA. In terms of the neural networks, research suggests that IJA and RJA may be supported by somewhat different neural networks (e.g., Mundy et al., 2000). Hence research on one or the other type of joint attention cannot provide a clear picture of either its cognitive or its neural network foundations. This argument is bolstered by the use of clever methods that have also begun to reveal that IJA and RJA involve similar and unique neural networks in adults.

Imaging, Motivation, and Joint Attention

In work with adults, several research groups have described methods for examining the cognitive processes and neural networks involved in IJA and RJA (e.g., Bayliss et al., 2013; Gordon et al., 2013; Kim & Mundy, 2012; Redcay et al., 2012; Schilbach et al., 2010). In these methods, research participants view a live video image of a social partner, or a virtual reality avatar, during task performance. In some conditions, the research participants follow the gaze of the social partner or avatar (RJA); in others, the video image of the social partner or avatar follows the gaze of the research participant, emulating the experience of IJA.

Schilbach et al. (2010) provided the first functional imaging study of *both* IJA and RJA. With the help of 21 adult volunteers, they observed that RJA and IJA were associated with a distributed neural network composed of the medial prefrontal cortex (including the rostral ACC), the medial orbital prefrontal cortex, the ventral striatum, the posterior cingulate cortex, and areas of the temporal and occipital cortex. In addition, the data in this study suggested that IJA was associated with significantly greater evidence of striatal activation than was RJA. Interestingly, striatal activation often appears to play a role in processing the reward contingencies associated with initiating behaviors. With respect to attention, a network involving the striatum, amygdala, ACC, and possibly insula is associated with *processing the predicted reward value of shifts of attention,* as well as with the processing of positive and negative reinforcement in learning (e.g., Gottfried, O'Doherty, & Dolan, 2003; Krebs, Boehler, Roberts, Song, & Woldorff, 2012; Niznikiewicz & Delgado, 2011). Thus the observations of Schilbach et al. (2010) were consistent with theory suggesting that that IJA may be distinguished from RJA on the basis of greater involvement of reward processing in guiding social attention allocation (Mundy, 1995, 2003).

It may also be noteworthy that the striatum is at least interconnected with, if not part of, the subcortical nonconscious emotional processing network that hypothetically is involved in the fast-track modulation of the eye contact effect (Senju & Johnson, 2009). Together, these observations raise the possibility that the experience of the eyes of the avatar following the research participants triggered processes related to the eye contact effect associated with striatal activation during IJA trials in the Schilbach et al. (2010) study. This hypothesis is consistent with the recent findings of Bayliss et al. (2013) that the experience of "gaze leading" of another person in IJA biases affective responses to the face of the social partner and the attended object.

Pfeiffer et al. (2014) have more directly replicated and extended the work of Schilbach et al. (2010) by demonstrating that striatal activation was more prominent in tasks where participants believed they were engaged in real-time IJA interactions controlled by another participant (human), rather than by a computer program. Other observations from an independent research group have also provided evidence of striatal activation as part of a broader neural network involved in IJA. Gordon et al. (2013) reported an fMRI study of 14 adults, each of whom were asked to try to get a screen character (Sally) to follow the participant's gaze to identical male characters positioned to the right and left of Sally. Sally followed the participant's gaze on some trials (IJA analogue trials), but not on others (non-IJA trials). As illustrated in Figure 7.6, this contrast revealed that the experience of IJA was associated with bilateral activations in the dorsal ACC, right fusiform gyrus, bilateral posterior parietal cortex, and right amygdala, as well as the bilateral striatum and parahippocampal regions.

An Expanded View of Neural Networks in Adult Joint Attention

In addition to providing further evidence of the role of striatal and possible reward processing in neural networks associated with IJA, the Gordon et al. (2013) study is noteworthy for at least three other reasons. The results revealed a bimodal distribution of activation versus inhibition of the ACC during IJA trials. This is additional evidence that is consistent with the idea that differences in ACC activation may play a role in the range of human joint attention proclivity we observe across both typical and autism spectrum development (Mundy, 2003). It is also consistent with the recent observation that neural organization within the ACC is significantly related to chimpanzees' tendency to initiate triadic social attention with a human tester (Hopkins & Taglialatela, 2013). Similarly, studies of pointing for joint attention (Brunetti et al., 2014) and related

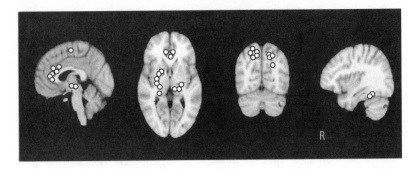

FIGURE 7.6. An illustration of the social, reward, and attention brain networks activated in an IJA task in adults. The far left cortical panel illustrates the activation of the anterior cingulate cortex (attention network) in processing attention to self in IJA and the ventral striatum (reward network) in processing attention to self in IJA. The activation of the ventral striatum (reward networks), in association with the amygdala and parahippocampal complex, can be seen in the bottom of the far left and center of the middle right panels. Bilateral parietal activation is illustrated in the middle right middle panel and fusiform activation can be seen in the far right panel. From Gordon, Eilbott, Feldman, Pelphrey, and Vander Wyk (2013). Copyright 2013 by Taylor & Francis. Reprinted by permission.

research on sharing attention in cooperative joint action (Chaminade, Marchant, Kilner, & Frith, 2012) provide evidence of the involvement of the ACC as part of the joint attention network, which includes prominent parietal components as well.

Second, the Gordon et al. (2013) data provide evidence of the involvement of neural systems that are central to memory and encoding. This evidence is consistent with the idea that the activation of the joint attention systems may be associated with effects on stimulus encoding and memory (e.g., Frischen & Tipper, 2004; Striano, Chen, et al., 2006; Striano, Reid, & Hoel, 2006). It also may indicate that current acts of joint attention involve elicitation of information encoded in previous episodes of shared reference. Recall that recent research also suggests that the experience of IJA may be more strongly associated with increases in stimulus encoding and memory in adults than is the experience of RJA (Kim & Mundy, 2012). This is not to say, though, that RJA does not affect information processing. An especially informative recent study indicates that the posterior superior temporal sulcus, adjacent to the parietal cortex, may play a central role in RJA information processing (Redcay et al., 2015).

Finally, Gordon et al. (2013) reported observations addressing the role of the fusiform face-processing cortical region in the joint attention network. The regions of the joint attention network observed in this study, such as the ACC, posterior parietal cortex, and right amygdala, displayed distinctly *different patterns* of positive activation to congruent joint attention trials and deactivation to incongruent trials. However, the fusiform gyrus displayed a *common pattern* of activation to both congruent and incongruent trials, albeit of different intensities. This suggests that the frontoparietal neural network and fusiform gyrus may make different functional contributions in joint attention information processing. So we should remain cautious about explaining the dimension of joint attention singularly in terms of neurobehavioral functions of the face-processing system.

Elizabeth Redcay at the University of Maryland has also significantly expanded the literature on the cognitive neuroscience of joint attention and its impairment in ASD. In one study, Redcay et al. (2012) used fMRI to examine the network correlates of joint attention in a relatively large sample of 41 adults. Consistent with previous adult and infant studies, they observed that IJA and RJA together were associated with a distributed frontal–parietal–temporal network. Within this paper, the research group also recognized the very considerable overlap of their observations on joint attention network with the networks for social cognition identified in the literature. They provided an instructive illustration of this overlap, as well as the overlap of joint attention network observations, with networks involved in the cognitive control of attention and visual information processing (Figure 7.7).

This overlap is curious in a way, because the joint attention tasks used by Redcay et al. (2012) do not explicitly require research participants to solve a problem that involves mentalizing the intensions, beliefs, or emotions of others. In the IJA condition, for example, the task demand was to look intentionally at a target. At the same time, visual information was provided to the participants to indicate that their behavior directed the gaze of a social partner. So this task involved the self-regulation of attention, the monitoring of another person's attention, and processing the contingency between one's own gaze and its deictic effect on the gaze of another person. These task demands would seem to be quite different from those of the conceptual problem-solving paradigms used in many imaging studies of social cognition (see Mahy et al., 2014). Yet these distinct types of paradigms recruit very similar neural network responses in adults. Understanding why this might this be is likely to be an informative quest for social-cognitive science, as well as for research on autism spectrum development.

Redcay et al. (2012) also observed evidence of the constituents of the joint attention neural network that differentiated IJA from RJA. The experience of RJA was associated with ventral orbital prefrontal and

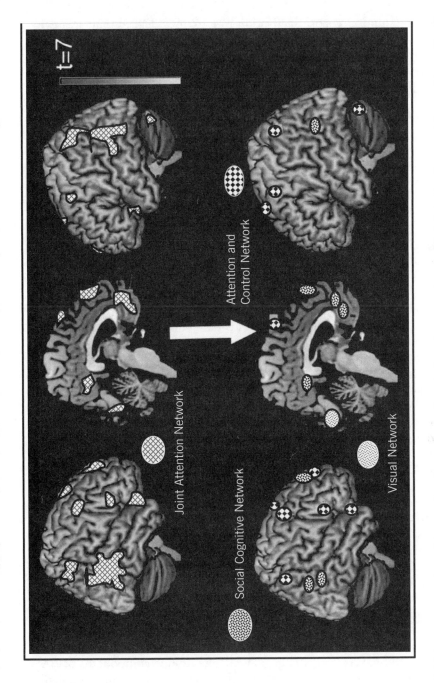

FIGURE 7.7. An illustration of the overlapping nature of cortical regions associated with joint attention, social cognition, attention and cognitive control, and visual information processing in adults. From Redcay, Kleiner, and Saxe (2012). Reprinted in accord with the open-access guidelines of the *Frontiers in Human Neuroscience* journal.

posterior temporal cortical activation to a greater degree than was evident for IJA. Alternatively, IJA was associated with activation of the dorsal and medial prefrontal cortex, inferior frontal cortex, and parietal cortex to a greater extent than was the case for RJA. Like those of Schilbach et al. (2010), these observations provided evidence of neurofunctional differences between IJA and RJA, but the details of these contrasts were different across the two studies. The studies were consistent in supporting the hypothesis that IJA and RJA reflect different as well as common aspects of joint attention (Mundy, 1995), but they also indicate that much more research is needed before we can more definitively describe and understand these differences.

One such contribution has come from Caruana, Brock, and Woolgar (2015), who directly tested the hypothesis that RJA and IJA are executed within partially independent yet parallel networks (e.g., Mundy & Jarrold, 2010; Mundy & Newell, 2007). This study used an innovative paradigm to gather imaging data on 13 adults. Participants interacted with an onscreen avatar who (they believed) was controlled by an unseen person named Alan. Each participant engaged in a cooperative game of finding a burglar inside a matrix of rows of small houses with blue or red doors. The avatar searched houses with blue doors, and the participant searched those with red doors. When a door was fixated, it opened briefly to reveal an empty house or one inhabited by the burglar. The avatar and participant searched all their houses and then returned to mutual gaze with each other. If the participant had not found the burglar, he or she next needed to follow the avatar's gaze to the correct door, which opened when the participant fixated the door. Conversely, on trials when the participant found the burglar, he or she had to use gaze to direct the avatar to look at the correct door, which would open after being fixated by the avatar. The former condition emulated RJA for the participant, while the latter was an analogue of IJA for the participant.

According to Caruana et al. (2015), the data from this study provided support for the hypothesis that in adulthood RJA and IJA shared common and distinctive neural network functions. They shared a right lateralized and distributed network hypothesized to reflect activation of representation of simultaneous self and other perspectives on attention. Specifically, Caruana et al. (2015) observed that the common components of IJA and RJA included activation across the temporoparietal junction, precuneous, posterior superior temporal sulcus, middle frontal gyrus, and middle temporal gyrus. However, IJA was also associated with specific frontal–temporal–parietal networks reflecting the additional, more volitional, goal-directed nature of IJA engagement. The unique components of IJA included activation of the superior frontal gyrus, ACC, middle cingulate cortex, cerebellum, and thalamus (Caruana et al., 2015).

The latter observations were consistent with theory about the neural networks that might be expected to distinguish IJA from RJA (Mundy, 2003; Mundy & Jarrold, 2010). Perhaps more importantly, they were very consistent with Gordon et al.'s (2013) observations of the specific involvement of ACC, middle cingulate, thalamic region, and cerebellum neural network activation in conjunction with IJA performance. The observation of thalamic activation is consistent with previous suggestions of the likelihood of basal ganglia and ACC reward processing in IJA (Gordon et al., 2013; Mundy, 2003; Pfeiffer et al., 2014; Schilbach et al., 2010). The now-repeated observations of possible cerebellar contributions to IJA may be one of the more important new observations in research on the neurodevelopment of joint attention. This is because research and theory have long suggested that differences in the cerebellar influence on spatial encoding of a location for an attentional shift and the subsequent gaze shift may play a role in the pathogenesis of ASD (Townsend et al., 1999).

This review of the emerging neuroscience of joint attention leads to several cautious but evidence-based conclusions. First, it is possible to examine the neurodevelopment of joint attention from early infancy through adulthood. Second, research suggests that elements of a joint attention network that includes frontal and temporal–amygdala poles are most easily detected in the first 6 months of life. By the second year, frontal and parietal components have been observed. There is also evidence of the differentiation of networks associated with IJA versus RJA, as well as the detection of both different and common cortical correlates of IJA and RJA.

Adult studies reveal a rather more distributed network of cortical involvement in joint attention. The dorsal medial frontal cortex, insula, and areas of the cingulate gyrus have most consistently been observed to be involved in joint attention, especially IJA. Temporal cortical areas most commonly involve the amygdala, superior temporal sulcus, and fusiform gyrus. Parietal network contributions most often involve the posterior parietal cortex and precuneous. Neural activation of these networks appears to be common to both RJA and IJA. Furthermore, activity in subcortical striatal regions, the adjacent parahippocampal region, and the cerebellum has been associated with joint attention. The striatal patterns of activation are consistent with the idea of a greater reward-processing component in IJA (Mundy, 1995, 2003). Some adult studies also suggest that the combination of striatal, parietal, and cerebellar involvement may be more pronounced in IJA, whereas activation of the superior temporal sulcus and orbital frontal cortex may be more common in RJA. Finally, *many components of the observed joint attention neural network in adults appear to be co-located with major components of the adult social-cognitive system or social brain, as well as neural networks associated with imitation.* This is consistent with the notion of ongoing functional relations among joint attention, imitation, and social cognition in mature social-cognitive neural networks.

Relative to these observations, the next sections of this chapter focus on three issues. The first is whether or not imaging studies with people affected by ASD provide meaningful information on differences in their experience of joint attention. The second addresses hypotheses about why a common neural network may be involved in joint attention, social cognition, and imitation in human development, including the development of ASD. The third examines joint attention and joint activity within current models of three superordinate distributed neural control networks.

Imaging Studies of Joint Attention in Autism Spectrum Development

To date, there have been relatively few imaging studies of joint attention that have also included samples of people affected by ASD. Nevertheless, at least four informative studies are available.

Mosconi, Cody-Hazlett, et al. (2009) reported a longitudinal imaging study of amygdala volume and joint attention in ASD. The study involved over 30 toddlers (ages 18–35 months) with ASD. It was designed to examine how well imaging measures of the amygdala volumes predicted joint attention measures on the same children obtained at 42–59 months of age. As a group, the children with ASD displayed larger amygdala volumes than developmental age-matched typical controls at both Time 1 and Time 2. However, both groups displayed similar levels of increases in amygdala volume across age. Twenty-one percent of the sample with ASD displayed IJA or RJA at Time 1; this increased to 39% at Time 2. Most importantly, at Time 2, lower amygdala volume in the sample with ASD was significantly associated with better RJA and IJA performance; there was evidence of a stronger association with RJA than with IJA.

It is likely that developing a better understanding of the functional links between the amygdala and joint attention is an important goal of the neuroscience of ASD. The amygdala is often most closely associated with the experience and perception of emotional states. More generally, it is thought to be involved in perceiving *biological significance*, or the importance of events for survival (Pessoa & Adolphs, 2010). However, the amygdala and its connections to the hippocampus also play an instrumental role in learning and memory, and in how these are affected by social influences in people (Amaral, 1987/2011; Edelson, Sharot, Dolan, & Dudai, 2011). The importance of understanding this in research on

ASD has been recently been emphasized in a recent longitudinal study of typical infant-to-preschool language development (Ortiz-Mantilla, Choe, Flax, Grant, & Benasich, 2010). This research group observed that infants with larger amygdala volumes at 6 months of age had significantly lower expressive and receptive language scores at 2 (r's = −.55 and −.51, respectively), 3, and 4 years of age. The authors noted that understanding the yet-unspecified role that that the amygdala plays in early language development may be a key to understanding an important part of autism spectrum development. My guess is that understanding its link to joint attention is one important path of inquiry in attempts to specify the link between the amygdala's roles in typical and atypical language development.

Another study (Pelphrey et al., 2005) did not reveal a link between the amygdala and joint attention in adults with ASD, but was informative with respect to their differences in gaze following. This study compared 10 adults affected by ASD to 9 adults with typical development. This imaging study was designed to examine neural network responses to trials when an avatar's gaze shifts directed participants' attention to a peripheral target (RJA), compared to trials when the avatar's gaze shifts did not direct the participants' attention to a target. In adults with typical development, this contrast revealed that RJA was associated with activation in the superior temporal sulcus, middle temporal gyrus, parietal lobe, middle frontal gyrus, and ACC. In adults with ASD, a more limited pattern of activations was observed in the middle temporal, occipital, inferior frontal, and insular cortices. The groups differed significantly in their patterns of activation in the superior temporal cortex, insula, and inferior frontal gyrus. Interestingly, behavioral and superior temporal sulcus imaging data suggested that individuals with ASD perceived and reacted at about the same speed to all of the avatar's shifts of gaze.

One of the more comprehensive studies of joint attention in individuals has been reported by Redcay, Dodell-Feder, et al. (2013). Recall that Redcay and colleagues use an imaging paradigm that presents participants with analogues of IJA as well as RJA. This study compared 13 adults with ASD, all of whom had full-scale IQs greater than 90, with an age- and IQ-comparable sample of 14 adults with typical development. Combined across IJA and RJA, the results indicated that those with typical development displayed significantly stronger activity in the dorsal medial prefrontal cortex and left posterior superior temporal cortex than individuals with ASD. Alternatively, both groups displayed patterns of activity in the right anterior insula and left inferior parietal cortex indicating greater responding to IJA than RJA, and greater responding to RJA than the attention control condition. The former neural network differences emerged even though there was little evidence of group differences in latency or accuracy of joint attention task performance.

This study also revealed specific diagnostic group differences on RJA but not IJA tasks. With respect to the former, the group with typical development displayed the often-observed pattern of greater anterior dorsal medial frontal and posterior superior temporal activation to RJA than in the group with ASD. Alternatively, the group with ASD displayed greater evidence of recruitment of the putamen, fusiform gyrus, and middle occipital gyrus on RJA trials than did those with typical development. These data indicated that the group with ASD differed in the organization of neural network responses to joint attention tasks: This group displayed less activation of key components of the social-cognitive network (dorsal medial prefrontal cortex and posterior superior temporal sulcus) during joint attention task performance, but greater activation of key components of the cortical visual–spatial processing system, face-processing system, and possibly motivation system (putamen, occipital, and fusiform cortex).

The lack of observed differences in IJA is at once surprising and yet consistent with some research. It is surprising because research on preschool children suggests that the delayed development of IJA may be more robust than the delay in RJA development. On the other hand, research also suggests that by 2 or more years of age, children with ASD may become sensitive to others' following their attention, and this may be a pivotal opening for effective intervention (e.g., Kasari et al., 2008). Of course, it is also plausible that the significant limits on the power of this study of 13 adults simply did not allow the researchers to observe all the joint attention diagnostic group differences that existed.

A fourth, but rather different, type of study has been provided by Mizuno et al. (2011). This study examined the neural basis of deictic shifting in linguistic perspective taking in children with higher-functioning autism. A bit of background may be useful in understanding the connection of this study to research on joint attention.

Deixis refers to linguistic, gestural, or other behaviors that help to establish the correct point of reference in communication. Joint attention enables preverbal children to establish the correct point of reference. Hence joint attention is thought to be integral to the development of deictic communication (Bruner, 1975; Tomasello, Carpenter, Call, et al., 2005). With the development of language, children subsequently develop the capacity to use words for deixis. One example is the use of personal pronouns, such as *I* and *you* to establish or shift between the first-person perspective and the second-person perspective of a common point of reference during social-communicative interactions (Dale & Crain-Thoreson,

1993). Developing the ability to remap personal perspective positions within referential communication is called *deictic shifting* (Dale & Crain-Thoreson, 1993). The development of deictic shifting is often a cognitive challenge in preschool development. Moreover, the development of the ability to shift between personal perspectives on a common point of reference (*I, you*) in spoken language and reading has long been recognized as unusually problematic for many individuals with ASD (e.g., Mizuno et al., 2011; O'Connor & Klein, 2004).

To better understand the neural systems that may contribute to linguistic deixis difficulties in ASD, Mizuno et al. (2011) examined functional connectivity during cognitive processing of pronoun shifts in 15 adults with ASD and 15 adults with typical development. During imaging, each participant was presented with scenes of "Sarah" holding open a two-page book with pictures on each page (e.g., a carrot and a house; see Figure 7.8). Sarah then folded the book so that she could see only one picture and the participant could only see one picture. Across a sequence of such presentations, conditions were presented that demanded engagement in a linguistic/joint attention deictic shift between self and other. Participants were required to answer the questions "What can you see now?" versus "What can I see now?" Other conditions were presented that required responses to similar but linguistically simpler tasks, using the participants and Sarah's proper names rather than pronouns (e.g., "What can John see now?", "What can Sarah see now?").

The adults with ASD displayed less evidence of functional connectivity between the precuneous (parietal lobe) and right insula cortex in response to pronoun cues for shifts between the perspectives of self and other, compared to individuals with typical development. Group differences, however, were not observed when proper names for Sarah and the research participants were used to cue shifts between the visual perspectives of self and other.

The degree to which functional connectivity was correlated with pronoun-cued deictic shifts was also examined. Individuals with ASD who exhibited lower evidence of functional connectivity between the precuneous and insula cortical regions displayed slower responses to pronomial cues to shift the self-reference visual perspective ("What do you see now?"). This association was significantly stronger in the sample with ASD than in the comparison sample.

In interpreting their data, the authors noted evidence for the role of the parietal (precuneous) region in processing information about the spatial relation between self and other external agents. They also noted evidence indicative of the insula's role in self-awareness and the integration of information about internally and externally referenced information.

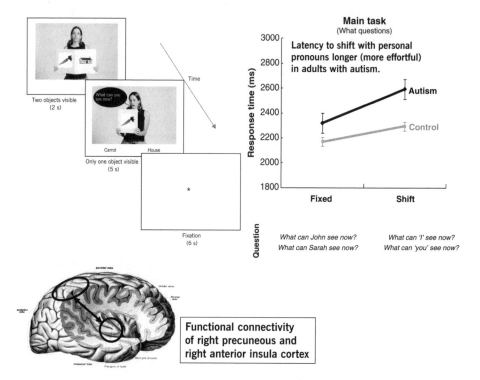

FIGURE 7.8. An illustration of the types of stimuli used to assess the rate of processing pronouns ("What can I see?") versus proper names ("What can Sarah see?") in a perspective-taking task (upper left) used to access the cortical network associated with deictic shifting in adults with and without ASD. The upper right panel illustrates the observation that adults with ASD required more time to process pronouns than proper names in this task. The illustration at the bottom of the figure illustrate the parietal and medial frontal cortical networks (insula cortex), which worked together less efficiently in many adults with ASD when they were processing pronouns. From Mizuno et al. (2011). Copyright 2011 by Oxford University Press. Reprinted by permission.

Based on this information, Mizuno et al. (2011) hypothesized that decreased functional connectivity between the parietal (precuneous) and insular brain systems may result in a disturbance in visual perspective taking, and especially in rapid shifting of the center of reference between self and other, in individuals with ASD. A very similar hypothesis has been raised about the role that a network involving the insula and parietal cortices may play in the typical and atypical self–other references in prelinguistic joint attention development (Mundy et al., 2010).

In summary, the current imaging and electrophysiological research literature provides an outline of evidence for the development of the neural network of joint attention. In the first year, this may include a fast-track modulator (Senju & Johnson, 2009) for emotional processing of visual information. The fast-track modulator involves the subcortical superior colliculus and pulvinar in interaction with the amygdala. Evidence indicates that dorsal and orbital ventral input, likely in conjunction with the amygdala, plays a role in the early phase (5–10 months) of joint attention or at least RJA development (e.g., Elison et al. 2013).

In studies of the second year, consistent evidence of amygdala, dorsal medial frontal, and posterior temporal and parietal cortical activation in joint attention has been reported. Evidence in the second year also indicates that frontoparietal neural networks are involved in triadic attention for declarative, experience-sharing functions to a greater degree than for imperative requesting functions. Moreover, evidence begins to emerge in the second year for different frontal and temporal contributions to IJA and RJA functions.

Adult imaging studies have provided more precise data on the mature joint attention neural network. This includes regions of the dorsal medial frontal cortex, including the ACC; the insula cortex; regions of ventral orbital frontal cortex and temporal cortex, including the amygdala as well as the posterior superior temporal region; the dorsal parietal (precuneous) cortex; and the striatal and possibly hippocampal subcortical regions of the basal ganglia (e.g., Mundy & Jarrold, 2010). Like several studies of the second year, some studies with adults reveal more evidence of frontoparietal activation in initiating pointing for joint attention rather than requesting. IJA and RJA also are differentiated in adult studies by the involvement of dorsal medial frontal, parietal, and striatal contributions to IJA, and ventral orbital frontal and superior temporal contributions to RJA.

Again, many nodes of the joint attention network overlap with nodes of networks activated in many imaging studies of adult social-cognitive responding and problem solving (e.g., Kennedy & Adolphs, 2012; Schilbach, Bzdok, et al., 2012). The nature and meaning of this overlap are considered below.

The Overlap between the Joint Attention and Social-Cognitive Networks

In contemporary social-cognitive neuroscience, the *social brain* is often conceptualized in terms of the interactions of multiple functional networks. Kennedy and Adolphs (2012), for example, have described the social brain in terms of four networks. One is a *mentalizing* network, consisting of the dorsal medial prefrontal cortex and the anterior and posterior temporal cortex. The second is a *salience* network, consisting of the amygdala, the anterior medial pole of the temporal cortex, and the ventral orbital prefrontal cortex; this network is involved in emotional responding and detecting socially salient stimuli. The third is an *empathizing* network, consisting of the insula and central cingulate cortex, and involving the capacity to perceive and resonate with others' emotional states. Finally, Kennedy and Adolphs's model includes a *mirror system/action perception* network that consists of the parietal and inferior frontal cortex, and that is involved in imitation and interpretations of the goals of others' behaviors.

A similar model of four distributed social brain networks has been proposed by Barrett and Satpute (2013), who also posit mentalizing, mirror, and salience networks. However, rather than an empathizing network, the Barrett and Satpute model includes an executive network. Both of these models provide useful guidance for advancing the neuroscience of atypical social cognition in ASD and other clinical differences in human mental development (Happé & Frith, 2014). However, the literature reviewed in this book suggests that these perspectives on the social brain may be significantly incomplete. This may be because they are based largely on the adult literature on social-cognitive neuroscience. A dynamic developmental model of social cognition may serve us better. That is, facets of social neurocognitive systems may be best appreciated by considering how typical and atypical social cognition develop across the lifespan, from infancy to adulthood.

Chapter 4 has raised the hypothesis that mentalizing in social cognition involves an internalized mental joint attention process. When we think about the content of other people's minds, we often consider what others have attended to and experienced, in order to mentalize what information another person has or does not have. At the same time, though, we must develop the capacity to keep this other-referenced information separate from our own history of attention, experience, and encoding of information, in order to identify valid or false beliefs in others (Leslie, 1987). At times, we must also draw upon our memory of our own and others' reactions to comparable information and experience, in order to estimate others' likely cognitive and emotional reactions to information and experiences. This internal information processing to arrive at social-cognitive knowledge flows, in part, across the joint attention network. This dynamic developmental process has been detailed to some extent in Chapter 4. Elements of this process are reviewed again in the next few pages, to fully inform the functional appraisal of the joint attention neural network in typical and atypical social cognition that is presented at the conclusion of this chapter.

The Dynamic Development of Behavior and Social-Cognitive Neural Systems

Recall from Chapter 4 the hypothesis that joint attention may have two phases of development that contribute to a particular social-cognitive executive function. The first has been called the *learning-to* phase, and the other the *learning-from* phase. In the first phase, the frontal, executive, cognitive control of joint attention begins to increase, and the cognitive load of engaging in joint attention decreases. Executive and cognitive control develops as repeated activation of the adaptive, goal-related behaviors involved in joint attention leads to frontal and subcortical maintenance of neural activation patterns that subsequently increase the efficiency of these adaptive behaviors (Miller & Cohen, 2001). If so, what elemental form of cognitive control guides the initial practice of joint attention behaviors early in infancy?

The above-described salience network is probably also at play early in the development of joint attention. This hypothesis begins with the idea that the early-onset fast-track modulator of the eye contact effect (Senju & Johnson, 2009) plays a role in kindling interest and information processing, which guide infants to begin practicing alternating looking between objects and people in the 2- to 6-month phase of development. This pathway hypothetically involves subcortical/striatal nodes, functioning in conjunction with an amygdalar–hippocampal–frontal–parietal circuit. Elison et al. (2013) have provided some evidence for the role of amygdala and frontal connectivity in early joint attention development. Joint attention theory and amygdala connectivity with the temporoparietal cortex, suggest the inclusion of the posterior cortical network connection as well.

Joint attention theory has long recognized the need to stipulate an initial control/guidance or motivation mechanism to understand how joint attention becomes organized in early development (e.g., Mundy, 1995; Tomasello, Carpenter, Call, et al., 2005). I believe that the confluence of ideas and evidence provided by Senju and Johnson (2009) and Elison et al. (2013) currently offers the best guess as to an outline of the specific nature of this mechanism. The particulars of this system, again, speak to the role of the amygdala in human learning. One shorthand way of describing the function of this system may be this: It ensures that, for many, what is attended to jointly acquires a level of intrinsic biological significance. This potentiates practice with joint attention early in life, and potentiates learning during joint attention throughout life.

The early practice of joint attention is essential to the dynamic process that sculpts its executive neural networks. The practice of joint attention involves the triadic processing of information about oneself, others' attention behaviors, and outcomes or referents. With maturation, it also involves processing information about past joint attention experience from episodic memory. Over time and repetitions, both processes update the representation of neural network activity that is optimal for flexible engagement in joint attention. That is, the frontal integration of current and past task-specific information into neural network activation gradually sculpts and improves neural network firing associated with successful joint attention goal-related behavior.

With maturation and dynamic developmental processes, the frontal cortex increasingly exerts cognitive control by providing bias signals to other brain structures. The net effect is to guide the flow of activity along neural pathways that establish the proper (most efficient) mappings between and among inputs, internal states, and outputs needed to perform joint attention (cf. Miller & Cohen, 2001). The bias signals are the essence of mature cognitive control, and they lead to a more efficient and precise automatic engagement of information-processing routines, such as joint attention. With increased efficiency of engagement, such information-processing routines can become internalized and integrated into more complex and flexibly adaptive cognitive applications.

According to this model of executive development, joint attention is not replaced by mature social-cognitive functions. Rather, joint attention becomes an integral executive routine in support of social cognition throughout the lifespan. This idea has been illustrated in Chapter 4 (see Figure 4.2).

Self–Other Processing, Joint Attention, and the Mirror Network

During infancy, increasing cognitive control enables better-integrated processing of (1) information about infants' own shifts of attention (internal *self-monitoring* of intentional goal-directed attention behavior); (2) information about the related attention behaviors of other people (external *monitoring of others'* attention); and (3) information about the common objects/events of attention (Mundy et al., 2010). This integrated processing of these streams of perception and action leads to differentiated and comparative representations of self and others as senders and receivers of information in social-communicative interactions. One outcome of this may be expected to be increasing conscious self-awareness (Mundy et al., 2010) or self-identification in infancy (Hobson, 2002). A current best guess is that a slow accretion in the dynamic interplay between experience and cognitive neurodevelopment gives rise to the increasing fidelity of self-awareness between 5 and 15 months of age (Kouider et al., 2013). This process presumably leads to the conscious awareness of participating in shared attention with other people, which Tomasello, Carpenter, Call, et al. (2005) have eloquently described as pivotal to the continuum of human development from joint attention to social cognition to cultural cognition.

In addition to increasing differentiation of self–other awareness, the learning-to phase of development also culminates in the gradual internalization of joint attention behaviors as *joint attention mental processes.* The process of internalization of overt perception and action patterns, such as those involved in joint attention, to covert cognitive operations or schemes is a major axis of cognitive development in the 4- to 24-month developmental time frame and beyond (Piaget, 1952). Cognitive internalization involves the capacity to represent a sequence of behavior mentally in order to recall it, examine it, and/or plan it, the better to achieve future goal-related success (e.g., Cruse, 2003).

Internalized representation of behavior theoretically involves frontohippocampal mediation of active patterns of neural activity associated with prior goal-directed behavioral actions as described by Miller and Cohen (2001), with the important addition of frontally mediated bias signals to inhibit the motor activation that initially accompanied the goal-directed behavior (Cruse, 2003; Rizzolatti & Arbib, 1998). That is, cognitive development often involves the increasing executive efficiency of neural execution of what were initially external goal-related behavior patterns, in conjunction with the inhibition of the motor expression of these behaviors. Thus the process of internalization in cognitive development may often involve what are referred to as *mirror neuron* phenomena (Rizzolatti & Arbib, 1998).

The mirror neuron system is thought to involve a distinct class of neurons that internally automatically activate and replicate the action patterns of others, without any other form of explicit neurocognitive mediation. Hypothetically, this allows us to directly understand the behavior and emotions of others (Gallese, Keysers, & Rizzolatti, 2004). However, a less nativist and more dynamic developmental perspective suggests that mirror neuron activation may be part of a generic system of function of translation of behavioral action into the cognitive representation of goal-related action (Cruse, 2003).

Accordingly, mirror neuron phenomena may be generic correlates of thinking, when *thinking* is conceptualized as the ability to mentally represent (mentalize) goal-directed actions without fully engaging in their associated motor patterns. This process plays a role in the internalization of joint attention behaviors, wherein children can begin to think about episodes of convergent and divergent attention with others without the *in vivo* experience of convergent or divergent attention with other people. This is likely to involve neural network activations that have been engaged in past overt joint attention behaviors, but with inhibition of the overt motor components of those behaviors. Thus theory should antici-pate some overlap between mirror neuron phenomena and the neural networks involved in covert mental joint attention functions.

Self-Awareness and Learning from Joint Attention

As internalized and self-aware joint attention blossoms, the learning-from phase of joint attention becomes more prominent. For example, in word learning, it is likely that toddlers need not as frequently track the atten-tion of another person to objects in the environment to engage in refer-ential mapping. As they can increasingly maintain an accurate representa-tion of the environment in memory, they should be able to use working memory to map information about the attention of others onto their cog-nitive map of the environment to map a word to an object. Hence we may expect to see a decrease in gaze following, or a decrease in the relations between gaze following and referential mapping, with age in novel word-learning paradigms.

In this phase, infants may also appear to begin using their own past or present experience of visual attention to make inferences about other people's attention capacities. As noted in Chapter 4, evidence here includes the elegant demonstrations of Meltzoff and Brooks (2008) that 18-month-olds appreciate the meaning of eye gaze in following the attention of others, rather than head direction, to a greater extent than 12-month-olds do. The older infants do not follow the head turn and "gaze direction" of a blindfolded social partner, but 12-month-olds do. However, if infants are given experience with blindfolds, memory for that infor-mation can be integrated into a joint attention trial so that they change their behavior in the context of a blindfolded partner and do not follow their head turns. Hence the 12-month-olds can learn information from self-referenced attention that enables them to make better interpretations of social perceptions in a possible joint attention episode. This learning from self with extrapolation or projection to explain the behavior of oth-ers is called *simulation* (Gordon, 1986). Theory and evidence suggest that the medial prefrontal cortex plays a significant role in simulation, and that simulation plays a significant role in social-cognitive development (Mitchell, Banaji, & Macrae, 2005).

The role of joint attention in social-cognitive mentalizing, however, may be best illustrated by the unique studies of Lee et al. (1998). Lee et al. (1998) reported four experiments comparing the ability of 2-, 3-, 4-, and 5-year-olds to make social-cognitive inferences about the desires of a social agent. In each experiment, a social agent (e.g., "Larry") was depicted on multiple trials as looking at four to six objects. Three different questions were asked of child research participants: "Where is Larry looking?" or "What is Larry looking at?", or the desire inference question, "What does Larry want?"

The results indicated that 4- and 5-year-olds could respond to the desire inference question, but younger children could not when the task involved a static picture of Larry's gaze direction in Experiments 1–3. However, younger children correctly answered questions about where and what Larry looked at. In the fourth experiment, though, video of the social agent's moving his gaze to a target was presented, and in this context 3- and even 2-year-olds demonstrated the capacity for mentalizing and correctly thinking about Larry's desires.

Lee et al. (1998) interpreted their findings to indicate that young children use eye gaze as well as pointing and head direction as directional cues to infer another's desire. That is, young children use attention cues as part of their decoding of the intentional states of others. Lee et al. (1998) were careful to say that attentional cues do not in and of themselves reveal the mental states of others. However, they play a vital role in social-cognitive mentalizing when processed in combination with other aspects of cognition, such as simulation or memory of one's own experience or goals in similar states of attention. Moreover, Lee et al.'s (1998) data indicated that the quality of the information about others' attention that is needed to contribute to mentalizing probably becomes more subtle or abstract over age and development. Four-year-olds could infer mental state from attention information provided in static pictures, whereas 2-year-olds still required the greater perceptual authenticity of eye movement video information.

A Functional Appraisal of the Joint Attention Neural Network

In summary, joint attention in infancy involves sharing attention and experiences with others. The reciprocal adoption of sender (IJA) and receiver (RJA) roles across episodes of sharing experience of common referents contributes to the mental capacity to simulate and/or represent what others may experience, based on attention to and information processing of a referent. However, it is expected that the role of joint attention in social-cognitive development is not limited to visual information. It also involves experience shared across socially coordinated auditory, gustatory, olfactory, and/or tactile attention and information processing (e.g., Nuku & Bekkering, 2008; Rossano, Carpenter, & Tomasello, 2012; Werner & Kaplan, 1963). Joint attention theory posits that with development, social-cognitive mentalizing builds on and incorporates joint attention processes, such that mentalizing often involves representing the episodic point of reference and attention of others, and what experience or information the others are likely to have encoded.

Admittedly, the conjectures above offer only one of several possible explanations for why joint attention and social-cognitive mentalizing may share common neural network support. Nevertheless, I believe that this rationale has a sufficient foundation in theory and evidence to support including the dimension of joint attention and related developmental theory in the next generation of models of typical and atypical human social-cognitive neuroscience. This is because joint attention theory raises the idea that *human social cognition is a class of functions, all of which are based on the dynamic development of neurocognitive networks for the goal-directed integration of self–other information processing.* In particular, joint attention may be regarded as a function of the interaction among three neural control networks. These include the default system, which is engaged in self-referenced processing; the dorsal attention system, which is engaged in the processing of information about other people; and a frontoparietal network, which allows for parallel and integrated processing of both sources of information in social interaction. Before I provide a review of these neural control networks in relation to joint attention theory, I present some of the specifics about the nature of self- and other-referenced processing addressed in this theory.

Throughout this volume, I have highlighted that the early development of joint attention involves the practice of parallel and ultimately integrated processing of interoceptive information (internally referenced) about one's own attention; exteroceptive information (externally referenced information) about another person's attention; and information about a common referent that exists physically or abstractly beyond the dyad. Moreover, the individual's processing of information about the common referent includes three types of information: sensory-perceptual or representational information concerning the characteristics of the common referent; proprioceptive and interoceptive information about the individual's experience of the common referent; and the person's experience of sharing attention and information processing with a social partner.

Interoception describes sensitivity to physiological information originating within the body, such as heart rate, respiration, autonomic arousal, respiration, and emotional states. *Proprioception* involves sensitivity to the position, location, orientation, and movement of the body. This includes monitoring of goal-directed body movements. The anterior insula is one important node of the neural systems involved in processing interoceptive information, and the dorsal medial prefrontal cortex, the ACC, and the parietal cortex play important roles in proprioceptive information processing about one's own goal-directed movement and orientation. These cortical systems also may be primary in integrating these two dimensions to yield adaptive, conscious, self-referenced human information processing (Craig, 2009; Balslev & Miall, 2008; Uddin & Menon, 2009). Another specific hypothesis stemming from comparative research is that the integration of interoception and proprioception may be more elaborated in humans via the von Economo neurons of the ACC than it is in in other primates and mammals (Allman et al., 2010; Craig, 2009).

In contrast to self-referenced information processing, *exteroception* describes the processing of information about the environment, including social partners, that is separate from the body. In addition to the primary sensory cortex, cortical networks in the parietal, temporal, and frontal lobes are thought to support the social-cognitive subclass of exteroception that involves processing of spatial/postural, behavioral, vocal, and affect-related information arising from other people (Decety & Sommerville, 2003; Emery, 2000; Northoff et al., 2006). Although partially overlapping, the self- and other-referenced information-processing networks are distinct. One idea is that developmental articulation of these systems both reflects and promotes the psychological differentiation of self from other in early development (cf. Decety & Sommerville, 2003; Northoff et al., 2006).

A previous discussion of the role of self- and other-referenced processing in the development of joint attention (Mundy, 2003) emphasized proprioceptive processes, but not interoceptive processes. A follow-up paper more explicitly elaborated and described the dual nature of proprioceptive and interoceptive self-referenced information processing in joint attention (Mundy et al., 2010). This included a discussion of the role of processing information about the arousal and positive, negative, or neutral valence of each participant's perceptions of the object or event, and the act of sharing attention, during joint attention. The general point made was that joint attention and shared reference engage as much self-referenced processing of internal sensory and affective experiences, as they do cognitive processing of other people's behavior or intentions. Hence joint attention theory emphasizes the need to study the dynamic interplay of self- and other-referenced information processing in the typical development of social-cognitive mentalizing, as well as its development in ASD (Mundy et al., 2010).

Of course, many important social behaviors involve integrated processing of self- and other-referenced information, such as empathy, facial emotional processing, imitation, and others. Each of these dimensions of behavior serves an important function in the complex development of social cognition. With repeated experience and practice with each function, the associated neural networks become increasingly consolidated and efficient. If the behaviors serve the same or very similar functions, the neural networks involved, and the associated biobehavioral developmental processes, may be expected to be the same (or nearly so). However, to the degree that there are goal-related functional differences between behaviors, their neurodevelopment and biobehavioral developmental processes are likely to differ in significant ways.

I, and many others before me, have argued that joint attention provides us with a window onto the development of a specific function of the human mind. That function is referential cognition. *Reference* in this context is the capacity to share or direct the attention and thoughts of other people with respect to a specific object or event in space, time, and/or our own minds. The capacity for shared reference is essential to human learning and language development. Sharing reference is also critical to the developmental continuity between joint attention and mature social cognition. We engage in mental referential processes (internalized joint attention) whenever we try to infer where other persons are directing their attention and thoughts. Often this type of inference is based on memory about where the other persons have previously directed their attention or thoughts. It also often involves integrating information about what we or others commonly experience in similar episodes of directed attention and thought. These internalized, joint-attention-related referential thought processes are essential to what is commonly referred to as *mentalizing* in social cognition.

Other important social behavior dimensions (face processing, imitation, empathy, etc.) do not involve the same functional level or quality of referential information processing. Therefore, they are not as formative in the cultivation of neural networks and functions associated with the internalized mental capacity for reference. There is no intent or need to argue that joint attention is more important than another dimension in social-cognitive development. However, it is important to recognize the significant developmental continuity among joint attention, the referential mind, language, and social cognition. To exclude joint attention from our models of social-cognitive development, or to relegate it to a subdomain of face processing, may not be valid; it may even be counterproductive in developmental science and in the science of ASD.

A marked difference in referential mental processes is characteristic of autism spectrum development, and we can observe the development of this difference with joint attention measures, language (especially deictic language) measures, and social-cognitive measures. It is difficult, though, to disentangle the essential nature of the referential process differences within the complexity of measure of language or social-cognitive processes. It may be simpler, though by no means easy, to peer more clearly and deeply into the nature of this axis of human nature and the human nature of ASD through a more intensive neurodevelopmental examination of specific types of joint attention behavior development across the lifespan. This focus within the science of ASD has only just begun. With all appropriate caution, due to the early days of this aspect of science, the next section of the chapter examines hypotheses about the functions of nodes of the joint attention/referential mind neural networks that may be better understood with future research.

The Model of Three Neural Control Networks

As outlined above, the current theory of joint attention is most at home with a model of the three superordinate brain networks that interact in the development of cognition (Spreng et al., 2013; see Figure 7.9). Again, these include the default network, which supports internal or self-referenced attention and cognition, and the dorsal attention system, which serves external and other-referenced attention and cognition. A third network—the frontoparietal control or executive network—serves to prioritization activation, inhibition, or integrated processing across the dorsal and default systems in a context- or goal-directed fashion.

The default and dorsal attention systems show little evidence of mutually positive activation connectivity, but they may directly conflict with or inhibit functions of the opposing network. Alternatively, the frontoparietal network has positive connectivity with both the default and dorsal attention networks. Hypothetically, the frontoparietal network can bring components of both the default and dorsal networks actively to bear in information processing, either simultaneously or rapidly sequentially. The goal-related deactivation of the default network and activation of the dorsal network to best meet external task demands is often envisioned as a primary function of cognitive control (Persson, Lustig, Nelson, & Reuter-Lorenz, 2007).

In this regard, though, it is noteworthy that Spreng et al. (2013) have identified *three different* types of nodes within the frontoparietal network: default-network-aligned nodes, dorsal-network-aligned nodes, and *dually aligned nodes*. All three types of nodes are thought to play a dynamic gatekeeping role in the balance of activating and inhibiting the default and dorsal networks in goal-directed attention and cognition. That is, they operate to mediate the adaptive equilibrium between internally and externally focused attention and cognition from moment to moment, to address different tasks most effectively across different contexts. Regarding the

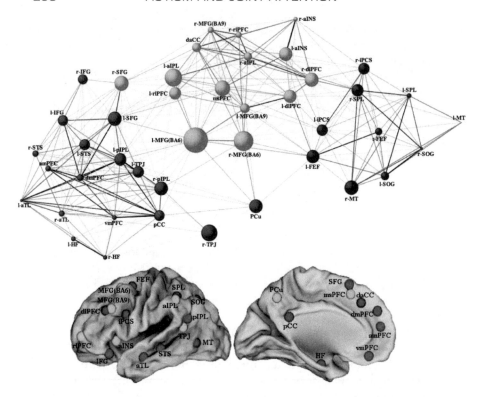

FIGURE 7.9. An illustration of the three cortical control networks described by Spreng and colleagues. amPFC, anterior medial prefrontal cortex; aTL, anterior temporal lobe; dmPFC, dorsal medial prefrontal cortex; HF, hippocampal formation; IFG, inferior frontal gyrus; pCC, posterior cingulate cortex; pIPL, posterior inferior parietal lobule; PCu, precuneus PCu; SFG, superior frontal gyrus; STS, superior temporal sulcus; TPJ, temporal parietal junction; vmPFC, ventral medial prefrontal cortex; FEF, frontal eye fields; iPCS, inferior precentral sulcus; MT, middle temporal motion complex; SOG, superior occipital gyrus; SPL, superior parietal lobule; aIPL, Anterior inferior parietal lobule; aINS, anterior insula aINS; daCC, dorsal anterior cingulate cortex daCC; dlPFC, dorsolateral prefrontal cortex; msPFC, medial superior prefrontal cortex; MFG (BA 6), middle frontal gyrus Brodmann's Area 6; MFG (BA 9), middle frontal gyrus Brodmann's Area 9; rlPFC, rostrolateral prefrontal cortex. From Spreng, Sepulcre, Turner, Stevens, and Schacter (2013). Copyright 2013 by The MIT Press. Reprinted by permission.

development of these network nodes, Spreng et al. (2013) note: "Evidence suggests that patterns of intrinsic connectivity are sculpted by a history of repeated task-driven coactivation of brain regions, which in turn facilitates efficient coupling within task-relevant networks during future task performance" (p. 82).

Table 7.1 provides an integration of the Spreng et al. (2013) model of superordinate brain systems of cognitive development with the results of several studies of the neurodevelopment of joint attention in infants and adults. Recognition of the current power and methodological limits of this small set of studies notwithstanding, the pattern of observations across the studies leads to a set of conjectures that may guide future research.

The first thing that struck me when composing Table 7.1 was that the three studies of the neurodevelopment of joint attention in the first 6 months of life all emphasized the role of cortical activation associated with the default and frontoparietal control networks (Spreng et al., 2013). It is also the case that the four diagnostic group comparative studies in Table 7.1 (Mizuno et al., 2011; Mosconi, Cody-Hazlett, et al., 2009; Pelphrey et al., 2005; Redcay, Dodell-Feder, et al., 2013) emphasize the role of differences in default and frontoparietal control network activation in differences between joint attention in ASD and in typical development. This is consistent with the idea that there may be important (but as yet poorly identified) links between anomalous default and frontoparietal control network development, and pivotal clinical and phenotypic differences in joint attention, in the development of ASD (Mundy, 2003; Mundy et al., 2010).

I have argued here and elsewhere that the lack of responsiveness to other people in ASD has led to an overemphasis in conceptualizations of autism on differences in attention to others, and too little emphasis on differences in self-referenced processing. This may be especially true in research and theory on joint attention and social cognition (Mundy, 2003; Mundy et al., 2010; Mundy & Jarrold, 2010). This idea is expressed, in part, in the concept of *inside-out social learning* in the development of joint attention. Inside-out learning is based on the assumption that there is a relatively large amount of self-referenced information available in early development, and that this plays a role in joint attention and social-cognitive development. In particular, the simulation or extrapolation of current or encoded self-referenced information to other people plays a significant role in the cognitive development of joint attention and understanding reference (Mundy et al., 2009). These ideas match well with evidence for the role of the default network in joint attention development and for differences in this area in autism spectrum development.

TABLE 7.1. Joint Attention Neural Network Components Identified in Studies from Infancy through Adulthood

Study	Developmental period	Type of joint attention	Neural system	Control network
Grossman & Johnson (2010)	5 months	RJA	Medial dorsal frontal	Default or FPC
Elison et al. (2013)	6 months	RJA	Connectivity: Temporal, amygdala, insula, orbital, ventromedial, frontal	Default & FPC
Lloyd-Fox et al. (2011)	5 months	RJA	PFC and temporoparietal	Default & FPC
Grossman et al. (2007)	12 months	RJA	MPFC, parietal	Default & FPC
Caplan et al. (1993)	13+ months	IJA	dMPFC	Default
Mundy et al. (2000)	14 months	IJA & RJA	dMPFC (BA 8)	Default & FPC
Henderson et al. (2002)	14 months	IJA (pointing)	dMPFC; orbital and dorsolateral frontal temporal cortex	Default, FPC, & dorsal attn.
Kühn-Popp et al. (2015)	15 months	IJA (pointing)	Medial frontal and dorsal central EEG coherence	Default, dorsal attn.
Mosconi, Cody-Hazlett, et al. (2009)	18+ months (TD vs. ASD)	IJA & RJA	Amygdala size	Default
Greene et al. (2011)	Children (TD vs. ASD)	RJA	Inferior frontal gyrus, middle frontal gyrus, middle temporal gyrus, occipital gyrus, supramarginal gyrus, superior temp. gyrus	Default & FPC
Vaidya et al. (2011)	Children (TD vs. ASD)	RJA	Superior temp. sulcus, ACC, striatal/caudate, dorsolateral frontal	Default, FPC, dorsal attn.

(continued)

TABLE 7.1. *(continued)*

Study	Developmental period	Type of joint attention	Neural system	Control network
Brunetti et al. (2014)	Adults	IJA (pointing)	dMPFC (ACC, temporoparietal cortex)	Dorsal attn., default, FPC
Williams et al. (2005)	Adults	RJA	dMPFC (BA 9, 10), cingulate cortex, precuneus (parietal), caudate nucleus	Default, dorsal attn., FPC
Schilbach et al. (2010)	Adults	IJA & RJA	dMPFC, ACC/posterior cingulate, medial orbital PFC, temporal and occipital cortex, striatum/caudate	Default, dorsal attn., FPC
Pfeiffer et al. (2014)	Adults	IJA	Striatal	Motivation & spatial processing of motor movement
Gordon et al. (2013)	Adults	IJA	ACC, right fusiform gyrus, parietal cortex, amygdala, striatum, hippocampus	Dorsal attn., default, FPC,
Caruana et al. (2014)	Adults	IJA & RJA	*Both IJA and RJA:* Temporoparietal juncture, precuneous, inferior frontal gyrus, middle frontal gyrus, middle temporal gyrus *IJA, not RJA:* Supplementary motor cortex, superior frontal gyrus, left temporal pole, thalamus, cerebellum	Default, FPC, dorsal attn.
Redcay et al. (2012)	Adults	IJA & RJA	MPFC, inferior frontal, parietal, ventral orbital frontal, temporal	Dorsal attn., default, FPC

(continued)

TABLE 7.1. *(continued)*

Study	Developmental period	Type of joint attention	Neural system	Control network
Pelphrey et al. (2005)	Adults (ASD vs. TD)	RJA	*TD:* Middle frontal gyrus, ACC, middle and superior temporal gyrus *ASD:* Less superior temporal; more insula, inferior frontal gyrus	Default & FPC
Redcay, Dodell-Feder, et al. (2013)	Adults (ASD vs. TD)	IJA & RJA	*TD > ASD on RJA:* dMPFC, superior temporal cortex *ASD > TD on RJA:* Putamen, fusiform gyrus, middle occipital gyrus *IJA > RJA:* Right anterior insula, left inferior parietal	Default, FPC, face processing, spatial processing
Mizuno et al. (2011)	Adults (ASD vs. TD)	RJA & IJA	*TD > ASD:* Deictic shift; precuneous and insula connectivity	Default & FPC

Note. TD, typical development; ASD, autism spectrum disorder/development; RJA, responding to joint attention; IJA, initiating joint attention; (dM)PFC, (dorsal medial) prefrontal cortex; BA, Brodmann's area; ACC, anterior cingulate cortex; FPC, frontoparietal control.
[a]Control network designations from Spreng et al. (2013).

The Default Network in Social Communication

Buckner, Andrews-Hanna, and Schacter's (2008) insightful synthesis of the research suggests that the default network is active when individuals are engaged in internally focused tasks, including autobiographical memory retrieval, envisioning the future, and *conceiving the perspectives of others*. They mention this last task without allusion to joint attention. They go on to suggest that the medial temporal lobe subsystem provides information from prior experiences in the form of memories and associations that are the building blocks of mental simulation. The medial prefrontal subsystem facilitates the flexible use of this (autobiographical) information during the construction of self-relevant mental simulations. More generally, the default system may be central to spontaneous cognition leading to covert ideation (imagination, planning, thought), and cognition leading to spontaneous behavior but including planned behavior.

This depiction of the functional role of the default network dovetails with the lack of organized spontaneous social behavior and imagination that is characteristic of many young children with ASD (e.g., Brown, Morris, Nida, & Baker-Ward, 2012; Jones et al., 2011). Not surprisingly, Buckner et al. (2008) also noted that differences in the default network may be central to several forms of psychopathology, including ASD.

Several studies have identified associations between autism spectrum development and differences in the default control network. One study observed that activity in medial prefrontal cortical and ventral ACC regions of the default network was reduced in 13 people with ASD relative to controls during tasks in which true–false judgments pertaining to psychological or behavioral characteristics were self-referenced or referenced to a familiar other (Kennedy & Courchesne, 2008).

Three recent reports have observed connections between patterns of activity in the default network and variation in symptom presentation in people with autism spectrum development. Weng et al. (2010) observed that 16 adolescents with ASD and IQs above 85, compared to adolescents with typical development, displayed similar but weaker patterns of connectivity among nodes of the default network. The default nodes in this study included the regions of dorsal and medial prefrontal cortex, temporal cortex and parahippocampal gyrus, retrosplenial cortex, posterior cingulate cortex, and inferior parietal cortex (angular gyrus). Within the group with ASD, poorer social functioning (as measured by parental report on the ADI-R; see Chapter 3) was significantly associated with weaker connectivity among the posterior cingulate, dorsal frontal, temporal, and parahippocampal regions. Weng et al. (2010) also reported that greater local right parietotemporal cortical connectivity in their sample with ASD was associated with evidence of poorer communication development. This pattern of results reminds us that both distal hypoconnectivity and local hyperconnectivity may play a role in ASD (Wass, 2011).

What appears to be a related pattern of findings has been reported by Lynch et al. (2013) in a study of 20 children ages 7–12 with ASD and higher IQs. Lynch et al. also observed evidence of greater hyperconnectivity in the parietal cortical regions of default systems in the children with ASD, compared to age- and IQ-matched control children. Moreover, they observed that greater social symptom intensity (measured with the ADOS) was associated with greater evidence of right-hemisphere local connectivity in the default networks of the sample with ASD. In this case, the critical path of hyperconnectivity was between the right posterior parahippocampal gyrus, left temporal pole, and left lingual gyrus (posterior temporal cortex).

Another study of adolescents with ASD and higher IQs reported a pattern of findings that both diverged from and converged with the results of these studies. Redcay, Moran, et al. (2013) observed little evidence of reduced connectivity in the default control network in a group of 14 higher-IQ adolescents with ASD, compared to adolescents with typical development. But, like Weng et al. (2010) and Lynch et al. (2013), these researchers reported evidence of *greater* parietal centrality (positive and negative connections) in the right-hemisphere default network of the adolescents with ASD. However, greater right-hemisphere connectivity was not associated with symptom presentation. Instead, evidence of less right-hemisphere functional connectivity from parietal to medial prefrontal cortex was associated with poorer Social Affect scores ADOS. This association was strongest for communication items within the Social Affect factor-based scale scores.

Together, Weng et al. (2010) and Lynch et al. (2013) have reported evidence that local hyperconnectivity in the right-hemisphere posterior default network is related to poorer social and communication development in ASD. Comparatively, Weng et al. (2010) and Redcay, Moran, et al. (2013) have also reported evidence that distal hypoconnectivity between the posterior and anterior nodes of the default network is associated with poor social communication in adolescents with ASD. We do not yet know to what degree observations of hypoconnectivity and hyperconnectivity within a control network may be reciprocal or related phenomena. However, the pattern of findings across studies motivates a closer look at this issue.

It is not clear from these studies whether the differences in default connectivity are causes or consequences of social-communicative disturbance in ASD. However, they are consistent in their implication of the default control network in both typical and atypical development of social communication. One specific component of such development associated with the default system appears to be joint attention. Seven studies in Table 7.1 link the default control network and its functions in self-referenced processing, such as interoception, proprioception, and simulation, to the early development of joint attention in both typical children and those who go on to develop ASD. These data are consistent with the theory that medial prefrontal cortical functions are integral to the types of self-referenced cognitive functions that are involved in dynamic development of the triadic self–other–referent processing in joint attention in typical development and autism spectrum development (Mundy, 2003; Mundy et al., 2010; Mundy & Jarrold, 2010).

The data in Table 7.1, and theory (e.g., Mundy, 2003), also specify that the frontoparietal control network may also be involved in early joint attention development. The role of this network in joint attention is considered next.

The Frontoparietal Control Network and Social Communication

Theory suggests that joint attention development involves the capacity to engage in the simultaneous, or very rapidly sequential, processing of both self-referenced and other-referenced information (Mundy et al., 2009; Mundy & Jarrold, 2010). In their model of superordinate neural control networks, Spreng et al. (2013) observe that a frontoparietal control network probably coordinates the interaction between internal or self-referenced processing (default network) and external information processing (dorsal attention), which would include other-referenced information processing. The frontoparietal control network is composed of regions of the superior and middle frontal gyrus, the ACC, the insula cortex, and the anterior inferior parietal cortex, as well as the medial superior parietal cortex or precuneous. This network has distinct nodes aligned with the default and dorsal attention networks. Presumably these play roles in relative activation or inhibition of internal self-referenced and external other-referenced information processing, depending on task-related goals.

Spreng et al. (2013), however, also reported evidence of frontoparietal network nodes that exhibited *dual alignment* with the default and dorsal control networks. Though Spreng et al. (2013) did not specify the function of these dual-alignment nodes, the logic of their model allows for the possibility that these are engaged when balanced or integrated activation of self-referenced and other-referenced processing is required in goal-directed task performance. Social tasks, and especially social communication, may be expected to be among the primary goal-related tasks that benefit from—or, indeed, require—integrated activation of both networks. Early in development, and throughout life, joint attention information processing is thought to place a high demand on this type of integrated processing (Mundy, 2003; Mundy et al., 2009; Mundy & Jarrold, 2010).

More details about such rapid integrated interoceptive (self-referenced) and exteroceptive (other-referenced) processing may be found in recent research and theory. The insula and ACC may be part of a network that serves a primary role in internal and external attention switching and integration (Allman et al., 2010; Menon & Uddin, 2010). Moreover, specific components of the frontoparietal control network (such as the ACC and insula), along with input and output relations with the frontal eye fields, have been recognized as playing a specific role in self–other information processing (Denny, Kober, Wager, & Ochsner, 2012), as well as joint attention development (Mundy, 2003; Mundy et al., 2010; Mundy & Jarrold, 2010).

Seven of the studies reviewed in Table 7.1 reported observations of ACC and/or insula activation associated with joint attention or joint attention differences in ASD. More impressive, perhaps, is a meta-analysis of 39 imaging studies in which Di Martino et al. (2009) reported that the most robust differences in social-cognitive paradigm performance were related to hypoactivation of pregenual ACC and anterior insula in individuals with ASD versus controls. Using an innovative fMRI procedure, one research group reported two studies that mapped ACC activation patterns associated with self-referenced activation during an interpersonal exchange game. They also reported observations from a third study indicating that adults with ASD displayed significantly less activation of these regions of the ACC when playing the game with a social partner (Chiu et al., 2008).

Hopkins and Taglialatela (2013) at the Yerkes National Primate Research Center recently tested the hypothesis that functions of the ACC are vital to joint attention. They did so by examining the morphometry of the ACC in chimpanzees, which either consistently or inconsistently engaged in triadic (referential) attention with human experimenters. They observed that the chimpanzees that performed more poorly on triadic attention tasks had greater ACC grey matter volumes than did those that displayed better triadic attention performance. Hopkins and Taglialatela (2013) concluded that these results provided comparative research support for the role of the ACC in human joint attention; they also suggested that the greater grey matter volumes might reflect lower white matter connectivity between the ACC and other cortical regions in the chimpanzees with poorer triadic attention ability.

Recent morphometric studies of anomalies of the ACC have also revealed that that hyperglutamatergic neurometabolic abnormality of the pregenual ACC may be characteristic of ASD (Bejjani et al., 2012). As mentioned above, the meta-analysis of Di Martino et al. (2009) indicated that relative hypoactivation of the pregenual ACC may be a neural network characteristic of social-cognitive processing in ASD (see also Dichter, Felder, & Bodfish, 2009). Within the frontoparietal control network, the pregenual ACC may play a significant role in learning to differentiate or maintaining differentiation between self-referenced and other-referenced cues (Shad, Brent, & Keshavan, 2011).

An equally important set of observations has recently provided evidence of decreased axon guidance proteins (PLXNA4 and ROBO2) in the ACC of people with ASD (Suda et al., 2011). This observation is important, because the ACC–insula axis of the frontoparietal control network is distinctively characterized by the development of von Economo neurons, the axons of which provide local and distal connectivity of the ACC–insula axis with other brain regions. These neurons are unique to postnatal development, appearing in the 36th week after conception and increasing during the first 8 months after birth (Allman et al., 2010). This characteristic makes the von Economo neurons amenable to a characteristic of intrinsic connectivity in control networks that Spreng et al. (2013) describe as "sculpted by a history of repeated task-driven co-activation of brain regions, which in turn facilitates efficient coupling within task-relevant networks during future task performance" (p. 80).

In this regard, Simms, Kemper, Timbie, Bauman, and Blatt (2009) observed that among nine individuals with autism spectrum development, three had significantly increased density of von Economo neurons in the ACC and six had reduced density, relative to controls. In a more recent study, Uppal et al. (2014) did not observe significant differences between individuals with ASD and controls, but did observe that the numbers of von Economo neurons and pyramidal neurons in layer V of the ACC were correlated with historical records of ADI-R symptom presentation in 4- to 8-year-olds affected by ASD (but not 13- to 21-year-olds).

The work of Spreng et al. (2013), and many others, suggests that the frontoparietal control network is complex. Therefore, it is risky to focus on one or the other component in ascribing a role to this network in autism spectrum development. Yet, at this point in our science, it may still be useful to note that the literature over the last decade points to the hypothesis that the ACC and insula may play an as yet poorly understood role in ASD (e.g., Allman et al., 2010; Mizuno et al., 2011; Uddin & Menon, 2009). In particular, it may play a role in joint attention development in ASD (Mundy, 2003). The risk here is to miscommunicate the suggestion that we should consider the "ACC hypothesis of ASD." It's probably best to explicitly avoid that type of region-of-interest framing of the issue. The goal here is to only to suggest some functional details with respect to a possible role of the ACC in the complex network of neurodevelopmental differences that we are beginning to understand as characteristic of autism spectrum development.

Summary and Conclusions

My 2003 paper concluded with a statement of the obvious: "The study of autism presents an enormously complex puzzle and, unfortunately, several of the pieces critical to the solution of the puzzle seem to be missing at this time" (Mundy, 2003, p. 805). The thesis of that paper was that the dorsal medial prefrontal cortex and ACC may play a role in the capacity to monitor proprioceptive information concerning self-action and to integrate this self-related information with exteroceptive perceptual information about the behavior of other people. A disturbance in these functions was hypothesized to be linked with the atypical development of intersubjectivity, joint attention, and social cognition that may impair the lives of people with autism. Thus impairment in the development of the dorsal medial prefrontal–ACC system may constitute a neural substrate for social-cognitive deficits in autism (Mundy, 2003).

Since that paper was published, several possible missing pieces of the puzzle related to the study of intersubjectivity and joint attention in autism spectrum development may have been found, or at least finding them may be on the horizon. The dorsal medial prefrontal cortex and ACC may be important in autism spectrum development, but only as part of the dynamic functions of a larger system of neural networks (cf. Devinsky & Luciano, 1993). The emergence of a neuroscience of joint attention and related deictic functions (e.g., Mizuno et al., 2011) provides one significant source of information to enable us to envision not only that larger system of neural networks, but their functional development and impact from infancy to adulthood.

What we see today includes the possibility of a subcortical–amygdalar–frontal network that potentiates the organization and development of joint attention in the first 6 months of life. It does so through the eye contact effect and the role of mutual gaze in arousing interest in attending to other people (Senju & Johnson, 2009). As volitional control of attention increases after 2 months of age, this early neurocognitive self-organizing mechanism increases the likelihood that when novelty draws the attention of infants to objects in the world, they will shift attention back to a social partner. So begins the development of joint attention. In addition to contributing to the organization of early joint attention development, the subcortical–amygdalar–frontal eye contact effect network plays a lifelong role in factors involved in stimulating information processing, encoding, and learning in the context of joint attention.

To learn from joint attention, though, requires more than a boost to information processing. It also requires the development of a complex executive system that enables humans to rapidly process and compare multiple strands of self-referenced and other-referenced information, in conjunction with information from a third focus of attention shared between two or more people. This type of information processing is effortful and takes years to become fully efficient. It emerges in the context of, and is dependent upon, maturational advances in the speed of information processing and working memory. However, it is not defined by those processes, important though they may be. Rather, the executive efficiency of joint attention engagement is defined by components of the development of a parietal–temporal–insula system *and* a dorsal medial prefrontal–ACC system, both of which enable the increasingly rapid integration of self, other, and object (triadic) information processing during social interactions. I should note that the relevant literature is beginning to suggest that a focus on the ACC in this network may be too limited, since there is reason to believe that functions of the posterior cingulate are involved as well (Leech & Sharp, 2014; Lynch et al., 2013).

The frequent and rapid integration of self-referenced and other-referenced processing is necessary, though not sufficient, to prompt the development of a cognitive mechanism for fluently adopting a common frame of references with others. Once the experience of a common frame becomes easy to establish and maintain, self–other comparative informa-tion processing and awareness of shifts between sender and receiver roles during the exchange of information about the common reference may occur. Subsequently, it even becomes possible to shift points of reference multiple times in the course of extended social-communicative interac-tions. This neurocognitive capacity to adopt a common point of reference with another, and to recognize when we have not adopted a common frame of reference, is essential to language learning and social-cognitive development. It begins in interactions involving a common referent in the world, but gradually becomes internalized as a mental capacity for shared reference, or deixis (e.g., Bruner, 1995). Differences in the initial phases and internalization of this dimension of human cognition are significant features of the path of human nature we describe with the label ASD. I think we need to know much more about the development of the neuro-cognitive system for joint attention to understand typical development, as well as to understand autism spectrum development.

Much of what has been described in this chapter is consistent with the conclusions of the NIMH RDoC Social Process Workshop Proceedings of February 27–28, 2012 (published online at *www.nimh.nih.gov/research-priorities/rdoc/social-processes-workshop-proceedings.shtml*). The workshop group members noted that social processes appear to be supported by the "default," "social," or "self" network and exteroceptive other-referenced processing, which they suggested is related to "action perception." How-ever, the group noted that the degree to which these networks are specific or separable was unclear at that time, and especially that it might not be possible to study them separately at all developmental time points.

The workshop group members went on to note that for the RDoC matrix, they focused on tasks that can reliably discriminate between the two networks. "However, the group also noted that this is not the only one way of studying these questions/constructs [related to the nature of social processes]. There may be tasks that jointly recruit multiple circuits, and they may be more interesting and/or ecologically valid" (p. 12). I couldn't agree more. I would add that joint attention epitomizes a dimen-sion that recruits multiple circuits (including cognitive control circuits), and that its measurement has relatively strong ecological validity in the study of social-communicative and social-cognitive development within the autism spectrum. Because of this characteristic, it may not be best to couch joint attention as a task that measures processes associated with one network (face processing) or another (action perception). Rather, it involves the phylogenetic and ontogenetic integration, synthesis, and ultimately redescription of the neural functions of these networks, to yield a higher-order neurocognitive social process. This social process is not as robustly observed in other animals, or is best studied with paradigms that implicitly reduce it to functions of one network or another.

Chapter 8

The Genetics of Joint Attention and Joint Engagement

An impressive amount of progress has been made in understanding autism in the last three to four decades. Much of this has taken the form of eliminating the types of simple explanatory models that tend to populate thinking at the starting point of any science. Simple models that describe autism as a developmental cascade from a single, circumscribed cause have been very difficult to verify. This is true regardless of whether the cause has been framed in terms of a single set of genes, neural networks, sensory/perceptual factors, psychological processes, or teratogenic environmental effects (including the iatrogenic effects of vaccines). We now understand that basic linear models of autism, where X leads inevitably to Y, do not provide the answer to the puzzle, even though their simplicity remains alluring.

Simple models do not apply, because we are trying to understand a particular path of human development—the autism path—and all paths of human development are dynamically complex. Just as human development is variable, the effects of autism on development are variable. Hence the development of autism can take many forms and is characterized by a *spectrum of developmental outcomes* that probably arise from related but not identical assemblages of genetic and epigenetic factors across individuals (e.g., Yuen et al., 2015).

Yet, even though autism syndrome development may arise from different combinations of factors, we can still perceive significant developmental commonalities across individuals. We can reliably observe the outline of a fuzzy but valid category of individuals who share a cluster of common phenotypic characteristics of human development. At the mildest detectable levels of characteristics of autism spectrum development, we refer to the *broad autism phenotype* (BAP), mentioned in earlier chapters. At the strongest levels, these characteristics are associated with significantly maladaptive outcomes and attenuations of quality of life. To identify this group we use the term *autism spectrum disorder* (ASD), to designate the need for therapeutic assistance to improve the quality of life for affected individuals. The implications of the term *disorder*, though, can be problematic.

It is possible for some people with higher levels of autism syndrome characteristics to experience very adaptive outcomes, either by way of systematically supportive environments in childhood (e.g., treatment), or through combinations of constitutional and environmental processes yet unknown. Yet they may clearly continue to display the characteristics of the autism syndrome. We think this may be because in some admixtures of human development, it is possible for characteristics of autism spectrum development—such as the tendency to pursue an idea or perception of the world very persistently—to give rise to thinking and motivation in some people that provides positive value not only to these individuals, but also to the community and culture at large. A prominent example here is the contribution of Temple Grandin to large-animal husbandry and the ethics of animal care. For this reason, among others, we will need to take great care with the exercise of precision medicine that may become possible in the next decades, based on the advances in the genetics of autism. To paraphrase Grandin (1995), in an ideal world scientists should find a method to prevent the most severe forms of autism, but allow the milder forms to survive. After all, the milder forms represent integral and valued aspects of human nature. They may be expressed in the less social but perseverative and single-minded paths of human lives that contribute great value to society in problem solving, science, and art.

The many complexities of autism spectrum development demand that we continue to refine our creative concepts and research to define the details of its common characteristics, even as they may be fluid and significantly change across the developmental course. Whatever its genesis or pathogenesis, we know that complex metabolic and neural systems of autism affect a finite number of pathways along which individual differences in viable human mental development can be expressed. We must cultivate research efforts that are more focused on examining the nature and genesis of each of these final common pathways or dimensions of mental development, so as to be able to create a clarified picture of the complex nature of autism (Cuthbert & Insel, 2013; Lord & Jones, 2012).

In this book, I have argued that one of these mental pathways or dimensions may be measured and conceptualized in terms of the development of joint attention in infancy *and its elaboration across the lifespan in human social cognition and social affiliation.* This is not a new claim (e.g., Mundy, 1995, 2003; Mundy & Sigman, 2006), but one that has (I hope) been elaborated here more fully and effectively than previously.

Like many others, I think that understanding the nature of joint attention involves conceiving of a broad dimension of social processes—a dimension that provides a bridge across concepts and theory on motivation, communication, and social cognition (e.g., Fuchs & De Jaegher, 2009; Hobson, 2002; Tomasello, Carpenter, Call, et al., 2005; Trevarthen, 1979; Tronick, 2005). Consequently, joint attention theory helps us to understand more fully how motivation, social attention coordination, and social cognition interact to play a role in the human nature of the social learning and social affect/engagement axes of ASD from infancy to adulthood (Mundy & Sigman, 2006; Mundy et al., 2009).

Joint Attention/Joint Engagement, Motivation, and Molecules

The dimension of joint attention is multifaceted, although its name, perhaps unfortunately, suggests that it should be operationally defined simply in terms of measures of orienting. Joint attention clearly involves mechanisms of orienting and attention allocation. However, from its inception, it has been as much about social information processing, social learning, and social cognition as it has been about orienting. Joint attention is a cognitive mechanism involved in the integrated processing of self-referenced and other-referenced information, as well as information about a common physical or mental referent. In short, joint attention is central to the lifetime development of the human propensity to engage in high-level *socially collaborative attention, cognition, and communication.*

Recall from Chapter 5 that another facet of joint attention involves social motivation. In terms of goal-related behavior, this has often been viewed as the human biobehavioral drive to experience the cognitive–emotional state of intersubjectivity with other people (Fuchs & De Jaegher, 2009; Hobson, 2002; Mundy et al., 1992; Mundy & Sigman, 2006; Tomasello, Carpenter, Call, et al. 2005; Trevarthen, 1979; Tronick, 2005). It is this aspect of theory that has begun to lend itself to guiding research about the genetic influences on joint attention development.

Theory has suggested that joint attention may be most specifically associated with two sets of molecular mechanisms and their genetic regulators. One involves promoting focused attention in order to engage in goal-related learning and information processing. An earlier paper (Mundy, 2003) recognized that this set of mechanisms and regulators

probably includes dopaminergic systems of reward regulation for directing attention for learning, especially as these involve ACC regulation of
choice and initiation of movement toward goal-related behaviors (e.g.,
Gray, 1987; Allman et al., 2010; Holroyd & Coles, 2002).

The other system involves the neuropeptide beta-endorphin and the
pentapeptide metenkephalin (Mundy, 1995). This proposal was based
on Sahley and Panksepp's (1987) theory of the role these peptides may
play in initiating social approach and engagement behaviors early in typical development, and in the attenuation of these behaviors in autism.
Contemporary research continues to show that these peptides may be
involved in the mediation of reward for social engagement, especially
as they are involved in systems of the nucleus accumbens (e.g., Trezza,
Damsteegt, Achterberg, & Vanderschuren, 2011). However, more recent
interest in the role of peptides in the application of social motivation
theory in autism and joint attention has shifted to examining the role of
the neurohypophyseal nonapeptides, oxytocin and vasopressin, in social
engagement (Stavropoulos & Carver, 2013).

A term most descriptive of functions of the social motivation facet
of joint attention was coined some time ago by Bakeman and Adamson
(1984): *joint engagement.* In this regard, joint attention is motivated by
a prosocial appetitive drive to engage with others to share information
and experience (Mundy, 1995), which is expressed in acts of joint attention across the life span (Mundy & Acra, 2006; Mundy & Sigman, 2006).
The recognition of this joint engagement function is well recognized in
the development of targeted intervention to improve joint attention in
children with ASD. Hence the name of the intervention currently most
steeped in joint attention theory is Joint Attention, Symbolic Play *Engagement* and Regulation (JASPER; Kasari et al., 2008; Kasari, Lawton, et al.,
2014; see Chapter 6). For the sake of brevity, the multiple facets of the
joint attention and joint engagement latent construct are referred to as
the JAJE dimension for the remainder of this chapter.

The motivation perspective on joint attention described over the
last few years shares many concepts with other formulations of a social
motivation theory of ASD (e.g., Chevallier et al., 2012: Dawson, Webb,
& McPartland, 2005). However, it also differs in several important ways.
First, it does not assume that differences in motivation systems provide a
full or satisfactory explanation of the nature or impact of the differences
in joint attention development that characterize children with ASD. Second, it does not assume that the motivational component of joint attention in autism spectrum development, or other paths of human development, can be precisely examined with any and all measures of reward
sensitivity (e.g., Neuhaus, Beauchaine, & Bernier, 2010). Rather, in joint
attention theory the motivation is conceptualized in terms of the reward

value of positive social engagement, especially as this is involved in sharing information (social learning), sharing experience (affiliation), and sharing intentions with others (e.g., Kim et al., 2014; Tomasello, Carpenter, Call, et al., 2005).

This conceptualization corresponds with theory on the role of motivation in human communication and language development. These theories converge on the notion that both joint attention and language development result from the evolution of a link between the corticostriatal learning system and a subcortical social motivation neural network (Syal & Finlay, 2011). They both involve the hypothesis that dopaminergic-related genetic variation may play a role in differences in language learning and development (e.g., Wong, Morgan-Short, Ettlinger, & Zheng, 2012) and in the learning and development of joint attention (Liu et al., 2011; Mundy, 2003) in the autism syndrome. The motivation account of JAJE is thus important for many reasons, not the least of which is that it raises specific hypotheses about genetic and molecular influences on joint attention development.

The Genetics of JAJE: An Overview

Joint attention is a cognitive facility that is conserved in varying qualitative and quantitative levels across different species, such as nonhuman primates, dogs, ravens, and dolphins. In mammals, joint attention appears to serve a common set of cognitive and social functions: It affects learning and collaborative behavior through the enhanced capacity of individuals to adopt a common frame of reference and share information with others, and/or to monitor other conspecifics' information processing about that referent (Bugnyar, Stöwe, & Heinrich, 2004; Gong & Shuai, 2012; Janik, 2013; MacLean & Hare, 2012; Soproni, Miklósi, Topál, & Csányi, 2001).

The observation of common adaptive cognitive-behavioral homologies across species raises the possibility that there are identifiable genes, or gene complexes, that influence the development of similar behaviors in different species (Reaume & Sokolowski, 2011). If so, then JAJE has the potential to contribute to the understanding of the metabolic and molecular pathogenesis of autism spectrum development. This potential is bolstered by the observation that our national research network already possesses large genetic databases, as well as the measures of variability in JAJE provided in Modules 1 and 2 of the ADOS (see Chapter 3). To motivate the exploitation of this combination of archival data, let us consider the scant but thought-provoking evidence to date on the genetics of joint attention.

Observations of the conserved nature of joint attention across species raise fundamental and stimulating questions about the dimension of joint attention. Are individual differences in joint attention heritable? If so, what metabolic (e.g., genetic) and molecular (e.g., neurotransmitter) factors influence these differences? Answers could contribute to a better understanding of the genetics of autism and other disorders character- ized by social-cognitive differences. Of course, the veridical identification of the genetics of mental differences and disorders is a monumental task. Many genes (perhaps 1,000 or more), interacting with each other, the epigenome, and the environment, are likely to be involved in the devel- opment of many if not most disorders, such as ASD (De Rubeis et al., 2014; Geschwind, 2011) and schizophrenia (Bilder, Howe, Novak, Sabb, & Parker, 2011).

So we cannot reasonably expect that an understanding of the genet- ics of joint attention will be tantamount to a full understanding of the genetics of ASD. Among the great strengths of the RDoC model (see Chapter 2), though, is that it encourages a circumscribed but targeted approach to research on the genetic bases of major forms of psychopa- thology. Describing the genetics of important individual dimensions of a syndrome will ultimately inform the genetic picture of the full syndrome. In research on autism, one path is to understand the genetic ontology of major dimensions of the cognitive phenotype of autism (e.g., Bilder et al., 2011; Lu, Yoon, Geschwind, & Cantor, 2013), specifically including joint attention (e.g., Liu et al., 2011; Stavropoulos & Carver, 2013). Lu et al. (2013) have referred to this approach as *quantitative trait locus* (QTL) studies. Alternatively, Bilder et al. (2011) have referred to this approach as investigations of *intermediate cognitive phenotypes*.

Although this research is in its very early stages of development, theory currently points most obviously to two families of genes that may influence joint attention development. One involves the DRD1 dopamine receptors and DRD2 receptor family (DRD2, DRD3, and DRD4), and per- haps the dopamine transporter gene (DAT) and the dopamine-tempering gene (COMT) as well. The other family involves the nanopeptide hor- mone receptor genes OXTR (oxytocin receptor) and AVPR1A and AVPR2 (arginine vasopressin receptors). The oxytocin and dopamine receptors may be expected to interact in effects related to social motivation and behavior, because the oxytocinergic circuit innervates the ventral tegmen- tal area and dopaminergic neurons that project to the nucleus accumbens of the striatum (Baskerville & Douglas, 2010).

QTL Linkage and Joint Attention

Lu et al. (2013) have outlined three criteria that need to be met in QTL studies of ASD. To qualify as valid for study, a quantitative trait such as

JAJE must (1) display evidence that the trait is heritable, (2) exhibit variation in individuals affected by ASD, and (3) correlate with the presence or absence of ASD. Evidence of the second and third criteria for the quantitative trait characteristics of JAJE has been presented elsewhere in this book. Liu et al. (2011) have reported evidence for the first criterion in a QTL study of JAJE in ASD.

Liu et al. (2011) employed factor analysis of parent report data from the ADI-R) to identify potential quantitative traits in a sample of 1,236 children with ASD from the Autism Genome Project (AGP). They replicated their findings with a second independent sample of 804 children from Phase 2 data collection of the AGP. These analyses identified and replicated the presence of a Joint Attention factor that was associated with 24.7% of the ADI-R parent report of phenotypic variance in initial sample. Eleven ADI-R items loaded onto this factor. Three had high face validity for the construct of JAJE: showing and directing attention, seeking to share enjoyment with others, and pointing to express interests. Six additional items had moderate face validity: direct gaze, social smiling, interest in children, appropriateness of social responses, quality of social overtures, and offering comfort. Two items, range of facial expressions used to communicate and conventional/instrumental gestures, had modest to low face validity. So the precision of quantitative trait assessment of joint attention in this study may have had some limitations. Nevertheless, 9 of these 11 items displayed moderate to high face validity for joint attention assessment. Therefore, at a minimum, this study provides proof of principles specific to the use of diagnostic assessment data in the genomic study of joint attention in ASD.

Significantly, Liu et al. (2011) reported analyses estimating that the Joint Attention factor was associated with a .50 heritability index in the linkage analysis. In other words, it was estimated that 50% of the variance in the phenotypic Joint Attention trait score in this sample with ASD was associated with genetic factors in this study.

Liu et al. (2011) also identified five other factors among the ADI-R parent report items. These were labeled Social Interaction and Communication (24.6% or the phenotypic variance, .49 heritability); Nonverbal Communication (16.6% of the phenotypic variance, .47 heritability); Repetitive Sensory–Motor Behavior (15% of the phenotypic variation, .54 heritability); Peer Interaction (12.8% of the phenotypic variation, .29 heritability); and Compulsion/Restricted Interests (6.3% of the phenotypic variation, .65 heritability). The identification and characteristics of all of the quantitative traits were replicated in a confirmatory factor analysis of the 804 children in the Phase 2 AGP data collection.

Liu et al. (2011) used the six ADI-R factors as quantitative traits in a genome-wide variance components linkage analysis across the two AGP samples. Evidence for linkage was obtained for only two factors after four covariates (gender, age at ADI-R assessment, verbal–nonverbal status, and estimated population origin) were considered. The Repetitive Sensory–Motor Behavior factor displayed evidence of linkage with chromosome region 19q13.3, and the Joint Attention factor displayed evidence for linkage with a region of 11q23 (q23.1 toq23.3; logarithm of the odds or LOD score = 4.0). The latter met the genome-wide suggestive linkage criteria "but was just short of [the] significant" linkage criteria (Liu et al., 2011, p. 691; see Figure 8.1). It is noteworthy, though, that an independent study has recently linked the 11q23.2–q23.3 region to variance in the BAP (Piven et al., 2013).

Liu et al. (2011) noted that the 11q23.1–q23.3 region associated with the Joint Attention factor contains 83 genes, including the neural cell adhesion molecule 1 gene (NCAM1), dopamine receptor D2 (DRD2), and 5-hydroxytryptamine (5-HT) receptors 3A and 3B (5-HTR3A and 5-HTR3B). Liu et al. also noted that other studies have reported links between ASD and some of these genes. For example, NCAM1 has been observed to be associated with heightened risk of ASD (e.g., Fujita et al., 2010).

The linkage observed between the Joint Attention factor and DRD2, though, was the one finding that was predictable on the basis of joint attention theory (e.g., Mundy, 2003). The dopaminergic system genes play significant roles in moderating attention development across age (e.g., Störmer, Passow, Biesenack, & Li, 2012). These genes are also characterized by numerous copy number variants and constitute one common

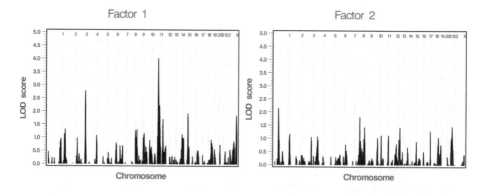

FIGURE 8.1. Comparison of the identification of the genetic loci underlying Factor 1 (Joint Attention) scores and Factor 2 (Social Interaction and Communication) scores from the Autism Diagnostic Interview–Revised (ADI-R). From Liu et al. (2011). Copyright 2011 by Lippincott Williams & Wilkins. Reprinted by permission.

pathway or vector by which the environment and genome interact in human development (Gatzke-Kopp, 2011). Both of these characteristics suggest that dopaminergic genes may be among the more important candidate or moderator genes to consider in attempts to understand heritable differences in typical and atypical joint attention development, as well as differences in joint attention development that may be potentiated by environmental processes.

Dopaminergic Pathways in Joint Attention Development

Although DRD2 has not been consistently linked to ASD in genome-wide studies, genes encoding for various elements of the dopaminergic system have been more clearly implicated in the pathogenesis of ASD (Nguyen et al., 2014). Some direct evidence of DRD2 involvement in ASD has also emerged. Hettinger et al. (2012) reported that DRD2 may contribute to relative risk for ASD in male-only sibling pairs. Indeed, their study reported that the DRD2 rs1800498 T allele was specifically associated with more severe ADI-R scores for reciprocal social interaction and verbal communication, as well as for repetitive and stereotyped behaviors. The potential importance of gender-specific findings is emphasized by recent related observations. DRD2 has been observed to interact with gender in its influence on attention switching with superior performance observed for males with the CC variant of the C957T polymorphism of this gene. However, superior performance was observed for females with the TT variant of this polymorphism (Gurvicj & Rossell, 2015).

There is also some evidence that different genes involved in dopaminergic system regulation, including DRD2, may be specifically related to social attention. Gong et al. (2013) have provided evidence that COMT Val158Met may contribute to trait attention bias to negative emotional expressions, but that DRD2 TaqlA was involved in trait bias for positive emotional expressions in 650 college students. This last finding is particularly interesting because a recent study suggests that an attenuation of positive response to positive facial expressions, rather than a pervasive attenuation of response to facial expressions, may be characteristic of higher-functioning children with ASD (Kim et al., 2014).

With regard to the relations of DRD2 to attention, it is also important to recall that IJA has repeatedly been observed to be associated with neural circuit activation of the striatal circuits of the basal ganglia (Caruana et al., 2015; Gordon et al., 2013; Schilbach et al., 2010). The striatum plays a major role in reward circuits of the brain (e.g., Báez-Mendoza & Schultz, 2013). These include specific ocular–motor visual attention control circuits that converge on the frontal eye fields of primates and humans (Shook, Schlag-Rey, & Schlag, 1991; Young, Neggers, Zandbelt, & Schall,

2014). These observations are consistent with the hypothesis that joint attention is affected by differences in reward circuits that regulate attention allocation in people. They may also help to explain the observation that activation of frontal eye fields of the superior frontal gyrus is often observed in imaging studies of social-cognitive and theory-of-mind task performance (Mundy, 2003).

The striatum constitutes a large part of the basal ganglia; it is composed of the caudate and the nucleus accumbens/ventral striatum. The striatum is highly interconnected with the reward circuit of the amygdala, orbitofrontal cortex, and ACC, as well as with the temporal and more dorsal networks of the parietal and frontal cortices (e.g., Báez-Mendoza & Schultz, 2013). The striatum plays a central role in integrating dopaminergic modulation of reward with sensory and cognitive information processing to facilitate learning and selection of goal-directed actions (Gerfen & Surmeier, 2011).

Dopaminergic effects on reward are largely orchestrated by the abundance of DRD1 and DRD2 receptors in the striatum. DRD1 appears to regulate direct and excitatory efferent neural pathways carrying information from the striatum to cortical networks. DRD2 appears to regulate indirect and inhibitory efferent pathways from the striatum to other brain regions (Gerfen & Surmeier, 2011). Although they affect distinct efferent circuits, cooperative activation of both the D1 and D2 pathways is likely to be necessary for many types of behavioral action selection and initiation, including the reward-based learning of social interaction behaviors and understanding of self- and other-agency (e.g., Macpherson, Morita, & Hikida, 2014; Báez-Mendoza & Schultz, 2013).

Finally, at least one experimental study also provides some evidence of the involvement of the dopaminergic system in joint attention development in some children with ASD. Jahromi et al. (2009) examined the impact of stimulant medication (methylphenidate) on joint attention and self-regulation in 29 children (ages 5–13 years) with ASD and symptoms of ADHD. Stimulants such as methylphenidate enhance dopaminergic system activity and are often effective in moderating symptoms ADHD. The results of the study indicated that the children who received methylphenidate, especially at the lowest of three dosage levels, displayed significantly better IJA and RJA scores in interaction with a tester who was unaware of their medication status than did children receiving a placebo. These observations cannot be interpreted as evidence of a specific effect of stimulant medication on joint attention in all children with ASD, in part because the stimulants may only have affected joint attention in a subset of children with ASD plus evidence of comorbid hyperactivity. Nevertheless, it provides one more line of evidence suggesting that understanding the regulator of the dopaminergic system may be important in understanding joint attention development in at least some children with ASD.

The Value of QTL Studies of Joint Attention

The one linkage study of Liu et al. (2011) does not provide the level of evidence necessary to form firm conclusions. However, the data in their innovative study do suggest that quantitative measures of joint attention may contribute to the identification of the complex matrix of ASD's genetic pathogenesis. At least two aspects of the data support this methodological assertion. First, this linkage study suggests that parent report data on the ADI-R may provide useful and valid quantitative trait measures of joint attention. Moreover, a significant portion of the variance in the ADI-R Joint Attention factor score used by Liu et al. was associated with genetic factors. This last observation comports well with increasing evidence that specific human social behaviors are heritable, and that the genetic factors involved can be distinguished from those involved in non-social behavior traits (e.g., Ebstein, Israel, Chew, Zhong, & Knafo, 2010; Ronald, Happé & Plomin, 2005). The fact that Liu et al. were able to observe useful information based only on one parent report index speaks to the strength of the "signal" provided by joint attention measures in ASD research. Improvement in the measurement will be likely to improve the strength of this signal. Such improvement may be realized by combining parent report measurement from the ADI-R with Joint Attention factor scores on young children from the ADOS (see Chapter 3) to yield more reliable measures of the latent construct of joint attention.

The data of Liu et al. (2011) also point to the potential for studies of joint attention (and social cognition more generally) to provide new information about the genetics of ASD and other forms of developmental psychopathology. For example, the hypothesis that differences in joint attention development among individuals affected by ASD may be moderated by a dopamine receptor gene is both consistent and inconsistent with information in the 2012 version of the NIMH RDoC Systems for Social Processes domain.

The current RDoC matrix notes that DRD2 and other dopamine regulators are candidate genes associated with the Affiliation and Attachment dimension of the Systems for Social Processes domain. However, attachment is not clearly an arena of impairment in autism, nor is attachment strongly related to typical or atypical joint attention (e.g., Sigman & Mundy, 1989; Naber et al., 2007). On the other hand, joint attention is a dimension of social behavior that plays a significant role in human affiliation and engagement (e.g., Mundy & Sigman, 2006; Sebanz et al., 2006). So perhaps joint attention should be included within this dimension of Systems for Social Processes. On the other hand, the contribution of the dopaminergic system (and the COMT gene) is also noted within the Reception of Facial Communication dimension, where joint attention is currently listed as a paradigm. This again raises the idea that joint attention may involve multiple social functions and systems and, consequently, is an ecologically valid dimension for the study of ASD.

Another interesting observation in the current RDoC description of Systems for Social Processes is that the dopaminergic genes are only noted for possible effects on Social Communication: Production or Reception of Facial and Non-Facial Communication. However, no genes are listed for Perception and Understanding of Self or for Perception and Understanding of Others dimensions. This is an important and even telling observation. It is indicative of just how little we know about the Systems for Social Processes domain and its constituent dimensions, even those (such as social cognition and self–other processing) that may be central to ASD. The theory and research described in this book support the argument that joint attention (and social cognition) may best be viewed as an integrated hybrid of self–other information processing. This hypothesis implies the possible utility of revising the current organization of the Systems for Social Processes domain of the RDoC. Perhaps more concerted research on joint attention and social cognition can contribute to such a revision. This will become more likely as the current gap in knowledge about genetic and molecular mechanisms involved in typical and atypical self- and other-awareness is addressed.

Lackner, Sabbagh, Hallinan, Liu, and Holden (2012) have reported observations related to narrowing this gap in knowledge. This research team examined the hypothesis that genetic regulators of dopamine may have an impact on individual differences in the preschool development of theory-of-mind ability. Theory-of-mind ability is part of Perception and Understanding of Others in the RDoC Systems for Social Processes. Seventy-three 4-year-olds were presented with a battery of three theory-of-mind tasks, as well as four non-social-cognitive control problem-solving tasks and four executive function control tasks. Saliva samples were collected, and DNA was extracted for genotyping of polymorphisms of the COMT, DAT1, and DRD4 genes. Notably, the theory-of-mind tasks included a deceptive pointing task. They also included two tasks that directly relied on the participants' processing of verbal or pictorial information concerning what another person had seen, and using this information to judge the other person's beliefs. Theory described in Chapter 4 suggests that these types of theory-of-mind tasks are likely to activate mental joint attention skills during social-cognitive problem solving.

Lackner et al. (2012) reported evidence that individuals with two shorter alleles (4 or fewer repeats) of 48 bp VNTR in exon III of DRD4 had significantly better total scores on the theory-of-mind battery than did children with one or two longer alleles (6 or more repeats; see Figure 8.2). No associations between COMT or DAT1 and theory-of-mind performance were observed, and no genetic associations with the problem-solving control tasks were observed. The DRD4 polymorphism was also associated with performance on the executive function battery. A mediation analysis, however, indicated that even after variance shared with executive function development was taken into account, DRD4 made a unique contribution to individual differences in preschool theory-of-mind development (Lackner et al., 2012).

As the foregoing discussion suggests, the contemporary research literature presents a compelling rationale for the investigation of the role of dopamine receptor and regulator genes in the typical development of JAJE and social cognition. Research and theory also suggest that dopamine receptor genes may potentially play roles in the broader range of phenotypic phenomena in autism. These include the role of dopamine regulators and the striatum in differences in associative learning, or flexibility in learning new strategies and suppressing old strategies (Macpherson et al., 2014; Yawata, Yamaguchi, Danjo, Hikida, & Nakanishi, 2012), as well as the role of dopamine and the stratum in the atypical movement patterns observed in some individuals with autism (Gerfen & Surmeier, 2011; Macpherson et al., 2014). Yet, when it comes to the extant contemporary literature on research on candidate genes for JAJE, the hypotheses

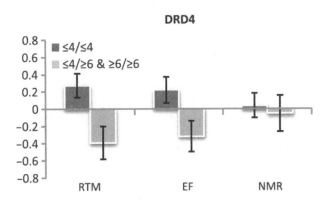

FIGURE 8.2. Illustration of the relation between variation in the dopamine receptor D4 gene (DRD4) and preschoolers' performance on a theory-of-mind task. From Lackner, Sabbagh, Hallinan, Liu, and Holden (2012). Copyright 2012 by Blackwell Publishing, Ltd. Reprinted by permission.

about the role of the hypophysiological peptide genes are of equal or greater prominence.

Oxytocin and Vasopressin Pathways and Joint Attention

In a recent review, Stavropoulos and Carver (2013) suggest that the role of the oxytocin receptor gene (OXTR) in social motivation makes it a prime candidate for metabolic research on JAJE in ASD. Oxytocin and vasopressin are members of a family of peptide hormones synthesized by the hypothalamus and secreted by the pituitary gland (Baskerville & Douglas, 2010). OXTR is involved in the regulation of systemic oxytocin availability, which appears to influence individual differences in a variety of social behaviors—including recognition of emotions, mutual gaze, social reinforcement sensitivity, and encoding of social memories (Hammock, 2015; Stavropoulos & Carver, 2013), as well as the development of cooperative behavior, theory of mind, and prosocial behavior in young children (Haas, Anderson, & Smith, 2013; Wu & Su, 2015).

There have also been observations of links between polymorphisms of OXTR and the vasopressin receptor 1A gene (AVPR1A) with ASD (Baskerville & Douglas; 2010; Stavropoulos & Carver, 2013). Some of this linkage evidence, though, has been inconsistent (Baskerville & Douglas, 2010; Hammock & Young, 2006).

Stavropoulos and Carver (2013) rely on the social motivation hypothesis of autism to envision a direct role for OXTR in the differences in JAJE that characterize autism spectrum development. As described in earlier chapters, the social motivation hypothesis suggests that an early attenuation of the quality of sensitivity to the reward value of social engagement leads to a cascade of differences in social information processing, social learning, and social brain development in ASD (e.g., Chevallier et al., 2012; Dawson, 2008; Kim et al., 2014; Mundy, 1995). Four possible patterns of differences in social reward sensitivity have been described by Kim et al. (2014): ASD may involve (1) aversion to social stimuli (negative reinforcement); (2) weak positive reinforcement or reward associated with social stimuli; (3) unusually high levels of intrinsic motivation for nonsocial stimuli (conflicting reinforcement/reward); and (4) subsets of individuals with each of these different motivation patterns, which lead to the common outcome of attenuated social information processing.

Stavropoulos and Carver (2013) describe an intuitive, plausible, and heuristic rationale for considering OTXR, and perhaps AVPR1A as well, in candidate gene studies of joint attention development. Moreover, recent research provides some evidence consistent with a role for OXTR and AVPR1A in the development of this dimension of social cognition.

OXTR in Joint Attention
and Social-Cognitive Development

Wade, Hoffman, Wigg, and Jenkins (2014) recently noted the parallels between measures of adult social cognition and infant measures of joint attention, cooperation, empathy, and self-regulation.[1] They developed a composite measure of these four behaviors in order to study the effects of maternal responsivity on social-cognitive development in 350 children 18 months of age. They also examined the degree to which four variants of the OXTR gene (single-nucleotide polymorphisms, or SNPs) influenced individual differences in this measure of social-cognitive development in this same sample of 18-month-olds. These SNPs included rs2254298, rs11131149, rs237897, and rs237899, which Wade et al. (2014, p. 604) noted have been implicated in autism and other conditions characterized by deficits in social cognition.[2]

The latent social-cognitive variable included the RJA measure from the ESCS (Mundy, Delgado, et al., 2003) and an empathy measure similar to that employed by Sigman, Kasari, Kwon, and Yirmiya (1992) in studies of children with autism. It also included a cooperation task described by Warneken, Chen, and Tomasello (2006). Finally, the composite measure of social cognition included a type of mirror–rouge self-recognition task that has previously been related to self-referenced processing in joint attention (Nichols et al., 2005). Joint attention (.64), self-recognition (.63), empathy (.44), and cooperation (.80) were all significantly correlated with the latent social-cognitive variable. Furthermore, the pairings of joint attention, social cooperation, self-recognition, and empathy were all significantly but weakly correlated (.14 to .23), with the exception of self-recognition and empathy (.07).

The primary results showed that variation on rs11131149 of the OXTR gene was significantly associated with infant individual differences on the latent social-cognitive variable. More copies of the major (G) allele were related to higher social-cognitive scores, and more copies of the minor (A) allele were associated with lower scores. Moreover, a GG haplotype (involving both G alleles, rs11131149 and rs2254298) was associated with

---

[1] Their arguments are consistent with those made about the connections among JAJE, cooperation, and social cognition made in Chapters 4 and 5.

[2] A recent study observed a significant association between OXTR SNP rs237887 SNP and imitation on the Childhood Autism Rating Scale—Tokyo Version in 111 individuals with ASD from 4 to 41 years of age (Egawa et al., 2013). Imitation ratings were lower for individuals who carried the minor A allele of re237887 than for those with the major G allele homozygotes. This is noteworthy because of the proximity of this OXTR SNP to those examined by Wade, Moore, Astington, Frampton, and Jenkins (2015).

better social-cognitive task performance, whereas the AG haplotype was associated with weaker performance. Wade et al. (2014, p. 608) have suggested that the AG haplotype may be a risk indicator for social-cognitive difficulties in childhood.

The data reported by Wade et al. (2014) dovetail with observations from studies of OXTR in adults (e.g., Haas et al., 2013). Moreover, a recent study by Wu and Su (2015) provides more direct evidence of an association between OXTR and social-cognitive development in preschool children. This research group examined the association of the rs53576 haplotype of OXTR with theory of mind and prosocial behavior in 87 children (ages 3–5 years). Prosocial behavior was measured with observations of child behavior on an empathy task, a comforting task that also involved empathy, and a helping task in which the tester used alternating gaze (joint attention) to elicit aid for the children. Theory of mind was measured with two false-belief tasks that involved understanding what another person had or had not seen. The results showed that children with two copies of the G allele (GG) performed better on the prosocial behaviors than children with one or two copies of the A allele. With respect to theory-of-mind performance, only children with two copies of the A allele (AA) performed worse than those with GG.

Similar data on prosocial behavior have been reported in adults. Tost et al. (2010) observed that the rs53576 variant of OXTR was associated with prosocial temperament in 309 nonaffected adult siblings of individuals with schizophrenia. OXTR was also associated with MRI data indicative of differences in the structural correlations between the hippocampus, amygdala, and anterior cingulate gyrus.

The observations of Wade et al. (2014), Wu and Su (2015), and Tost et al. (2010) on the relations of OXTR to latent measures of social cognition and prosocial behavior do not specifically link OXTR to joint attention per se. However, these studies raise the hypothesis that a specific link to joint attention development may exist. This assertion is supported by three observations that link joint attention and social cognition. First, infant joint attention development is a significant predictor of subsequent theory-of-mind development in childhood (e.g., Kristen et al., 2011; see Chapter 4). Second, joint attention and social cognition involve the activation of overlapping cortical neural networks (see Chapter 7). Third, several longitudinal studies provide evidence of significant and unique paths of association between infant joint attention development and later childhood development of prosocial behavior patterns, both in children with typical development (Parlade et al., 2009; Vaughan Van Hecke et al., 2007), and in impoverished children at risk for less than optimal behavioral outcomes (Sheinkopf et al., 2004).

Animal Models of Joint Attention

Current research on human development is suggestive of a specific link between the hypophysiological peptides and JAJE. In comparative primate research, more direct evidence of this linkage has recently been reported.

Primates, as well as many other animals, follow conspecifics' line of visual regard or engage in RJA (e.g., Tomasello, Hare, & Fogleman, 2001). Primates such as chimpanzees display RJA, but they also display significant individual differences in RJA development (e.g., Leavens & Racine, 2009). To begin to examine the factors that might influence these differences, Hopkins, Keebaugh, et al. (2014) worked with a sample of 232 chimpanzees. They estimated the heritability of differences in RJA in the chimpanzees and examined the influence of a candidate gene on these differences. They selected AVPR1A because, like OXTR, AVPR1A has repeatedly been linked to differences in social behavior in animals and people, especially in males.

RJA was assessed in the chimpanzees with three types of trials. In one type of trial, a human tester elicited mutual gaze and then looked behind a chimpanzee for 5 seconds. If the chimpanzee responded correctly within 15 seconds, it received a score of 3. Subsequent trials involved gaze and pointing behind the chimpanzee (score of 2) and calling the chimpanzee's name, pointing, and gazing behind (score of 3). Two sets of trials were presented on different occasions. A control task for spatial memory for food was also presented.

Of the 232 chimpanzees, 190 displayed consistent evidence of RJA, but the other 42 did not. RJA performance was associated with a significant heritability estimate in the chimpanzees ($h^2 = .25$). Moreover, males with the DupB+/– polymorphism of AVPR1A did significant better on the RJA tasks than did males with the DupB–/– polymorphism. However, there was no evidence for an effect of this AVPR1A polymorphism on the RJA performance of female chimpanzees (see Figure 8.3). There was also no evidence for an influence of AVPR1A on the nonsocial spatial memory task for either male or female chimpanzees. The significance of the observations in this paper is emphasized by research indicating that AVPR1A, like OXTR, may play a role in autism (e.g., Yirmiya et al., 2006) and that the effects of these genes may vary with the gender of affected children (Miller et al., 2013).

Aside from the significance of their observation of the association between AVPR1A and chimpanzee RJA, Hopkins, Keebaugh, et al. (2014) provided additional data on the heritability of JAJE. Their heritability (h^2) estimate of .25 was significant. Recall that Liu et al. (2011) reported

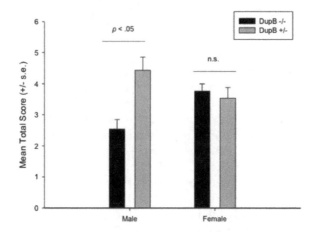

FIGURE 8.3. Illustration of the relation between variations in a polymorphism of the arginine vasopressin V1a receptor gene (AVPR1A) and RJA in male chimpanzees. Males with one DupB+ allele performed significantly better on RJA than did males who were homozygous for the DupB– deletion. From Hopkins, Keebaugh, et al. (2014). Copyright 2014 by the Nature Publishing Group. Reprinted by permission, through a Creative Commons 3.0 Unported License.

a significant heritability estimate of h^2 = .50 for a multiple-item parent report measure of JAJE in a sample of children with ASD. Neither estimate is likely to be precise. Nevertheless, the evidence for significant JAJE heritability across these studies emphasizes the validity of research on the metabolic and molecular influences of this dimension of human nature and the nature of autism spectrum development and ASD. Such research is likely to inform the next iteration of the NIMH RDoC Systems for Social Processes domain, or its ilk. Moreover, it may help us to understand how the complex human capacity for integrated self-referenced, other-referenced, and common-referent information processing comes to pass and plays a pivotal role in human learning and cognitive development. In that regard, though, how would research on the genetics of JAJE be best pursued? Stavropoulos and Carver (2013) have emphasized that investigations of the interaction of the oxytocin and dopamine systems in social motivation may constitute the best path to understanding the role of each system in JAJE. I think there is every reason to follow their advice.

In another line of comparative research, Nakako et al. (2014) have recently discussed the importance of incorporating animal models of joint attention into programmatic research on ASD. This research group, however, noted that rodent models may be incapable of capturing important features of autism, such as joint attention. This may be because many features of autism, including joint attention, may involve neurocognitive functions of the human prefrontal and frontal cortex that may not easily be modeled in rodents. Instead, this research group suggests that work on joint attention with highly social monkeys (such as marmosets) may complement work on joint attention with apes (such as chimpanzees).

Nakako et al. (2014) offer proof of this principle in a study of ketamine-induced joint attention dysfunction in common marmosets as a possible animal model of ASD. The first part of this study showed that marmosets could readily learn to follow a tester's eye gaze and pointing gesture to find food systematically in one of four containers. Citing theory on the role of *N*-methyl-D-aspartate (NMDA) receptor dysfunction in ASD (e.g., Carlson, 2012; Gandal, Anderson, Billingslea, Roberts, & Siegel, 2012), Nakako et al. then demonstrated that administration of ketamine, an NMDA antagonist, significantly reduced the marmosets' performance in the joint attention task. Finally, they also demonstrated that lurasidone, a drug that enhances NMDA receptor-mediated synaptic responses, rescued joint attention task performance in the ketamine-exposed marmosets. The specificity of effects in this study was supported by the inclusion of a condition controlling for the possibility that ketamine induced an effect on memory, rather than joint attention, that impaired the marmosets' food task performance.

The mechanism by which lurasidone reversed ketamine-induced joint attention impairments in this study was not clear. Nevertheless, Nakako et al. (2014) noted that lurasidone has been observed to have potent binding affinity for dopamine D2 receptors, especially in the frontal cortex (Ishibashi et al., 2010). The literature cited previously in this chapter raises the possibility that lurasidone may have rescued joint attention, at least in part, through the up-regulation of frontal dopamine in the marmosets. Alternatively, or perhaps in addition, lurasidone has an affinity for serotonin receptors (i.e., 5-HTR1A and 5-HTR7) (Ishibashi et al., 2010), and antagonists of these receptors have improved social behaviors in studies using rodent models of autism and schizophrenia (Nakako et al., 2014). The possible influence of serotonin receptors on joint attention was also noted in the QTL study of Liu et al. (2011). Hence Nakako and colleagues argued that this might be the path through which lurasidone rescued joint attention performance in their study of marmosets.

In the discussion of their results, Nakako et al. (2014) also made a well-informed observation about the nature of joint attention and the related limits of their animal model. First, they explicitly recognized the difference between the type of RJA bids they examined in their study and IJA. They also noted that research suggests that IJA deficits may be a longer-lasting and more diagnostically important facet of the ASD phenotype. Consequently, a marmoset model of joint attention may provide valuable information on one element of joint attention development in ASD, but not necessarily a comprehensive model of such development.

This points to an important issue in comparative research on the social communication phenotype of ASD: It is difficult to model all of the more important features of ASD in comparative research. Even in primate models, critical components of behavioral dimensions of ASD, such as the IJA component of joint attention, may not be part of typical neurocognitive development in these species (Tomasello, Carpenter, & Hobson, 2005). In part, this may be so because a major axis of the differences among humans, primates, and other mammals is likely to involve the repurposing of genetic, molecular, and cognitive neurodevelopmental factors as part of the evolution of social-communicative abilities. If nothing else, ASD is a disturbance of fundamental aspects of the nature of human social-communicative development. This is an important concept to keep in mind as we search for valid animal models, or as we search for the genetic and molecular bases of ASD. It may be fortuitous to mention this here, as the next part of the chapter addresses the possible implications of joint attention research for illuminating those genetic and molecular processes.

Joint Attention, Gene Interactions, and Genetic Repurposing

I have no great expertise in genetics. Nevertheless, we all try to keep up with literature in disciplines that lie beyond our expertise, in order to be more aware of the complexities of understanding autism spectrum development and ASD. When I read the research on genetics, I am struck by the prominence of a *main-effects* model in studies of autism. That is, research most often consists of technologically sophisticated searches for and measurements of the individual impact of genes in the development of autism. Even when it is successful, this research has thus far always revealed that any single gene has only a small direct or main effect in the pathogenesis of autism. Of course, other approaches are possible, but as yet they have been less frequently applied.

One of these approaches is suggested by recognition of the phenomenon of *epistasis*. Epistasis refers to the observation that the phenotypic expression of one gene can be affected by the presence of another gene. This moderating effect of one gene on another is referred to as a *genetic interaction* or GI (e.g., Ryan et al., 2012). According to Frost et al. (2012, p. 1339), measuring GIs is an unbiased way of determining functional relationships that has proven to be a powerful technique for discovering genes' functions, grouping genes into complexes, and organizing them into pathways.

Looking for GIs in research on neurodevelopmental disorders, though, is challenging. It may not be possible to rely on technology alone to identify important GIs among the possible permutations of the 20,000–25,000 genes in the human genome. Instead, it may be necessary to combine technology, statistics, and a priori knowledge or theory in pathway analyses to identify GIs associated with complex human traits and disorders (e.g., Backes et al., 2014). Moreover, to develop theoretical guidance for pathway analyses in ASD, it may be useful to be aware of another phenomenon recognized in contemporary genomics: the phenomenon known as *repurposing*, in which orthologous (ancestral) sets of genes come to take on new functions and partnerships across species and evolution. Frost et al. (2012) suggest that it is useful to anticipate that GIs may be repurposed across species when we are trying to understand gene–phenotype relations.

These notions suggest that studying one or another family of genes in research on JAJE development may not be as revealing as the study of the interactions of these genes and metabolic pathways. This may be undertaken in both human and comparative animal research. However, the phenomenon of repurposing raises the possibility that pathways may have changed in human phylogeny, in ways that support a different adaptive level of integrated functionality of attention and affiliation in the development of social learning, affiliation, and cognition. If so, the phenotype and pathways of the JAJE dimension observed in human research may display important differences from those observed in comparative research.

Another caveat is that research on a GI model of joint attention involving dopamine and neurohypophyseal peptides can be significant and informative, without being fully explanatory. This model, at best, would probably only describe one of several sets of GI and pathway complexes that may be involved in joint attention, let alone autism spectrum development or ASD. It would be expected to account for a substantial portion of the variance in typical and atypical JAJE development, but not necessarily all of the meaningful developmental variance in this dimension. These caveats notwithstanding, research has begun to support the validity of a GI research model for the investigating the genetics of JAJE.

Several papers discuss the need to recognize probable interaction of OXTR with other genes, and especially dopaminergic system regulators, in influencing social behaviors (e.g., Baskerville & Douglas, 2010; Chang et al., 2014; Churchland & Winkielman, 2012; Hammock, 2015). Indeed, Romero-Fernandez, Borroto-Escuela, Agnati, and Fuxe (2013,

p. 850) have reported experimental evidence supporting the hypothesis that D2R–OXTR interactions in the nucleus accumbens may represent a significant part of the molecular mechanisms for oxytocin-induced changes in social and emotional behavior. Several studies of humans suggest that dopamine–oxytocin interactions play a role in several behavior disorders (Baskerville & Douglas, 2010). More recently, a study led to the observation that OXTR genotypes interact with striatal dopamine transporter availability in a manner that is meaningfully related to human social behavior and personality (Chang et al., 2014). Again, recall that activations of the nucleus accumbens and/or ventral striatal and associated thalamic structures have been observed in association with the experience of joint attention in adults in multiple studies (Caruana et al., 2015; Gordon et al., 2013; Schilbach et al., 2010).

Research also indicates that both OXTR and DRD2 mediate attention to positive facial expressions (Gamer, Zurowski, & Büchel, 2010; Gong et al., 2013), via effects on the ventral striatum and amygdala. Positive appetitive social approach, including attention to positive facial expressions but not necessarily negative facial expressions, may play a role in joint attention development (Mundy, 1995). Moreover, attenuated approach to positive facial and vocal affective expressions, rather than an atypical response to negative facial/vocal emotions, may typify a central difference in social motivation of children with autism spectrum development (Kim et al., 2014).

Gong et al. (2013) have also reported evidence that the presence of the Taql A DRD2 polymorphism was positively related to a strength of the tendency to shift attention to faces with positive affect, measured in terms of reaction time and resistance to inhibition of return, in a sample of 650 college students. By contrast, the presence of the COMT Val158Met polymorphism (which affects availability of dopamine) was associated with a stronger tendency to shift to faces with negative affect. Previous research suggested that the effect on shifting attention to positive affect is likely to involve the role of DRD2 in regulating input and/or output from the ventral striatum, but not the fusiform gyrus (e.g., Cacioppo, Norris, Decety, Monteleone, & Nusbaum, 2008).

A similar set of findings has been reported with respect to an experimental study of the effects of intranasal oxytocin on attention via the amygdala. Gamer et al. (2010) reported that intranasal oxytocin in 45 men decreased amygdala activation of lateral and dorsal regions of the amygdala to faces with negative emotions, but enhanced activation to happy emotions. Of course, this study does not constitute a direct investigation of OXTR mediation of attention. This is because little detailed knowledge exists about how variations in OXTR relate to observed responses to intranasal oxytocin (Haas et al., 2013). However, at least one study has reported evidence that intranasal enhancement of a preference for attention to infant faces was observed in, and limited to, adults who were homozygous for the re53576 OXTR allele (Marsh et al., 2012).

Observations that both DRD2 and OXTR may play differential roles in motivation for attention to positive versus negative facial expression is consistent with the hypothesis that DRD2–OXTR interactions play a significant part in the molecular mechanisms for oxytocin-induced changes in social and emotional behavior (Romero-Fernandez et al., 2013). Of course, the current understanding of the complex interactions between dopaminergic system genes and neurohypophyseal peptides in the social brain is meager (Skuse & Gallagher, 2009). Research on how a subset of these interactions may play a specific role in JAJE will constitute an important part of the new frontier of autism science, as well as social-cognitive neuroscience.

Informing the Dimensional Approach to Autism

Understanding the genetic, molecular, and neural circuit mechanisms involved in the development of social processes, social learning, social cognition, and social affiliation in humans is likely to require new ways of thinking. We must anticipate that some if not many of the genetic, molecular, and neural networks revealed in animal research on social processes have been repurposed into novel functions in human development through duplication, subfunctionalization, and other processes (e.g., Fu, Giavalisco, Liu, Catchpole, et al. 2011; Vallender, Mekel-Bobrov, & Lahn, 2008; Anderson & Finlay, 2013). Defining and understanding the Systems for Social Processes dimensions included in current and future versions of the RDoC more clearly and deeply than we do now is essential to the science of ASD and the broader sciences of human nature. I hope this book has raised the awareness that a deeper understanding of JAJE is a means to this end. In addition to the burgeoning literature and theory on the role of joint attention in social cognition, I think that the incipient but intriguing work on the genetics of joint attention makes a final point in this argument rather well.

To understand the Systems for Social Processes dimensions, though, I think we would do well to recognize that neither joint attention, nor any other cognitive dimension of the human mind, develops in isolation. One hypothesis raised here is that many if not all aspects of social cognition are likely to share a neurocognitive foundation in integrated self–other information processing and social-cognitive control. This hypothesis may help us to appreciate the commonalities, such as input and output associations, between JAJE and information processing involved in biological motion perception, the development of agency, processing invariance in self–other facial expressions, and imitation. However, in the search for the central behavioral tendency of the phenotype of ASD, no one of these aspects of social cognition may be primary. There is no single psychological dimension, gene, or neuroanatomical feature or neural circuit at the heart of the pathogenesis of autism spectrum development. We must have patience in the path of discovery. We must be curious about system interactions and dynamic models. Across generations, we can build blocks of knowledge that, though imperfect, are substantial enough for progress. The whole point of this book has been to argue that the knowledge we now have on joint attention constitutes one substantial building block for the science of autism. We should not seek to explain it away. Rather, at this point in the still-early years of our science, we need to put this block of knowledge to good use as we work toward better understanding the complexity of the human nature of autism.

References

Abreu, C. S. D., Cardoso-Martins, C., & Barbosa, P. G. (2014). The relationship between joint attention and theory of mind: A longitudinal study. *Psicologia: Reflexão e Crítica, 27*(2), 409–414.

Abuelo, D. N. (1991). Genetic disorders. In J. Matson & J. Mulick (Eds.), *Handbook of mental retardation* (pp. 97–114). Oxford, UK: Pergamon Press.

Achenbach, T. M. (1966). The classification of children's psychiatric symptoms: A factor-analytic study. *Psychological Monographs: General and Applied, 80*(7), 1–37.

Adamson, L. B. (1995). *Communication development during infancy.* Madison, WI: Brown & Benchmark.

Adamson, L., Bakeman, R., & Deckner, D. (2004). The development of symbol-infused joint engagement. *Child Development, 75,* 1171–1187.

Aldred, C., Green, J., & Adams, C. (2004). A new social communication intervention for children with autism: Pilot randomised controlled treatment study suggesting effectiveness. *Journal of Child Psychology and Psychiatry, 45*(8), 1420–1430.

Aldred, C., Phillips, R., Pollard, C., & Adams, C. (2001). Multidisciplinary social communication intervention for children with autism and pervasive developmental disorder: The Child's Talk project. *Educational and Child Psychology, 18*(2), 76–87.

Allman, J. M., Tetreault, N. A., Hakeem, A. Y., Manaye, K. F., Semendeferi, K., Erwin, J. M., . . . Hof, P. R. (2010). The von Economo neurons in frontoinsular and anterior cingulate cortex in great apes and humans. *Brain Structure and Function, 214*(5–6), 495–517.

Amaral, D. G. (2011). Memory: Anatomical organization of candidate brain regions. *Comprehensive Physiology.* Retrieved from *www.comprehensivephysiology.com/*

WileyCDA/CompPhysArticle/refId-cp010507.html (Original work published 1987)

American Psychiatric Association. (1952). *Diagnostic and statistical manual of mental disorders.* Washington, DC: Author.

American Psychiatric Association. (1968). *Diagnostic and statistical manual of mental disorders* (2nd ed.). Washington, DC: Author.

American Psychiatric Association. (1980). *Diagnostic and statistical manual of mental disorders* (3rd ed.). Washington, DC: Author.

American Psychiatric Association. (1987). *Diagnostic and statistical manual of mental disorders* (3rd ed., rev.). Washington, DC: Author.

American Psychiatric Association. (1994). *Diagnostic and statistical manual of mental disorders* (4th ed.). Washington, DC: Author.

American Psychiatric Association. (2000). *Diagnostic and statistical manual of mental disorders* (4th ed., text rev.). Washington, DC: Author.

American Psychiatric Association. (2013). *Diagnostic and statistical manual of mental disorders* (5th ed.). Arlington, VA: Author.

Anderson, M. L., & Finlay, B. L. (2013). Allocating structure to function: The strong links between neuroplasticity and natural selection. *Frontiers in Human Neuroscience, 7,* 918.

Asada, K., & Itakura, S. (2012). Social phenotypes of autism spectrum disorders and Williams syndrome: Similarities and differences. *Frontiers in Psychology, 3,* 247.

Asperger, H. (1944). Die 'Autistischen Psychopathen' im Kindesalter. *Archiv für Psychiatrie und Nervenkrankheiten, 117,* 76–136.

Atkinson, J., Hood, B., Wattam-Bell, J., & Braddick, O. (1992). Changes in infants' ability to switch attention in the first three months of life. *Perception, 21,* 643–653.

Backes, C., Rühle, F., Stoll, M., Haas, J., Frese, K., Franke, A., . . . Keller, A. (2014). Systematic permutation testing in GWAS pathway analyses: Identification of genetic networks in dilated cardiomyopathy and ulcerative colitis. *BMC Genomics, 15*(1), 622.

Báez-Mendoza, R., & Schultz, W. (2013). The role of the striatum in social behavior. *Frontiers in Neuroscience, 7,* 233.

Bahrick, L. E., & Lickliter, R. (2000). Intersensory redundancy guides attentional selectivity and perceptual learning in infancy. *Developmental Psychology, 36*(2), 190–201.

Bakeman, R., & Adamson, L. B. (1984). Coordinating attention to people and objects in mother–infant and peer–infant interaction. *Child Development, 55*(4), 1278–1289.

Baker, M. J. (2000). Incorporating the thematic ritualistic behaviors of children with autism into games increasing social play interactions with siblings. *Journal of Positive Behavior Interventions, 2*(2), 66–84.

Baldwin, D. (1995). Understanding the link between joint attention and language. In C. Moore & P. Dunham (Eds.), *Joint attention: Its origins and role in development* (pp. 131–158). Hillsdale, NJ: Erlbaum.

Baldwin, J. M. (1894). Personality-suggestion. *Psychological Review, 1*(3), 274–279.

Balslev, D., & Miall, R. C. (2008). Eye position representation in human anterior parietal cortex. *Journal of Neuroscience, 28*(36), 8968–8972.

Bandura, A. (1962). Social learning through imitation. In M. R. Jones (Ed.), *Nebraska Symposium on Motivation: 1962* (pp. 211–274). Lincoln: University of Nebraska Press.

Baron-Cohen, S. (1989). Joint attention deficits in autism: Towards a cognitive analysis. *Development and Psychopathology, 3*, 185–190.

Baron-Cohen, S. (1995). *Mindblindness.* Cambridge, MA: MIT Press.

Baron-Cohen, S. (2002). The extreme male brain theory of autism. *Trends in Cognitive Sciences, 6*(6), 248–254.

Baron-Cohen, S., Baldwin, D. A., & Crowson, M. (1997). Do children with autism use the speaker's direction of gaze strategy to crack the code of language? *Child Development, 68*(1), 48–57.

Baron-Cohen, S., Cox, A., Baird, G., Swettenham, J., Nightingale, N., Morgan, K., . . . Charman, T. (1996). Psychological markers in the detection of autism in infancy in a large population. *British Journal of Psychiatry, 168*(2), 158–163.

Baron-Cohen, S., Leslie, A. M., & Frith, U. (1985). Does the autistic child have a "theory of mind"? *Cognition, 21*(1), 37–46.

Barrett, L. F., & Satpute, A. B. (2013). Large-scale brain networks in affective and social neuroscience: Towards an integrative functional architecture of the brain. *Current Opinion in Neurobiology, 23*(3), 361–372.

Barton, S. (1994). Chaos, self-organization, and psychology. *American Psychologist, 49*(1), 5–21.

Baskerville, T. A., & Douglas, A. J. (2010). Dopamine and oxytocin interactions underlying behaviors: Potential contributions to behavioral disorders. *CNS Neuroscience and Therapeutics, 16*(3), e92–e123.

Bassett, D. S., & Gazzaniga, M. S. (2011). Understanding complexity in the human brain. *Trends in Cognitive Sciences, 15*(5), 200–209.

Bates, E. (1976). *Language and context: The acquisition of performatives.* New York: Academic Press.

Bates, E. (1993). Comprehension and production in early language development. *Monographs of the Society for Research in Child Development, 58*(3–4, Serial No. 233), 222–242.

Bates, E., Benigni, L., Bretherton, I., Camaioni, L., & Volterra, V. (1979). *The emergence of symbols: Cognition and communication in infancy.* New York: Academic Press.

Bates, E., Camaioni, L., & Volterra, V. (1975). The acquisition of performatives prior to speech. *Merrill-Palmer Quarterly, 21*(3), 205–226.

Bayliss, A. P., Murphy, E., Naughtin, C. K., Kritikos, A., Schilbach, L., & Becker, S. I. (2013). "Gaze leading": Initiating simulated joint attention influences eye movements and choice behavior. *Journal of Experimental Psychology: General, 142*(1), 76–92.

Bayliss, A. P., Paul, M., Cannon, P., Tipper, S. (2006). Gaze cuing and affective judgments of objects: I like what you look at. *Psychonomic Bulletin and Review, 13*, 1061–1066.

Bayliss, A. P., Pellegrino, G. D., & Tipper, S. P. (2005). Sex differences in eye gaze and symbolic cueing of attention. *Quarterly Journal of Experimental Psychology, 58*(4), 631–650.

Becchio, C., Bertone, C., & Castiello, U. (2008). How the gaze of others influences object processing. *Trends in Cognitive Sciences, 12*(7), 254–258.

Bedford, R., Elsabbagh, M., Gliga, T., Pickles, A., Senju, A., Charman, T., & Johnson, M. H. (2012). Precursors to social and communication difficulties in infants at-risk for autism: Gaze following and attentional engagement. *Journal of Autism and Developmental Disorders, 42*(10), 2208–2218.

Beglinger, L., & Smith, T. (2005). Concurrent validity of social subtype and IQ after early intensive behavioral intervention in children with autism: A preliminary investigation. *Journal of Autism and Developmental Disorders, 35*(3), 295–303.

Behne, T., Liszkowski, U., Carpenter, M., & Tomasello, M. (2012). Twelve-month-olds' comprehension and production of pointing. *British Journal of Developmental Psychology, 30*(3), 359–375.

Bejjani, A., O'Neill, J., Kim, J. A., Frew, A. J., Yee, V. W., Ly, R., . . . Levitt, J. G. (2012). Elevated glutamatergic compounds in pregenual anterior cingulate in pediatric autism spectrum disorder demonstrated by 1H MRS and 1H MRSI. *PLoS One, 7*(7), e38786.

Belmonte, M. K., Allen, G., Beckel-Mitchener, A., Boulanger, L. M., Carper, R. A., & Webb, S. J. (2004). Autism and abnormal development of brain connectivity. *Journal of Neuroscience, 24*(42), 9228–9231.

Benga, O. (2005). Intentional communication and the anterior cingulate cortex. *Interaction Studies, 6*(2), 201–221.

Bengston, M. (2013). Types of schizophrenia. *Psych Central.* Retrieved from *http://psychcentral.com/lib/types-of-schizophrenia.*

Bertalanffy, L. von. (1968). *General system theory: Foundations, development, applications.* New York: Braziller.

Bertone, A., Mottron, L., Jelenic, P., & Faubert, J. (2005). Enhanced and diminished visuo-spatial information processing in autism depends on stimulus complexity. *Brain, 128*(10), 2430–2441.

Bettelheim, B. (1959). Joey: A "mechanical boy." *Scientific American, 200,* 117–126.

Beuker, K. T., Rommelse, N. N., Donders, R., & Buitelaar, J. K. (2013). Development of early communication skills in the first two years of life. *Infant Behavior and Development, 36*(1), 71–83.

Bigelow, A. (2003). The development of joint attention in blind infants. *Development and Psychopathology, 15,* 259–275.

Bilder, R. M., Howe, A., Novak, N., Sabb, F. W., & Parker, D. S. (2011). The genetics of cognitive impairment in schizophrenia: A phenomic perspective. *Trends in Cognitive Sciences, 15*(9), 428–435.

Blakemore, S. J., & Frith, C. (2003). Self-awareness and action. *Current Opinion in Neurobiology, 13,* 219–224.

Blanc, J. M., Dodane, C., & Dominey, P. F. (2003). Temporal processing for syntax acquisition: A simulation study. In *Proceedings of the 25th Annual Meeting of the Cognitive Science Society,* pp. 145–150. Retrieved from *http://csjarchive.cogsci.rpi.edu/proceedings/2003/pdfs/48.pdf.*

Böckler, A., Knoblich, G., & Sebanz, N. (2011). Giving a helping hand: Effects of joint attention on mental rotation of body parts. *Experimental Brain Research, 211*, 531–545.

Böckler, A., Knoblich, G., & Sebanz, N. (2012). Effects of a coactor's focus of attention on task performance. *Journal of Experimental Psychology: Human Perception and Performance, 38*(6), 1404–1415.

Böckler, A., Timmermans, B., Sebanz, N., Vogeley, K., & Schilbach, L. (2014). Effects of observing eye contact on gaze following in high-functioning autism. *Journal of Autism and Developmental Disorders, 44*(7), 1651–1658.

Bondy, A. S., & Frost, L. A. (1994). The Picture Exchange Communication System. *Focus on Autism and Other Developmental Disabilities, 9*(3), 1–19.

Bono, M., Daley, T., & Sigman, M. (2004). Joint attention moderates the relation between intervention and language development in young children with autism. *Journal of Autism and Developmental Disorders, 34*, 495–505.

Boothby, E. J., Clark, M. S., & Bargh, J. A. (2014). Shared experiences are amplified. *Psychological Science, 25*(12), 2209–2216.

Bornstein, M., & Sigman, M. (1986). Continuity in mental development from infancy. *Child Development, 57*, 251–274.

Bottema-Beutel, K., Yoder, P. J., Hochman, J. M., & Watson, L. R. (2014). The role of supported joint engagement and parent utterances in language and social communication development in children with autism spectrum disorder. *Journal of Autism and Developmental Disorders, 44*(9), 2162–2174.

Bregman, J. D., Dykens, E., Watson, M., Ort, S. I., & Leckman, J. F. (1987). Fragile-X syndrome: Variability of phenotypic expression. *Journal of the American Academy of Child and Adolescent Psychiatry, 26*(4), 463–471.

Brenner, L., Turner, K., & Muller, R. (2007). Eye movement and visual search: Are there elementary abnormalities in autism? *Journal of Autism and Developmental Disorders, 37*, 1289–1309.

Bretherton, I. (1991). Intentional communication and the development of an understanding of mind. In D. Frye & C. Moore (Eds.), *Children's theories of mind: Mental states and social understanding* (pp. 49–75). Hillsdale, NJ: Erlbaum.

Bristol, M. M., Cohen, D. J., Costello, E. J., Denckla, M., Eckberg, T. J., Kallen, R., . . . Spence, M. A. (1996). State of the science in autism: A report to the National Institutes of Health. *Journal of Autism and Developmental Disorders, 26*(2), 121–154.

Brooks, R., & Meltzoff, A. (2002). The importance of eyes: How infants interpret adult looking behavior. *Developmental Psychology, 38*, 958–966.

Brooks, R., & Meltzoff, A. N. (2015). Connecting the dots from infancy to childhood: A longitudinal study connecting gaze following, language, and explicit theory of mind. *Journal of Experimental Child Psychology, 130*, 67–78.

Brown, B. T., Morris, G., Nida, R. E., & Baker-Ward, L. (2012). Brief report: Making experience personal: Internal states language in the memory narratives of children with and without Asperger's disorder. *Journal of Autism and Developmental Disorders, 42*(3), 441–446.

Brownell, C. A., Ramani, G. B., & Zerwas, S. (2006). Becoming a social partner with peers: Cooperation and social understanding in one- and two-year-olds. *Child Development, 77*(4), 803–821.

Bruce, S. M. (2005). The impact of congenital deafblindness on the struggle to symbolism. *International Journal of Disability, Development and Education, 52*(3), 233–251.

Bruner, J. S. (1975). From communication to language: A psychological perspective. *Cognition, 3*, 255–287.

Bruner, J. S. (1977). Early social interaction and language acquisition. In H. Schaffer (Ed.), *Studies in mother–infant interaction* (pp. 271–289). New York: Academic Press.

Bruner, J. S. (1995). From joint attention to the meeting of minds: An introduction. In C. Moore & P. J. Dunham (Eds.), *Joint attention: Its origins and role in development* (pp. 1–14). Hillsdale, NJ: Erlbaum.

Bruner, J. S., Goodnow, J. J., & Austin, G. A. (1956). *A study of thinking.* New York: Wiley.

Bruner, J. S., & Sherwood, V. (1983). Thought, language and interaction in infancy. In J. Call, E. Galenson, & R. Tyson (Eds.), *Frontiers of infant psychiatry* (pp. 38–55). New York: Basic Books.

Brunetti, M., Zappasodi, F., Marzetti, L., Perrucci, M. G., Cirillo, S., Romani, G. L., . . . Aureli, T. (2014). Do you know what I mean?: Brain oscillations and the understanding of communicative intentions. *Frontiers in Human Neuroscience, 8*, 36.

Buckner, R. L., Andrews-Hanna, J. R., & Schacter, D. L. (2008). The brain's default network. *Annals of the New York Academy of Sciences, 1124*(1), 1–38.

Bugnyar, T., Stöwe, M., & Heinrich, B. (2004). Ravens, *Corvus corax,* follow gaze direction of humans around obstacles. *Proceedings of the Royal Society of London: Series B. Biological Sciences, 271*(156), 1331–1336.

Burnette, C. P., Henderson, H. A., Inge, A. P., Zahka, N. E., Schwartz, C. B., & Mundy, P. C. (2011). Anterior EEG asymmetry and the modifier model of autism. *Journal of Autism and Developmental Disorders, 41*(8), 1113–1124.

Butterworth, B., & Kovas, Y. (2013). Understanding neurocognitive developmental disorders can improve education for all. *Science, 340*(6130), 300–305.

Butterworth, G., & Jarrett, N. (1991). What minds have in common is space: Spatial mechanisms in serving joint visual attention in infancy. *British Journal of Developmental Psychology, 9*, 55–72.

Byom, L. J., & Mutlu, B. (2013). Theory of mind: Mechanisms, methods, and new directions. *Frontiers in Human Neuroscience, 7*, 413.

Cacioppo, J. T., Norris, C. J., Decety, J., Monteleone, G., & Nusbaum, H. (2009). In the eye of the beholder: Individual differences in perceived social isolation predict regional brain activation to social stimuli. *Journal of Cognitive Neuroscience, 21*(1), 83–92.

Cahill, L. (2006). Why sex matters for neuroscience. *Nature Reviews Neuroscience, 7*(6), 477–484.

Calder, A. J., Beaver, J. D., Winston, J. S., Dolan, R. J., Jenkins, R., Eger, E., & Henson, R. N. (2007). Separate coding of different gaze directions in the superior temporal sulcus and inferior parietal lobule. *Current Biology, 17*(1), 20–25.

Camaioni, L., Perucchini, P., Bellagamba, F., & Colonnesi, C. (2004). The role of declarative pointing in developing a theory of mind. *Infancy, 5*(3), 291–308.

Canfield, R., & Kirkham, N. (2001). Infant cortical development and the prospective control of saccadic eye movements. *Infancy, 2,* 197–211.

Caplan, R., Chugani, H., Messa, C., Guthrie, D., Sigman, M., de Traversay, J., & Mundy, P. (1993). Hemispherectomy for early onset intractable seizures: Presurgical cerebral glucose metabolism and postsurgical nonverbal communication. *Developmental Medicine and Child Neurology, 35,* 582–592.

Capps, L., Sigman, M., & Mundy, P. (1994). Attachment security in children with autism. *Development and Psychopathology, 6*(2), 249–261.

Carlin, J. D., & Calder, A. J. (2013). The neural basis of eye gaze processing. *Current Opinion in Neurobiology, 23*(3), 450–455.

Carlson, G. C. (2012). Glutamate receptor dysfunction and drug targets across models of autism spectrum disorders. *Pharmacology, Biochemistry and Behavior, 100*(4), 850–854.

Caruana, N., Brock, J., & Woolgar, A. (2015). A frontotemporoparietal network common to initiating and responding to joint attention bids. *NeuroImage, 108,* 34–46.

Carver, C. S., & White, T. L. (1994). Behavioral inhibition, behavioral activation, and affective responses to impending reward and punishment: The BIS/BAS scales. *Journal of Personality and Social Psychology, 67*(2), 319–333.

Castellanos, F. X., Sonuga-Barke, E. J., Milham, M. P., & Tannock, R. (2006). Characterizing cognition in ADHD: Beyond executive dysfunction. *Trends in Cognitive Sciences, 10*(3), 117–123.

Cavalli-Sforza, L. L., & Feldman, M. W. (1983). Paradox of the evolution of communication and of social interactivity. *Proceedings of the National Academy of Sciences USA, 80*(7), 2017–2021.

Centers for Disease Control and Prevention (CDC). (2014, March 28). Prevalence of autism spectrum disorder among children aged 8 years–Autism and Developmental Disabilities Monitoring Network, 11 sites, United States, 2010. *Morbidity and Mortality Weekly Report, 63*(SS02), 1–21.

Chaminade, T., Marchant, J. L., Kilner, J., & Frith, C. D. (2012). An fMRI study of joint action–varying levels of cooperation correlates with activity in control networks. *Frontiers in Human Neuroscience, 6,* 179.

Chang, W. H., Lee, I. H., Chen, K. C., Chi, M. H., Chiu, N. T., Yao, W. J., . . . Chen, P. S. (2014). Oxytocin receptor gene rs53576 polymorphism modulates oxytocin–dopamine interaction and neuroticism traits—A SPECT study. *Psychoneuroendocrinology, 47,* 212–220.

Charlop, M. H., Schreibman, L., & Tryon, A. S. (1983). Learning through observation: The effects of peer modeling on acquisition and generalization in autistic children. *Journal of Abnormal Child Psychology, 11*(3), 355–366.

Charman, T. (2003). Why is joint attention a pivotal skill in autism? *Philosophical Transactions of the Royal Society of London: Series B. Biological Sciences, 358,* 315–324.

Charman, T., Baron-Cohen, S., Swettenham, J., Baird, G., Cox, A., & Drew, A. (2000). Testing joint attention, imitation, and play infancy precursors to language and theory of mind. *Cognitive Development, 15,* 481–498.

Chechlacz, M., & Gleeson, J. G. (2003). Is mental retardation a defect of synapse structure and function? *Pediatric Neurology, 29*(1), 11–17.

Cheng, Y., & Huang, R. (2012). Using virtual reality environment to improve joint attention associated with pervasive developmental disorder. *Research in Developmental Disabilities, 33*(6), 2141–2152.

Chess, S. (1977). Follow-up report on autism in congenital rubella. *Journal of Autism and Childhood Schizophrenia, 7*(1), 69–81.

Chevallier, C., Kohls, G., Troiani, V., Brodkin, E. S., & Schultz, R. T. (2012). The social motivation theory of autism. *Trends in Cognitive Sciences, 16*(4), 231–239.

Chiu, P. H., Kayali, M. A., Kishida, K. T., Tomlin, D., Klinger, L. G., Klinger, M. R., & Montague, P. R. (2008). Self responses along cingulate cortex reveal quantitative neural phenotype for high-functioning autism. *Neuron, 57*(3), 463–473.

Chlebowski, C., Robins, D. L., Barton, M. L., & Fein, D. (2013). Large-scale use of the Modified Checklist for Autism in low-risk toddlers. *Pediatrics, 131*(4), e1121–e1127.

Chomsky, N. (1959). A review of B. F. Skinner's *Verbal Behavior. Language, 35*, 26–58.

Churchland, P. S., & Winkielman, P. (2012). Modulating social behavior with oxytocin: How does it work? What does it mean? *Hormones and Behavior, 61*(3), 392–399.

Clark, P., & Rutter, M. (1981). Autistic children's responses to structure and to interpersonal demands. *Journal of Autism and Developmental Disorders, 11*(2), 201–217.

Clifford, S. M., Hudry, K., Elsabbagh, M., Charman, T., Johnson, M. H., & BASIS Team. (2013). Temperament in the first 2 years of life in infants at high-risk for autism spectrum disorders. *Journal of Autism and Developmental Disorders, 43*(3), 673–686.

Clohessy, A. B., Posner, M. I., & Rothbart, M. K. (2001). Development of the functional visual field. *Acta Psychologica, 106*(1), 51–68.

Cohen, D. J., Caparulo, B. K., & Shaywitz, B. A. (1978). Neurochemical and developmental models of childhood autism. In G. Serban (Ed.), *Cognitive defects in the development of mental illness* (pp. 66–100). New York: Brunner/Mazel.

Cohen, H., Amerine-Dickens, M., & Smith, T. (2006). Early intensive behavioral treatment: Replication of the UCLA model in a community setting. *Journal of Developmental and Behavioral Pediatrics, 27*(2), S145–S155.

Cohen, I. (2007). A neural network model of autism: Implication for theory and treatment. In D. Mareschal, S., Sylvain, & G. Westerman (Eds.), *Neuroconstructivism II: Perspectives and prospects* (pp. 231–264). New York: Oxford University Press.

Cohen, N. J., Menna, R., Vallance, D. D., Barwick, M. A., Im, N., & Horodezky, N. B. (1998). Language, social cognitive processing, and behavioral characteristics of psychiatrically disturbed children with previously identified and unsuspected language impairments. *Journal of Child Psychology and Psychiatry, 39*(6), 853–864.

Coleman, M., & Gillberg, C. (2012). *The autisms.* New York: Oxford University Press.

Colombi, C., Liebal, K., Tomasello, M., Young, G., Warneken, F., & Rogers, S. J. (2009). Examining correlates of cooperation in autism Imitation, joint attention, and understanding intentions. *Autism, 13*(2), 143–163.

Colombo, J. (1993).. *Sage series on individual differences and development: Vol. 5. Infant cognition: Predicting later intellectual functioning.* Thousand Oaks, CA: Sage.

Colombo, J., Mitchell, D. W., & Horowitz, F. D. (1988). Infant visual attention in the paired-comparison paradigm: Test–retest and attention–performance relations. *Child Development, 59*(5), 1198–1210.

Colonnesi, C., Rieffe, C., Koops, W., & Perucchini, P. (2008). Precursors of a theory of mind: A longitudinal study. *British Journal of Developmental Psychology, 26*(4), 561–577.

Colonnesi, C., Stams, G. J. J., Koster, I., & Noom, M. J. (2010). The relation between pointing and language development: A meta-analysis. *Developmental Review, 30*(4), 352–366.

Corbetta, M., Patel, G., & Shulman, G. L. (2008). The reorienting system of the human brain: from environment to theory of mind. *Neuron, 58*(3), 306–324.

Corkum, V., & Moore, C. (1998). The origins of joint visual attention in infants. *Developmental Psychology, 34*(1), 28–38.

Cornew, L., Dobkins, K. R., Akshoomoff, N., McCleery, J. P., & Carver, L. J. (2012). Atypical social referencing in infant siblings of children with autism spectrum disorders. *Journal of Autism and Developmental Disorders, 42*(12), 2611–2621.

Courchesne, E., Campbell, K., & Solso, S. (2011). Brain growth across the life span in autism: Age-specific changes in anatomical pathology. *Brain Research, 1380*, 138–145.

Courchesne, E., & Pierce, K. (2005). Why the frontal cortex in autism might be talking only to itself: Local over-connectivity but long distance disconnection. *Current Opinion in Neurology, 15*, 225–230.

Couture, S. M., Penn, D. L., & Roberts, D. L. (2006). The functional significance of social cognition in schizophrenia: A review. *Schizophrenia Bulletin, 32*(Suppl. 1), S44–S63.

Cowan, N., Elliott, E. M., Saults, J. S., Morey, C. C., Mattox, S., Hismjatullina, A., & Conway, A. R. (2005). On the capacity of attention: Its estimation and its role in working memory and cognitive aptitudes. *Cognitive Psychology, 51*(1), 42–100.

Craig, A. (2009). How do you feel—now?: The anterior insula and human awareness. *Nature Reviews Neuroscience, 10*(1), 59–70.

Cruse, H. (2003). The evolution of cognition—A hypothesis. *Cognitive Science, 27*(1), 135–155.

Curcio, F. (1978). Sensorimotor functioning and communication in mute autistic children. *Journal of Autism and Developmental Disorders, 8*, 281–292.

Cuthbert, B. N., & Insel, T. R. (2013). Toward the future of psychiatric diagnosis: The seven pillars of RDoC. *BMC Medicine, 11*(1), 126.

Dale, P. S., & Crain-Thoreson, C. (1993). Pronoun reversals: Who, when, and why? *Journal of Child Language, 20*(3), 573–589.

Dawson, G. (2008). Early behavioral intervention, brain plasticity and the prevention of autism spectrum disorders. *Development and Psychopathology, 20,* 775–804.

Dawson, G., & Adams, A. (1984). Imitation and social responsiveness in autistic children. *Journal of Abnormal Child Psychology, 12*(2), 209–226.

Dawson, G., Jones, E. J., Merkle, K., Venema, K., Lowy, R., Faja, S., . . . Webb, S. J. (2012). Early behavioral intervention is associated with normalized brain activity in young children with autism. *Journal of the American Academy of Child and Adolescent Psychiatry, 51*(11), 1150–1159.

Dawson, G., & McKissick, F. C. (1984). Self-recognition in autistic children. *Journal of Autism and Developmental Disorders, 14,* 383–394.

Dawson, G., Meltzoff, A., Osterling, J., Rinaldi, J., & Brown, E. (1998). Children with autism fail to orient to naturally occurring social stimuli. *Journal of Autism and Developmental Disorders, 28,* 479–485.

Dawson, G., Munson, J., Estes, A., Osterling, J., McPartland, J., Toth, K., . . . Abbott, R. (2002). Neurocognitive function and joint attention ability in young children with autism spectrum disorder versus developmental delay. *Child Development, 73*(2), 345–358.

Dawson, G., Osterling, J., Rinaldi, J., Carver, L., & McPartland, J. (2001). Brief report: Recognition memory and stimulus–reward associations: Indirect support for the role of ventromedial prefrontal dysfunction in autism. *Journal of Autism and Developmental Disorders, 31,* 337–341.

Dawson, G., Rogers, S., Munson, J., Smith, M., Winter, J., Greenson, J., . . . Varley, J. (2010). Randomized, controlled trial of an intervention for toddlers with autism: The Early Start Denver Model. *Pediatrics, 125*(1), e17–e23.

Dawson, G., Toth, K., Abbott, R., Osterling, J., Munson, J., Estes, A., & Liaw, J. (2004). Early social attention impairments in autism: Social orienting, joint attention, and attention in autism. *Developmental Psychology, 40,* 271–283.

Dawson, G., Webb, S. J., & McPartland, J. (2005). Understanding the nature of face processing impairment in autism: Insights from behavioral and electrophysiological studies. *Developmental Neuropsychology, 27*(3), 403–424.

Decety, J., & Grèzes, J. (2006). The power of simulation: Imagining one's own and other's behavior. *Brain Research, 1079*(1), 4–14.

Decety, J., & Sommerville, J. (2003). Shared representations between self and other: A social cognitive neuroscience view. *Trends in Cognitive Sciences, 7,* 527–533.

DeMyer, M. K., Alpern, G. D., Barton, S., DeMyer, W. E., Churchill, D. W., Hingtgen, J., & Kimberlin, C. (1972). Imitation in autistic, early schizophrenic, and non-psychotic subnormal children. *Journal of Autism and Childhood Schizophrenia, 2*(3), 264–287.

Denny, B. T., Kober, H., Wager, T. D., & Ochsner, K. N. (2012). A meta-analysis of functional neuroimaging studies of self- and other judgments reveals a spatial gradient for mentalizing in medial prefrontal cortex. *Journal of Cognitive Neuroscience, 24*(8), 1742–1752.

D'Entremont, B., Hains, S., & Muir, D. (1997). A demonstration of gaze following in 3- to 6- month-olds. *Infant Behavior and Development, 20,* 569–572.

Devinsky, O., & Luciano, D. (1993). The contributions of the cingulate cortex to human behavior. In B. Vogt & M. Gabriel (Eds.), *Neurobiology of the cingulate cortex and limbic thalamus: A comprehensive handbook* (pp. 527–556). Boston, MA: Birkhauser.

Dichter, G. S., Felder, J. N., & Bodfish, J. W. (2009). Autism is characterized by dorsal anterior cingulate hyperactivation during social target detection. *Social Cognitive and Affective Neuroscience, 4*(3), 215–226.

Diessel, H. (2006). Demonstratives, joint attention, and the emergence of grammar. *Cognitive Linguistics, 17*(4), 463–489.

Di Martino, A., Ross, K., Uddin, L. Q., Sklar, A. B., Castellanos, F. X., & Milham, M. P. (2009). Functional brain correlates of social and nonsocial processes in autism spectrum disorders: An activation likelihood estimation meta-analysis. *Biological Psychiatry, 65*(1), 63–74.

Doane, J. A., West, K. L., Goldstein, M. J., Rodnick, E. H., & Jones, J. E. (1981). Parental communication deviance and affective style: Predictors of subsequent schizophrenia spectrum disorders in vulnerable adolescents. *Archives of General Psychiatry, 38*, 679–685.

Dunlosky, J., Hertzog, C., & Powell-Moman, A. (2005). The contribution of mediator-based deficiencies to age differences in associative learning. *Developmental Psychology, 41*(2), 389–400.

Dykstra Steinbenner, J., & Watson, L. (2015). Student engagement in the classroom: The impact of the classroom, teacher, and student factors. *Journal of Autism and developmental Disorders, 45*, 2392–2410.

Ebstein, R. P., Israel, S., Chew, S. H., Zhong, S., & Knafo, A. (2010). Genetics of human social behavior. *Neuron, 65*(6), 831–844.

Edelson, M., Sharot, T., Dolan, R. J., & Dudai, Y. (2011). Following the crowd: Brain substrates of long-term memory conformity. *Science, 333*(6038), 108–111.

Edwards, G., Stephenson, L., Dalmaso, M., & Bayliss, A. (2015). Social orienting in gaze leading: A mechanism for shared attention. *Proceedings of the Royal Society of London: Series B. Biological Sciences, 282*.

Egawa, J., Watanabe, Y., Endo, T., Tamura, R., Masuzawa, N., & Someya, T. (2013). Association between OXTR and clinical phenotypes of autism spectrum disorders. *Psychiatry Research, 208*(1), 99–100.

Egel, A., Richman, G., & Koegel, R. (1981). Normal peer models and autistic children's learning. *Journal of Applied Behavior Analysis, 14*, 3–12.

Eisenberg, N., Fabes, R. A., Shepard, S. A., Murphy, B. C., Guthrie, I. K., Jones, S., . . . Maszk, P. (1997). Contemporaneous and longitudinal prediction of children's social functioning from regulation and emotionality. *Child Development, 68*(4), 642–664.

Elison, J. T., Wolff, J. J., Heimer, D. C., Paterson, S. J., Gu, H., Hazlett, H. C., . . . Piven, J. (2013). Frontolimbic neural circuitry at 6 months predicts individual differences in joint attention at 9 months. *Developmental Science, 16*(2), 186–197.

Elman, J. (2005). Connectionist models of cognitive development: Where next? *Trends in Cognitive Sciences, 9*, 111–117.

Emery, N. (2000). The eyes have it: The neuroethology, function, and evolution of social gaze. *Neuroscience and Biobehavioral Reviews, 24*, 581–604.

Emmorey, K., Thompson, R., & Colvin, R. (2009). Eye gaze during comprehension of American Sign Language by native and beginning signers. *Journal of Deaf Studies and Deaf Education, 14*(2), 237–243.

Escalona, A., Field, T., Nadel, J., & Lundy, B. (2002). Brief report: Imitation effects on children with autism. *Journal of Autism and Developmental Disorders, 32*(2), 141–144.

Estes, A., Rivera, V., Bryan, M., Cali, P., & Dawson, G. (2011). Discrepancies between academic achievement and intellectual ability in higher-functioning school-aged children with autism spectrum disorder. *Journal of Autism and Developmental Disorders, 41*(8), 1044–1052.

Ezell, S., Field, T., Nadel, J., Newton, R., Murrey, G., Siddalingappa, V., . . . Grace, A. (2012). Imitation effects on joint attention behaviors of children with autism. *Psychology, 3*(9), 681–685.

Fagan, J. F., III, & Detterman, D. K. (1992). The Fagan test of infant intelligence: A technical summary. *Journal of Applied Developmental Psychology, 13*(2), 173–193.

Falck-Ytter, T., Thorup, E., & Bölte, S. (2014). Brief report: Lack of processing bias for the objects other people attend to in 3-year-olds with autism. *Journal of Autism and Developmental Disorders, 45*(6), 1897–1904.

Farrant, B. M., & Zubrick, S. R. (2011). Early vocabulary development: The importance of joint attention and parent–child book reading. *First Language, 32*, 343–364.

Farroni, T., Csibra, G., Simion, F., & Johnson, M. H. (2002). Eye contact detection in humans from birth. *Proceedings of the National Academy of Sciences USA, 99*(14), 9602–9605.

Farroni, T., Mansfield, E. M., Lai, C., & Johnson, M. H. (2003). Infants perceiving and acting on the eyes: Tests of an evolutionary hypothesis. *Journal of Experimental Child Psychology, 85*(3), 199–212.

Farroni, T., Massaccesi, S., & Francesca, S. (2002). Can the direction of gaze of another person shift the attention of a neonate? *Giornale Italiano di Psicologia, 29*, 857–864.

Farroni, T., Massaccesi, S., Menon, E., & Johnson, M. H. (2007). Direct gaze modulates face recognition in young infants. *Cognition, 102*(3), 396–404.

Farroni, T., Massaccesi, S., Pividori, D., & Johnson, M. H. (2004). Gaze following in newborns. *Infancy, 5*(1), 39–60.

Fausto-Sterling, A., Coll, C. G., & Lamarre, M. (2012a). Sexing the baby: Part 2— What do we really know about sex differentiation in the first three years of life? *Social Science and Medicine, 74*(11), 1684–1692.

Fausto-Sterling, A., Coll, C. G., & Lamarre, M. (2012b). Sexing the baby: Part 2—Applying dynamic systems theory to the emergences of sex-related differences in infants and toddlers. *Social Science and Medicine, 74*(11), 1693–1702.

Fein, D., Stevens, M., Dunn, M., Waterhouse, L., Allen, D., Rapin, I., & Feinstein, C. (1999). Subtypes of pervasive developmental disorders: Clinical characteristics. *Child Neuropsychology, 5*, 1–23.

Feldman, J., & Narayanan, S. (2004). Embodied meaning in a neural theory of language. *Brain and Language, 89*, 385–392.

Field, T., Lasko, D., Mundy, P., Henteleff, T., Kabat, S., Talpins, S., & Dowling,

M. (1997). Autistic children's attentiveness and responsivity improved after touch therapy. *Journal of Autism and Developmental Disorders, 27,* 333–338.

Fields, R. D. (2008). White matter matters. *Scientific American, 298*(3), 54–61.

Findlay, J., & Gilchrist, I. (2003). *Active vision: The psychology of looking and seeing.* New York: Oxford University Press.

Fombonne, E. (1999). The epidemiology of autism: A review. *Psychological Medicine, 29*(4), 769–786.

Fraser, A. G., & Marcotte, E. M. (2004). A probabilistic view of gene function. *Nature Genetics, 36*(6), 559–564.

Freeman, R., Fast, D., Burd, L., Kerbeshian, J., Robertson, M., & Sandor, P. (2000). An international perspective on Tourette syndrome: Selected findings from 3500 individuals in 22 countries. *Developmental Medicine and Child Neurology, 42,* 436–447.

Freeman, S. F., Gulsrud, A., & Kasari, C. (2015). Brief report: Linking early joint attention and play abilities to later reports of friendships for children with ASD. *Journal of Autism and Developmental Disorders, 45,* 2259–2266.

Frischen, A., & Tipper, S. P. (2004). Orienting attention via observed gaze shift evokes longer term inhibitory effects: Implications for social interactions, attention, and memory. *Journal of Experimental Psychology: General, 133*(4), 516–533.

Friston, K. J. (1994). Functional and effective connectivity in neuroimaging: A synthesis. *Human Brain Mapping, 2*(1–2), 56–78.

Frith, C. D., & Frith, U. (1999). Interacting minds—a biological basis. *Science, 286*(5445), 1692–1695.

Frith, U. (1989). *Autism: Explaining the enigma.* Oxford, UK: Blackwell.

Frith, U., & Frith, C. (2001). The biological basis of social interaction. *Current Directions in Psychological Science, 10*(5), 151–155.

Frost, A., Elgort, M. G., Brandman, O., Ives, C., Collins, S. R., Miller-Vedam, L., . . . Weissman, J. S. (2012). Functional repurposing revealed by comparing *S. pombe* and *S. cerevisiae* genetic interactions. *Cell, 149*(6), 1339–1352.

Fu, X., Giavalisco, P., Liu, X., Catchpole, G., Fu, N., Ning, Z. B., . . . Khaitovich, P. (2011). Rapid metabolic evolution in human prefrontal cortex. *Proceedings of the National Academy of Sciences USA, 108*(15), 6181–6186.

Fuchs, T., & De Jaegher, H. (2009). Enactive intersubjectivity: Participatory sense-making and mutual incorporation. *Phenomenology and the Cognitive Sciences, 8*(4), 465–486.

Fujita, E., Dai, H., Tanabe, Y., Zhiling, Y., Yamagata, T., Miyakawa, T., . . . Momoi, T. (2010). Autism spectrum disorder is related to endoplasmic reticulum stress induced by mutations in the synaptic cell adhesion molecule, CADM1. *Cell Death and Disease, 1*(6), e47.

Gable, S. L., Reis, H. T., Impett, E. A., & Asher, E. R. (2004). What do you do when things go right?: The intrapersonal and interpersonal benefits of sharing positive events. *Journal of Personality and Social Psychology, 87*(2), 228–245.

Gallese, V., Keysers, C., & Rizzolatti, G. (2004). A unifying view of the basis of social cognition. *Trends in Cognitive Sciences, 8*(9), 396–403.

Gamer, M., Hecht, H., Seipp, N., & Hiller, W. (2011). Who is looking at me?: The cone of gaze widens in social phobia. *Cognition and Emotion, 25*(4), 756–764

Gamer, M., Zurowski, B., & Büchel, C. (2010). Different amygdala subregions mediate valence-related and attentional effects of oxytocin in humans. *Proceedings of the National Academy of Sciences USA, 107*(20), 9400–9405.

Gandal, M. J., Anderson, R. L., Billingslea, E. N., Carlson, G. C., Roberts, T. P., & Siegel, S. J. (2012). Mice with reduced NMDA receptor expression: more consistent with autism than schizophrenia? *Genes, Brain and Behavior, 11*(6), 740–750.

Gangi, D. N., Ibañez, L. V., & Messinger, D. S. (2014). Joint attention initiation with and without positive affect: Risk group differences and associations with ASD symptoms. *Journal of Autism and Developmental Disorders, 44*(6), 1414–1424.

Garon, N., Bryson, S. E., Zwaigenbaum, L., Smith, I. M., Brian, J., Roberts, W., & Szatmari, P. (2009). Temperament and its relationship to autistic symptoms in a high-risk infant sib cohort. *Journal of Abnormal Child Psychology, 37*(1), 59–78.

Garrido, M. I. (2012). Brain connectivity: The feel of blindsight. *Current Biology, 22*(15), R599–R600.

Gatzke-Kopp, L. M. (2011). The canary in the coalmine: The sensitivity of mesolimbic dopamine to environmental adversity during development. *Neuroscience and Biobehavioral Reviews, 35*(3), 794–803.

Gavrilov, Y., Rotem, S., Ofek, R., & Geva, R. (2012). Socio-cultural effects on children's initiation of joint attention. *Frontiers of Human Neuroscience, 6*, 286.

Gerfen, C. R., & Surmeier, D. J. (2011). Modulation of striatal projection systems by dopamine. *Annual Review of Neuroscience, 34*, 441–466.

Geschwind, D. H. (2011). Genetics of autism spectrum disorders. *Trends in Cognitive Sciences, 15*(9), 409–416.

Geschwind, D. H., & Levitt, P. (2007). Autism spectrum disorders: Developmental disconnection syndromes. *Current Opinion in Neurobiology, 17*, 103–111.

Gillespie-Lynch, K., Elias, R., Escudero, P., Hutman, T., & Johnson, S. P. (2013). Atypical gaze following in autism: A comparison of three potential mechanisms. *Journal of Autism and Developmental Disorders, 43*(12), 2779–2792.

Gillespie-Lynch, K., Sepeta, L., Wang, Y., Marshall, S., Gomez, L., Sigman, M., & Hutman, T. (2012). Early childhood predictors of the social competence of adults with autism. *Journal of Autism and Developmental Disorders, 42*(2), 161–174.

Gleick, J. (1987). *Chaos: Making a new science.* New York: Viking Penguin.

Gong, P., Shen, G., Li, S., Zhang, G., Fang, H., Lei, L., . . . Zhang, F. (2013). Genetic variations in COMT and DRD2 modulate attentional bias for affective facial expressions. *PloS One, 8*(12), e8144.

Gong, T., & Shuai, L. (2012). Modelling the coevolution of joint attention and language. *Proceedings of the Royal Society of London: Series B. Biological Sciences, 279*(1747), 4643–4651.

Goods, K. S., Ishijima, E., Chang, Y. C., & Kasari, C. (2013). Preschool based JASPER intervention in minimally verbal children with autism: Pilot RCT. *Journal of Autism and Developmental Disorders, 43*(5), 1050–1056.

Gordon, I., Eilbott, J. A., Feldman, R., Pelphrey, K. A., & Vander Wyk, B. C.

(2013). Social, reward, and attention brain networks are involved when online bids for joint attention are met with congruent versus incongruent responses. *Social Neuroscience, 8*(6), 544–554.

Gordon, R. (1986). Folk psychology as simulation. *Mind and Language, 1*, 158–171.

Gotham, K., Risi, S., Dawson, G., Tager-Flusberg, H., Joseph, R., Carter, A., . . . Lord, C. (2008). A replication of the Autism Diagnostic Observation Schedule (ADOS) revised algorithms. *Journal of the American Academy of Child and Adolescent Psychiatry, 47*(6), 642–651.

Gotham, K., Risi, S., Pickles, A., & Lord, C. (2007). The Autism Diagnostic Observation Schedule: Revised algorithms for improved diagnostic validity. *Journal of Autism and Developmental Disorders, 37*(4), 613–627.

Gottfried, J. A., O'Doherty, J., & Dolan, R. J. (2003). Encoding predictive reward value in human amygdala and orbitofrontal cortex. *Science, 301*(5636), 1104–1107.

Grandin, T. (1995). *Thinking in pictures: Reports from my life with autism*. New York: Doubleday.

Gray, J. A. (1981). A critique of Eysenck's theory of personality. In H. Eysenck (Ed.), *A model for personality* (pp. 246–277). Berlin: Springer.

Gray, J. A. (1987). *The psychology of fear and stress*. Cambridge, UK: Cambridge University Press.

Gredebäck, G., Fikke, L., & Melinder, A. (2010). The development of joint visual attention: A longitudinal study of gaze following during interactions with mothers and strangers. *Developmental Science, 13*(6), 839–848.

Greene, D. J., Colich, N., Iacoboni, M., Zaidel, E., Bookheimer, S. Y., & Dapretto, M. (2011). Atypical neural networks for social orienting in autism spectrum disorders. *NeuroImage, 56*(1), 354–362.

Greenough, W., Black, J., & Wallace, C. (1987). Experience and brain development. *Child Development, 58*, 539–559.

Grice, S. J., Halit, H., Farroni, T., Baron-Cohen, S., Bolton, P., & Johnson, M. H. (2005). Neural correlates of eye-gaze detection in young children with autism. *Cortex, 41*(3), 342–353.

Griffith, E., Pennington, B., Wehner, E., & Rogers, S. (1999). Executive functions in young children with autism. *Child Development, 70*, 817–832.

Grossmann, T., & Johnson, M. H. (2010). Selective prefrontal cortex responses to joint attention in early infancy. *Biology Letters, 6*(4), 540–543.

Grossmann, T., Johnson, M. H., Farroni, T., & Csibra, G. (2007). Social perception in the infant brain: Gamma oscillatory activity in response to eye gaze. *Social Cognitive and Affective Neuroscience, 2*, 284–291.

Gulsrud, A. C., Hellerman, G., Freeman, S., & Kasari, C. (2014). Two to ten years: Developmental trajectories of joint attention in children with ASD who received targeted social communication interventions. *Autism Research, 7*(2), 207–215.

Gulsrud, A. C., Kasari, C., Freeman, S., & Paparella, T. (2007). Children with autism's response to novel stimuli while participating in interventions targeting joint attention or symbolic play skills. *Autism, 11*(6), 535–546.

Guo, J., & Feng, G. (2013). How eye gaze feedback changes parent–child joint attention in shared storybook reading. In Y. A. Nakano, C. Conati, & T. Bader (Eds.), *Eye gaze in intelligent user interfaces* (pp. 9–21). London, UK: Springer.

Gurvich, C., & Rossell, S. L. (2015). Dopamine and cognitive control: Sex-by-genotype interactions influence the capacity to switch attention. *Behavioural Brain Research, 15,* 96–101.

Gutstein, S. E., Burgess, A. F., & Montfort, K. (2007). Evaluation of the relationship development intervention program. *Autism, 11*(5), 397–411.

Haas, B. W., Anderson, I. W., & Smith, J. M. (2013). Navigating the complex path between the oxytocin receptor gene (OXTR) and cooperation: An endophenotype approach. *Frontiers in Human Neuroscience, 7,* 801.

Hale, C. M., & Tager-Flusberg, H. (2003). The influence of language on theory of mind: A training study. *Developmental Science, 6*(3), 346–359.

Hall, S. S., Lightbody, A. A., Hirt, M., Rezvani, A., & Reiss, A. L. (2010). Autism in fragile X syndrome: A category mistake? *Journal of the American Academy of Child and Adolescent Psychiatry, 49*(9), 921–933.

Hammock, E. A. (2015). Developmental perspectives on oxytocin and vasopressin. *Neuropsychopharmacology, 40*(1), 24–42.

Hammock, E. A., & Young, L. J. (2006). Oxytocin, vasopressin and pair bonding: Implications for autism. *Philosophical Transactions of the Royal Society of London: Series B. Biological Sciences, 361*(1476), 2187–2198.

Hani, H. B., Gonzalez-Barrero, A. N. A., & Nadig, A. S. (2013). Children's referential understanding of novel words and parent labeling behaviors: Similarities across children with and without autism spectrum disorders. *Journal of Child Language, 40*(05), 971–1002.

Hanna, J. E., & Brennan, S. E. (2007). Speakers' eye gaze disambiguates referring expressions early during face-to-face conversation. *Journal of Memory and Language, 57*(4), 596–615.

Happé, F., & Frith, U. (2014). Annual research review: Towards a developmental neuroscience of atypical social cognition. *Journal of Child Psychology and Psychiatry, 55*(6), 553–577.

Happé, F., Ronald, A., & Plomin, R. (2006). Time to give up on a single explanation for autism. *Nature Neuroscience, 9*(10), 1218–1220.

Hart, S. A., Petrill, S. A., Willcutt, E., Thompson, L. A., Schatschneider, C., Deater-Deckard, K., & Cutting, L. E. (2010). Exploring how symptoms of attention-deficit/hyperactivity disorder are related to reading and mathematics performance general genes, general environments. *Psychological Science, 21*(11), 1708–1715.

Hazlett, H. C., Poe, M. D., Lightbody, A. A., Gerig, G., MacFall, J. R., Ross, A. K., . . . Piven, J. (2009). Teasing apart the heterogeneity of autism: Same behavior, different brains in toddlers with fragile X syndrome and autism. *Journal of Neurodevelopmental Disorders, 1*(1), 81–90.

Hebb, D. (1949). *The organization of behavior.* New York: Wiley.

Henderson, L., Yoder, P., Yale, M., & McDuffie, A. (2002). Getting the point: Electrophysiological correlates of protodeclarative pointing. *International Journal of Developmental Neuroscience, 20,* 449–458.

Hermelin, B., & O'Connor, N. (1970). *Psychological experiments with autistic children*. Oxford, UK: Pergamon Press.

Hernandez, L. M., Rudie, J. D., Green, S. A., Bookheimer, S., & Dapretto, M. (2015). Neural signatures of autism spectrum disorders: Insights into brain network dynamics. *Neuropsychopharmacology, 40*(1), 171–189.

Hettinger, J. A., Liu, X., Hudson, M. L., Lee, A., Cohen, I. L., Michaelis, R. C., . . . Holden, J. J. (2012). DRD2 and PPP1R1B (DARPP-32) polymorphisms independently confer increased risk for autism spectrum disorders and additively predict affected status in male-only affected sib-pair families. *Behavioral and Brain Functions, 8*, 19.

Hirotani, M., Stets, M., Striano, T., & Friederici, A. D. (2009). Joint attention helps infants learn new words: Event-related potential evidence. *NeuroReport, 20*(6), 600–605.

Hobson, J., & Hobson, R. P. (2007). Identification: The missing link between joint attention and imitation. *Development and Psychopathology, 19*, 411–431.

Hobson, R. P. (2002). *The cradle of thought: Exploring the origins of thinking*. London, UK: Macmillan.

Hobson, R. P. (2005). What puts the "jointness" into joint attention? In N. Eilan, C. Hoerl, T. McCormack, & J. Roessler (Eds.), *Joint attention: Communication and other minds. Issues in philosophy and psychology* (pp. 185–204). Oxford, UK: Clarendon Press.

Hobson, R. P., Lee, A., & Brown, R. (1999). Autism and congenital blindness. *Journal of Autism and Developmental Disorders, 12*, 45–66.

Hobson, R. P., Ouston, J., & Lee, A. (1988). What's in a face?: The case of autism. *British Journal of Psychology, 79*(4), 441–453.

Holroyd, C., & Coles, M. (2002). The neural basis of human error processing: Reinforcement learning, dopamine and the error related negativity. *Psychological Review, 109*, 679–709.

Hood, B. M., Macrae, C. N., Cole-Davies, V., & Dias, M. (2003). Eye remember you: The effects of gaze direction on face recognition in children and adults. *Developmental Science, 6*(1), 67–71.

Hood, B. M., Willen, J., & Driver, J. (1998). Adult's eyes trigger shifts of visual attention in human infants. *Psychological Science, 9*, 131–134.

Hooker, C. I., Paller, K. A., Gitelman, D. R., Parrish, T. B., Mesulam, M. M., & Reber, P. J. (2003). Brain networks for analyzing eye gaze. *Cognitive Brain Research, 17*(2), 406–418.

Hopkins, W. D., Keebaugh, A. C., Reamer, L. A., Schaeffer, J., Schapiro, S. J., & Young, L. J. (2014). Genetic influences on receptive joint attention in chimpanzees (*Pan troglodytes*). *Scientific Reports, 4*, 3774.

Hopkins, W. D., Misiura, M., Reamer, L. A., Schaeffer, J. A., Mareno, M. C., & Schapiro, S. J. (2014). Poor receptive joint attention skills are associated with atypical gray matter asymmetry in the posterior superior temporal gyrus of chimpanzees (*Pan troglodytes*). *Frontiers in Psychology, 5*, 7.

Hopkins, W. D., & Taglialatela, J. P. (2013). Initiation of joint attention is associated with morphometric variation in the anterior cingulate cortex of chimpanzees (*Pan troglodytes*). *American Journal of Primatology, 75*(5), 441–449.

Howlin, P. (1978). The assessment of social behavior. In M. Rutter & E. Schopler (Eds.), *Autism: A reappraisal of concepts and treatment* (pp. 63–69). New York: Plenum Press.

Howlin, P. (1986). An overview of social behavior in autism. In E. Schopler & G. Mesibov (Eds.), *Social behavior in autism* (pp. 103–131). New York: Plenum Press.

Huemer, S. V., & Mann, V. (2010). A comprehensive profile of decoding and comprehension in autism spectrum disorders. *Journal of Autism and Developmental Disorders, 40*(4), 485–493.

Hughes, C., & Leekam, S. (2004). What are the links between theory of mind and social relations?: Review, reflections and new directions for studies of typical and atypical development. *Social Development, 13*(4), 590–619.

Hughes, C., & Russell, J. (1993). Autistic children's difficulty with mental disengagement from an object: Its implications for theories of autism. *Developmental Psychology, 29*(3), 498–510.

Humphreys, G. W., & Bedford, J. (2011). The relations between joint action and theory of mind: A neuropsychological analysis. *Experimental Brain Research, 211*(3–4), 357–369.

Hunt, E. (1999). Intelligence and human resources: Past, present and future. In P. Ackerman, P. Kyllonen, & R. Roberts (Eds.), *Learning and individual differences* (pp. 3–30). Washington, DC: American Psychological Association.

Hwang, B., & Hughes, C. (2000). The effects of social interactive training on early social communicative skills of children with autism. *Journal of Autism and Developmental Disorders, 30*(4), 331–343.

Iacoboni, M. (2005). Neural mechanisms of imitation. *Current Opinion in Neurobiology, 15*(6), 632–637.

Ibañez, L. V., Grantz, C. J., & Messinger, D. S. (2013). The development of referential communication and autism symptomatology in high-risk infants. *Infancy, 18*(5), 687–707.

Ingersoll, B. (2012). Brief report: Effect of a focused imitation intervention on social functioning in children with autism. *Journal of Autism and Developmental Disorders, 42*(8), 1768–1773.

Ingersoll, B., & Lalonde, K. (2010). The impact of object and gesture imitation training on language use in children with autism spectrum disorder. *Journal of Speech, Language, and Hearing Research, 53*(4), 1040–1051.

Ingersoll, B., & Schreibman, L. (2006). Teaching reciprocal imitation skills to young children with autism using a naturalistic behavioral approach: Effects on language, pretend play, and joint attention. *Journal of Autism and Developmental Disorders, 36*(4), 487–505.

Insel, T., Cuthbert, B., Garvey, M., Heinssen, R., Pine, D. S., Quinn, K., . . . Wang, P. (2010). Research Domain Criteria (RDoC): Toward a new classification framework for research on mental disorders. *American Journal of Psychiatry, 167*(7), 748–751.

Isaksen, J., & Holth, P. (2009). An operant approach to teaching joint attention skills to children with autism. *Behavioral Interventions, 24*(4), 215–236.

Ishibashi, T., Horisawa, T., Tokuda, K., Ishiyama, T., Ogasa, M., Tagashira, R., . . .

Nakamura, M. (2010). Pharmacological profile of lurasidone, a novel antipsychotic agent with potent 5-hydroxytryptamine 7 (5-HT7) and 5-HT1A receptor activity. *Journal of Pharmacology and Experimental Therapeutics, 334*(1), 171–181.

Jahromi, L. B., Kasari, C. L., McCracken, J. T., Lee, L. S., Aman, M. G., McDougle, C. J., . . . Posey, D. J. (2009). Positive effects of methylphenidate on social communication and self-regulation in children with pervasive developmental disorders and hyperactivity. *Journal of Autism and Developmental Disorders, 39*(3), 395–404.

Jamison, K. (1995). *An unquiet mind: A memoir of moods and madness.* New York: Knopf.

Janik, V. M. (2013). Cognitive skills in bottlenose dolphin communication. *Trends in Cognitive Sciences, 17*(4), 157–159.

Jarrold, W., Mundy, P., Gwaltney, M., Bailenson, J., Hatt, N., McIntyre, N., . . . Swain, L. (2013). Social attention in a virtual public speaking task in higher functioning children with autism. *Autism Research, 6*(5), 393–410.

Järvinen-Pasley, A., Bellugi, U., Reilly, J., Mills, D., Galaburda, A., Reiss, A., & Korenberg, J. (2008). Defining the social phenotype in Williams syndrome: A model for linking gene, the brain, and behavior. *Development and Psychopathology, 20*(1), 1–35.

Jocham, G., Klein, T. A., Neumann, J., von Cramon, D. Y., Reuter, M., & Ullsperger, M. (2009). Dopamine DRD2 polymorphism alters reversal learning and associated neural activity. *Journal of Neuroscience, 29*(12), 3695–3704.

Johnson, M. H. (1990). Cortical maturation and the development of visual attention in early infancy. *Journal of Cognitive Neuroscience, 2*, 81–95.

Johnson, M. H. (1995). The inhibition of automatic saccades in early infancy. *Developmental Psychobiology, 28*, 281–291.

Johnson, M. H., Dziurawiec, S., Ellis, H., & Morton, J. (1991). Newborns' preferential tracking of face-like stimuli and its subsequent decline. *Cognition, 40*(1), 1–19.

Johnson, M. H., Griffin, R., Csibra, G., Halit, H., Farroni, T., de Haan, M., . . . Richards, J. (2005). The emergence of the social brain network: Evidence from typical and atypical development. *Development and Psychopathology, 17*, 599–619.

Johnson, M. H., Grossmann, T., & Kadosh, K. C. (2009). Mapping functional brain development: Building a social brain through interactive specialization. *Developmental Psychology, 45*(1), 151–159.

Johnson, M. H., & Mareschal, D. (2001). Cognitive and perceptual development during infancy. *Current Opinion in Neurobiology, 11*(2), 213–218.

Jones, C. R., Happé, F., Golden, H., Marsden, A. J., Tregay, J., Simonoff, E., . . . Charman, T. (2009). Reading and arithmetic in adolescents with autism spectrum disorders: Peaks and dips in attainment. *Neuropsychology, 23*(6), 718–739.

Jones, C. R., Happé, F., Pickles, A., Marsden, A. J., Tregay, J., Baird, G., . . . Charman, T. (2011). 'Everyday memory' impairments in autism spectrum disorders. *Journal of Autism and Developmental Disorders, 41*(4), 455–464.

Jones, E. A. (2009). Establishing response and stimulus classes for initiating joint attention in children with autism. *Research in Autism Spectrum Disorders, 3*(2), 375–389.

Jones, E. A., Carr, E., & Feeley, K. (2006). Multiple effects of joint attention intervention for children with autism. *Behavior Modification, 30*, 782–834.

Jones, E. A., & Feeley, K. M. (2007). Parent implemented joint attention intervention for preschoolers with autism. *Journal of Speech–Language Pathology and Applied Behavior Analysis, 2*(3), 253–268.

Jones, E. J., Gliga, T., Bedford, R., Charman, T., & Johnson, M. H. (2014). Developmental pathways to autism: A review of prospective studies of infants at risk. *Neuroscience and Biobehavioral Reviews, 39*, 1–33.

Jones, W., & Klin, A. (2013). Attention to eyes is present but in decline in 2–6-month-old infants later diagnosed with autism. *Nature, 504*(7480), 427–431.

Just, M. A., Cherkassky, V. L., Keller, T. A., Kana, R. K., & Minshew, N. J. (2007). Functional and anatomical cortical underconnectivity in autism: Evidence from an FMRI study of an executive function task and corpus callosum morphometry. *Cerebral Cortex, 17*(4), 951–961.

Just, M. A., Keller, T. A., Malave, V. L., Kana, R. K., & Varma, S. (2012). Autism as a neural systems disorder: A theory of frontal–posterior underconnectivity. *Neuroscience and Biobehavioral Reviews, 36*(4), 1292–1313.

Kaale, A., Fagerland, M. W., Martinsen, E. W., & Smith, L. (2014). Preschool-based social communication treatment for children with autism: 12-month follow-up of a randomized trial. *Journal of the American Academy of Child and Adolescent Psychiatry, 53*(2), 188–198.

Kaale, A., Smith, L., & Sponheim, E. (2012). A randomized controlled trial of preschool-based joint attention intervention for children with autism. *Journal of Child Psychology and Psychiatry, 53*(1), 97–105.

Kaiser, A. P., Hancock, T. B., & Nietfeld, J. P. (2000). The effects of parent-implemented enhanced milieu teaching on the social communication of children who have autism. *Early Education and Development, 11*(4), 423–446.

Kanner, L. (1943). Autistic disorder of affective contact. *Nervous Child, 2*, 217–250.

Kanner, L. (1949). Problems of nosology and psychodynamics of early infantile autism. *American Journal of Orthopsychiatry, 19*, 416–426.

Kaplan, A. (1964). *The conduct of inquiry: Methodology for behavioral science.* New York: Harper & Row.

Kaplan, P., Wang, P., & Francke, U. (2001). Williams (Williams Beuren) syndrome: A distinct neurobehavioral disorder. *Journal of Child Neurology, 16*(3), 177–190.

Karlsgodt, K. H., Sun, D., Jimenez, A. M., Lutkenhoff, E. S., Willhite, R., van Erp, T. G., & Cannon, T. D. (2008). Developmental disruptions in neural connectivity in the pathophysiology of schizophrenia. *Development and Psychopathology, 20*(4), 1297–1327.

Karmel, B., Gardner, J., Swensen, L., Lennon, E., & London, E. (2008, March). *Contrasts of medical and behavioral data from NICU infants suspect and non-suspect for autism spectrum disorder (ASD).* Paper presented at the International Conference on Infant Studies, Vancouver, British Columbia, Canada.

Karmiloff-Smith, A. (1995). *Beyond modularity: A developmental perspective on cognitive science.* Cambridge, MA: MIT Press.

Kasari, C., Freeman, S. F., & Paparella, T. (2000). Early intervention in autism: Joint attention and symbolic play. *International Review of Research in Mental Retardation, 23,* 207–237.

Kasari, C., Freeman, S., & Paparella, T. (2006). Joint attention and symbolic play in young children with autism: A randomized controlled intervention study. *Journal of Child Psychology and Psychiatry, 47,* 611–620.

Kasari, C., Freeman, S., & Paparella, T. (2007, April). *The UCLA RCT on play and joint attention.* Paper presented at the Biennial Conference of the Society for Research on Child Development, Boston, MA.

Kasari, C., Gulsrud, A., Freeman, S., Paparella, T., & Hellemann, G. (2012). Longitudinal follow-up of children with autism receiving targeted interventions on joint attention and play. *Journal of the American Academy of Child and Adolescent Psychiatry, 51*(5), 487–495.

Kasari, C., Gulsrud, A., Hellemann, P. H., & Berry, K. (2015). Randomized comparative efficacy study of parent-mediated intervention for toddlers with ASD. *Journal of Consulting and Clinical Psychology, 83*(3), 554–563.

Kasari, C., Gulsrud, A. C., Wong, C., Kwon, S., & Locke, J. (2010). Randomized controlled caregiver mediated joint engagement intervention for toddlers with autism. *Journal of Autism and Developmental Disorders, 40*(9), 1045–1056.

Kasari, C., Kaiser, A., Goods, K., Nietfeld, J., Mathy, P., Landa, R., . . . Almirall, D. (2014). Communication interventions for minimally verbal children with autism: A sequential multiple assignment randomized trial. *Journal of the American Academy of Child and Adolescent Psychiatry, 53*(6), 635–646.

Kasari, C., Lawton, K., Shih, W., Barker, T. V., Landa, R., Lord, C., . . . Senturk, D. (2014). Caregiver-mediated intervention for low-resourced preschoolers with autism: An RCT. *Pediatrics, 134*(1), e72–e79.

Kasari, C., Paparella, T., Freeman, S., & Jahromi, L. B. (2008). Language outcome in autism: Randomized comparison of joint attention and play interventions. *Journal of Consulting and Clinical Psychology, 76*(1), 125–137.

Kasari, C., Sigman, M., Mundy, P., & Yirmiya, N. (1990). Affective sharing in the context of joint attention interactions of normal, autistic, and mentally retarded children. *Journal of Autism and Developmental Disorders, 20,* 87–100.

Kaushal, P., Mohan, N., & Sandhu, P. S. (2010). Relevancy of fuzzy concept in mathematics. *International Journal of Innovation, Management, and Technology, 1*(3), 312–315.

Kawashima, R., Sugiura, M., Kato, T., Nakamura, A., Hatano, K., Ito, K., . . . Nakamura, K. (1999). The human amygdala plays an important role in gaze monitoring. *Brain, 122*(4), 779–783.

Keehn, B., Wagner, J. B., Tager-Flusberg, H., & Nelson, C. A. (2013). Functional connectivity in the first year of life in infants at-risk for autism: A preliminary near-infrared spectroscopy study. *Frontiers in Human Neuroscience, 7,* 444.

Kennedy, D. P., & Adolphs, R. (2012). The social brain in psychiatric and neurological disorders. *Trends in Cognitive Sciences, 16*(11), 559–572.

Kennedy, D. P., & Courchesne, E. (2008). Functional abnormalities of the default network during self- and other-reflection in autism. *Social Cognitive and Affective Neuroscience, 3*(2), 177–190.

Keysers, C., & Perrett, D. (2004). Demystifying social cognition: A Hebbian perspective. *Trends in Cognitive Sciences, 8*, 501–507.

Khan, S., Gramfort, A., Shetty, N. R., Kitzbichler, M. G., Ganesan, S., Moran, J. M., . . . Kenet, T. (2013). Local and long-range functional connectivity is reduced in concert in autism spectrum disorders. *Proceedings of the National Academy of Sciences USA, 110*(8), 3107–3112.

Kim, H. I., & Johnson, S. P. (2014). Detecting 'infant-directedness' in face and voice. *Developmental Science, 17*(4), 621–627.

Kim, K., & Mundy, P. (2012). Joint attention, social cognition and recognition memory in adults. *Frontiers in Human Neuroscience, 6*, 172.

Kim, K., Rosenthal, M. Z., Gwaltney, M., Jarrold, W., Hatt, N., McIntyre, N., . . . Mundy, P. (2014). A virtual joy-stick study of emotional responses and social motivation in children with autism spectrum disorder. *Journal of Autism and Developmental Disorders.* [Epub ahead of print]

Kingstone, A., Friesen, C. K., & Gazzaniga, M. S. (2000). Reflexive joint attention depends on lateralized cortical connections. *Psychological Science, 11*(2), 159–166.

Kiyonaga, A., & Egner, T. (2014). The working memory Stroop effect when internal representations clash with external stimuli. *Psychological Science, 25*(8), 1619–1629.

Klein, J. L., MacDonald, R. P., Vaillancourt, G., Ahearn, W. H., & Dube, W. V. (2009). Teaching discrimination of adult gaze direction to children with autism. *Research in Autism Spectrum Disorders, 3*(1), 42–49.

Klein, P. S. (2003). A mediational approach to early intervention: Israel. In S. L. Odom, M. J. Hanson, J. A. Blackman, & S. Kaul (Eds.), *Early intervention practices around the world* (pp. 69–80). Baltimore, MD: Brookes.

Klein-Tasman, B. P., Mervis, C. B., Lord, C., & Phillips, K. D. (2007). Sociocommunicative deficits in young children with Williams syndrome: Performance on the Autism Diagnostic Observation Schedule. *Child Neuropsychology, 13*(5), 444–467.

Klin, A. (1991). Young autistic children's listening preferences in regard to speech: A possible characterization of the symptom of social withdrawal. *Journal of Autism and Developmental Disorders, 21*(1), 29–42.

Klin, A., Jones, W., Schultz, R., & Volkmar, F. (2004). The enactive mind, or from actions to cognition: Lessons from autism. In U. Frith & E. L. Hill (Eds.), *Autism: Mind and brain* (pp. 127–159). Oxford, England: Oxford University Press.

Klin, A., Jones, W., Schultz, R., Volkmar, F., & Cohen, D. (2002a). Visual fixation patterns during viewing of naturalistic social situations as predictors of social competence in individuals with autism. *Archives of General Psychiatry, 59*(9), 809–816.

Klin, A., Jones, W., Schultz, R., Volkmar, F., & Cohen, D. (2002b). Defining and quantifying the social phenotype in autism. *American Journal of Psychiatry, 159*, 895–908.

Klin, A., Sparrow, S. S., de Bildt, A., Cicchetti, D. V., Cohen, D. J., & Volkmar, F. R.

(1999). A normed study of face recognition in autism and related disorders. *Journal of Autism and Developmental Disorders, 29*(6), 499–508.

Koegel, L., Carter, C., & Koegel, R. (2003). Teaching children with autism self-initiations as a pivotal response. *Topics in Language Disorders, 23*, 134–145.

Koegel, R. L., Dyer, K., & Bell, L. K. (1987). The influence of child-preferred activities on autistic children's social behavior. *Journal of Applied Behavior Analysis, 20*(3), 243–252.

Konopka, G., & Geschwind, D. H. (2010). Human brain evolution: Harnessing the genomics of evolution to link genes, cognition, and behavior. *Neuron, 68*(2), 231–244.

Konrad, K., & Eickhoff, S. B. (2010). Is the ADHD brain wired differently?: A review on structural and functional connectivity in attention deficit hyperactivity disorder. *Human Brain Mapping, 31*(6), 904–916.

Kopp, F., & Lindenberger, U. (2011). Effects of joint attention on long-term memory in 9-month-old infants: An event-related potentials study. *Developmental Science, 14*(4), 660–672.

Kouider, S., Stahlhut, C., Gelskov, S. V., Barbosa, L. S., Dutat, M., De Gardelle, V., . . . Dehaene-Lambertz, G. (2013). A neural marker of perceptual consciousness in infants. *Science, 340*(6130), 376–380.

Krebs, R. M., Boehler, C. N., Roberts, K. C., Song, A. W., & Woldorff, M. G. (2012). The involvement of the dopaminergic midbrain and cortico–striatal–thalamic circuits in the integration of reward prospect and attentional task demands. *Cerebral Cortex, 22*(3), 607–615.

Kristen, S., Sodian, B., Thoermer, C., & Perst, H. (2011). Infants' joint attention skills predict toddlers' emerging mental state language. *Developmental Psychology, 47*(5), 1207–1219.

Krstovska-Guerrero, I., & Jones, E. A. (2013). Joint attention in autism: Teaching smiling coordinated with gaze to respond to joint attention bids. *Research in Autism Spectrum Disorders, 7*(1), 93–108.

Kuban, K. C., O'Shea, T. M., Allred, E. N., Tager-Flusberg, H., Goldstein, D. J., & Leviton, A. (2009). Positive screening on the Modified Checklist for Autism in Toddlers (M-CHAT) in extremely low gestational age newborns. *Journal of Pediatrics, 154*(4), 535–540.

Kühn-Popp, N., Kristen, S., Paulus, M., Meinhardt, J., & Sodian, B. (2015). Left hemisphere EEG coherence in infancy predicts infant declarative pointing and preschool epistemic language. *Social Neuroscience.* [Epub ahead of print 1-11]

Kwisthout, J., Vogt, P., Haselager, P., & Dijkstra, T. (2008). Joint attention and language evolution. *Connection Science, 20*(2–3), 155–171.

Lachat, F., Hugueville, L., Lemaréchal, J. D., Conty, L., & George, N. (2012). Oscillatory brain correlates of live joint attention: A dual-EEG study. *Frontiers in Human Neuroscience, 6*, 156.

Lackner, C., Sabbagh, M. A., Hallinan, E., Liu, X., & Holden, J. J. (2012). Dopamine receptor D4 gene variation predicts preschoolers' developing theory of mind. *Developmental Science, 15*(2), 272–280.

Lacreuse, A., Russell, J. L., Hopkins, W. D., & Herndon, J. G. (2014). Cognitive and motor aging in female chimpanzees. *Neurobiology of Aging, 35*(3), 623–632.

Laing, E., Butterworth, G., Ansari, D., Gsödl, M., Longhi, E., Panagiotaki, G., . . . Karmiloff-Smith, A. (2002). Atypical development of language and social communication in toddlers with Williams syndrome. *Developmental Science, 5*(2), 233–246.

Landa, R. J., Gross, A. L., Stuart, E. A., & Faherty, A. (2013). Developmental trajectories in children with and without autism spectrum disorders: The first 3 years. *Child Development, 84*(2), 429–442.

Landa, R. J., Holman, K. C., O'Neill, A. H., & Stuart, E. A. (2011). Intervention targeting development of socially synchronous engagement in toddlers with autism spectrum disorder: A randomized controlled trial. *Journal of Child Psychology and Psychiatry, 52*(1), 13–21.

Landry, R., & Bryson, S. (2004). Impaired disengagement of attention in young children with autism. *Journal of Child Psychology and Psychiatry, 45*, 1115–1122.

Langdell, T. (1978). Recognition of faces: An approach to the study of autism. *Journal of Child Psychology and Psychiatry, 19*, 255–268.

Lawton, K., & Kasari, C. (2012). Teacher-implemented joint attention intervention: Pilot randomized controlled study for preschoolers with autism. *Journal of Consulting and Clinical Psychology, 80*(4), 687–693.

Leavens, D., & Racine, T. P. (2009). Joint attention in apes and humans: Are humans unique? *Journal of Consciousness Studies, 16*(6–8), 240–267.

Lee, K., Eskritt, M., Symons, L. A., & Muir, D. (1998). Children's use of triadic eye gaze information for "mind reading." *Developmental Psychology, 34*(3), 525–539.

Leech, R., & Sharp, D. J. (2014). The role of the posterior cingulate cortex in cognition and disease. *Brain, 137*(1), 12–32.

Leekam, S. (2005). Why do children with autism have joint attention impairment? In N. Eilan, C. Hoerl, T. McCormack, & J. Roessler (Eds.), *Joint attention: Communication and other minds. Issues in philosophy and psychology* (pp. 205–229). Oxford, UK: Oxford University Press.

Leslie, A. M. (1987). Pretense and representation: The origins of "theory of mind." *Psychological Review, 94*(4), 412–426.

Leslie, A. M., & Happé, F. (1989). Autism and ostensive communication: The relevance of metarepresentation. *Development and Psychopathology, 1*(3), 205–212.

Lewis, J., & Elman, J. (2008). Growth-related neural organization and the autism phenotype: A test of the hypothesis that altered brain growth leads to altered connectivity. *Developmental Science, 11*, 135–155.

Lewy, A., & Dawson, G. (1992). Social stimulation and joint attention in young autistic children. Journal *of Abnormal Child Psychology, 20*, 555–566.

Lincoln, A. J., Searcy, Y. M., Jones, W., & Lord, C. (2007). Social interaction behaviors discriminate young children with autism and Williams syndrome. *Journal of the American Academy of Child and Adolescent Psychiatry, 46*(3), 323–331.

Liu, X. Q., Georgiades, S., Duku, E., Thompson, A., Devlin, B., Cook, E. H., . . . Szatmari, P. (2011). Identification of genetic loci underlying the phenotypic constructs of autism spectrum disorders. *Journal of the American Academy of Child and Adolescent Psychiatry, 50*(7), 687–696.

Lloyd-Fox, S., Blasi, A., Everdell, N., Elwell, C. E., & Johnson, M. H. (2011).

Selective cortical mapping of biological motion processing in young infants. *Journal of Cognitive Neuroscience, 23,* 2521–2532.

Lord, C. (1984). The development of peer relations in children with autism. *Applied Developmental Psychology, 1,* 165–230.

Lord, C., & Jones, R. M. (2012). Annual research review: Re-thinking the classification of autism spectrum disorders. *Journal of Child Psychology and Psychiatry, 53*(5), 490–509.

Lord, C., Floody, H., Anderson, D., & Pickles, A. (2003, April). *Social engagement in very young children with autism: Differences across contexts.* Paper presented at the Biennial Meeting of the Society for Research in Child Development, Tampa, FL.

Lord, C., Risi, S., Lambrecht, L., Cook, E., Leventhal, B., DiLavore, P., . . . Rutter, M. (2000). The Autism Diagnostic Observation Schedule—Generic: A standard measure of social communication deficits associated with the spectrum of autism. *Journal of Autism and Developmental Disorders, 30,* 205–223.

Lord, C., Rutter, M., DiLavore, P., & Risi, S. (1999). *Autism Diagnostic Observation Schedule–WPS edition.* Los Angeles, CA: Western Psychological Services.

Lord, C., Rutter, M., Dilavore, P., Risi, S., Gotham, K., & Bishop, S. (2002). *Autism Diagnostic Observation Schedule, Second Edition, WPS edition.* Los Angeles, CA: Western Psychological Services.

Lord, C., Rutter, M., Goode, S., Heemsbergen, J., Jordan, H., Mawhood, L., & Schopler, E. (1989). Autism Diagnostic Observation Schedule: A standardized observation of communicative and social behavior. *Journal of Autism and Developmental Disorders, 19*(2), 185–212.

Lord, C., Rutter, M., & Le Couteur, A. (1994). Autism Diagnostic Interview—Revised: A revised version of a diagnostic interview for caregivers of individuals with possible pervasive developmental disorders. *Journal of Autism and Developmental Disorders, 24*(5), 659–685.

Lovaas, O. I. (1987). Behavioral treatment and normal educational and intellectual functioning in young autistic children. *Journal of Consulting and Clinical Psychology, 55*(1), 3–9.

Loveland, K., & Landry, S. (1986). Joint attention and language in autism and developmental language delay. *Journal of Autism and Developmental Disorders, 16,* 335–349.

Lu, A. T., Yoon, J., Geschwind, D. H., & Cantor, R. M. (2013). QTL replication and targeted association highlight the nerve growth factor gene for nonverbal communication deficits in autism spectrum disorders. *Molecular Psychiatry, 18*(2), 226–235.

Luyster, R. J., Kadlec, M. B., Carter, A., & Tager-Flusberg, H. (2008). Language assessment and development in toddlers with autism spectrum disorders. *Journal of Autism and Developmental Disorders, 38*(8), 1426–1438.

Luyster, R., & Lord, C. (2009). Word learning in children with autism spectrum disorders. *Developmental Psychology, 45*(6), 1774.

Lynch, C. J., Uddin, L. Q., Supekar, K., Khouzam, A., Phillips, J., & Menon, V. (2013). Default mode network in childhood autism: Posteromedial cortex heterogeneity and relationship with social deficits. *Biological Psychiatry, 74*(3), 212–219.

Macari, S. L., Campbell, D., Gengoux, G. W., Saulnier, C. A., Klin, A. J., & Chawarska, K. (2012). Predicting developmental status from 12 to 24 months in infants at risk for autism spectrum disorder: A preliminary report. *Journal of Autism and Developmental Disorders, 42*(12), 2636–2647.

MacDuff, J. L., Ledo, R., McClannahan, L. E., & Krantz, P. J. (2007). Using scripts and script-fading procedures to promote bids for joint attention by young children with autism. *Research in Autism Spectrum Disorders, 1*(4), 281–290.

MacLean, E. L., & Hare, B. (2012). Bonobos and chimpanzees infer the target of another's attention. *Animal Behaviour, 83*(2), 345–353.

Macpherson, T., Morita, M., & Hikida, T. (2014). Striatal direct and indirect pathways control decision-making behavior. *Frontiers in Psychology, 5*, 1301.

Mahy, C. E., Moses, L. J., & Pfeifer, J. H. (2014). How and where: Theory-of-mind in the brain. *Developmental Cognitive Neuroscience, 9*, 68–81.

Maljaars, J., Noens, I., Scholte, E., & van Berckelaer-Onnes, I. (2012). Language in low-functioning children with autistic disorder: Differences between receptive and expressive skills and concurrent predictors of language. *Journal of Autism and Developmental Disorders, 42*(10), 2181–2191.

Mareschal, D., Johnson, M., Sirois, S., Spratling, S., Thomas, M., & Wasserman, G. (2007). *Neuroconstructivism: Vol. 1. How the brain constructs cognition.* New York: Oxford University Press.

Marsh, A. A., Henry, H. Y., Pine, D. S., Gorodetsky, E. K., Goldman, D., & Blair, R. J. R. (2012). The influence of oxytocin administration on responses to infant faces and potential moderation by OXTR genotype. *Psychopharmacology, 224*(4), 469–476.

Martin, R. C., & Caramazza, A. (1980). Classification in well-defined and ill-defined categories: Evidence for common processing strategies. *Journal of Experimental Psychology: General, 109*(3), 320–334.

Martins, M. P., & Harris, S. L. (2006). Teaching children with autism to respond to joint attention initiations. *Child and Family Behavior Therapy, 28*(1), 51–68.

Masten, A. S., & Coatsworth, J. D. (1998). The development of competence in favorable and unfavorable environments: Lessons from research on successful children. *American Psychologist, 53*(2), 205–220.

McAdoo, W. G., & DeMyer, M. K. (1978). Personality characteristics of parents. In M. Rutter & E. Schopler (Eds.), *Autism: A reappraisal of concepts and treatment* (pp. 251–267). New York: Plenum Press.

McCleery, J. P., Akshoomoff, N., Dobkins, K. R., & Carver, L. J. (2009). Atypical face versus object processing and hemispheric asymmetries in 10-month-old infants at risk for autism. *Biological Psychiatry, 66*(10), 950–957.

McCleery, J. P., Allman, E., Carver, L., & Dobkins, K. (2007). Abnormal magnocellular pathway visual processing in infants at risk for autism. *Biological Psychiatry, 62*, 1007–1014.

McClelland, J. L., Rumelhart, D. E., & Hinton, G. E. (1986). The appeal of parallel distributed processing. In D. E. Rumelhart, J. L. McClelland, & the PDP Research Group (Eds.), *Parallel distributed processing: Explorations in the microstructure of cognition* (Vol. 1, pp. 3–44). Cambridge, MA: MIT Press.

McDuffie, A., Kover, S. T., Hagerman, R., & Abbeduto, L. (2013). Investigating word learning in fragile X syndrome: A fast-mapping study. *Journal of Autism And Developmental Disorders, 43*(7), 1676–1691.

McDuffie, A., Thurman, A. J., Hagerman, R. J., & Abbeduto, L. (2015). Symptoms of autism in males with fragile X syndrome: A comparison to nonsyndromic ASD using current ADI-R scores. *Journal of Autism and Developmental Disorders, 45*(7), 1925–1937.

McEvoy, R. E., Rogers, S. J., & Pennington, B. F. (1993). Executive function and social communication deficits in young autistic children. *Journal of Child Psychology and Psychiatry, 34*(4), 563–578.

McIntyre, N., Mundy, P., Solomon, M., Oswald, T., Swain-Lerro, L., & Novotny, S. (2015, March). *The impact of attention disturbance and language impairment on reading comprehension in school-aged children with ASD.* Paper presented at the Biennial Meeting of the Society for Research in Child Development, Philadelphia, PA.

Meehl, P. E. (1995). Bootstraps taxometrics: Solving the classification problem in psychopathology. *American Psychologist, 50*(4), 266–275.

Meindl, J. N., & Cannella-Malone, H. I. (2011). Initiating and responding to joint attention bids in children with autism: A review of the literature. *Research in Developmental Disabilities, 32*(5), 1441–1454.

Meins, E., Fernyhough, C., Arnott, B., Vittorini, L., Turner, M., Leekam, S. R., & Parkinson, K. (2011). Individual differences in infants' joint attention behaviors with mother and a new social partner. *Infancy, 16*(6), 587–610.

Meltzoff, A. (2007). 'Like me': A foundation for social cognition. *Developmental Science, 10*, 126–134.

Meltzoff, A., & Brooks, R. (2008). Self experiences a mechanism for learning about others: A training study in social cognition. *Developmental Psychology, 44*, 1–9.

Menon, V., & Uddin, L. Q. (2010). Saliency, switching, attention and control: A network model of insula function. *Brain Structure and Function, 214*(5–6), 655–667.

Mervis, C., & Becerra, A. (2007). Language and communicative development in Williams syndrome. *Mental Retardation and Developmental Disabilities Research Reviews, 13*(1), 3–15.

Miller, E. K., & Cohen, J. D. (2001). An integrative theory of prefrontal cortex function. *Annual Review of Neuroscience, 24*, 167–202.

Miller, G. A. (1956). The magical number seven, plus or minus two: Some limits on our capacity for processing information. *Psychological Review, 63*(2), 81–97.

Miller, G. A. (2003). The cognitive revolution: A historical perspective. *Trends in Cognitive Sciences, 7*(3), 141–144.

Miller, M., Bales, K. L., Taylor, S. L., Yoon, J., Hostetler, C. M., Carter, C. S., & Solomon, M. (2013). Oxytocin and vasopressin in children and adolescents with autism spectrum disorders: Sex differences and associations with symptoms. *Autism Research, 6*(2), 91–102.

Milligan, K., Astington, J. W., & Dack, L. A. (2007). Language and theory of mind: Meta-analysis of the relation between language ability and false-belief understanding. *Child Development, 78*(2), 622–646.

Mišić, B., Doesburg, S. M., Fatima, Z., Vidal, J., Vakorin, V. A., Taylor, M. J., & McIntosh, A. R. (2014). Coordinated information generation and mental flexibility: Large-scale network disruption in children with autism. *Cerebral Cortex, 25*(9), 2815–2827. [Epub ahead of print]

Mitchell, J. P., Banaji, M. R., & Macrae, C. N. (2005). The link between social cognition and self-referential thought in the medial prefrontal cortex. *Journal of Cognitive Neuroscience, 17*(8), 1306–1315.

Mizuno, A., Liu, Y., Williams, D. L., Keller, T. A., Minshew, N. J., & Just, M. A. (2011). The neural basis of deictic shifting in linguistic perspective-taking in high-functioning autism. *Brain, 134*, 2422–2435.

Moore, C. (2012). Homology in the development of triadic interaction and language. *Developmental Psychobiology, 55*, 59–66.

Morales, M., Mundy, P., & Rojas, J. (1998). Following the direction of gaze and language development in 6-month olds. *Infant Behavior and Development, 21*, 373–377.

Morales, M., Mundy, P., Crowson, M., Neal, R., & Delgado, C. (2005). Individual differences in infant attention skills, joint attention, and emotion regulation behavior. *International Journal of Behavioral Development, 29*, 259–263.

Morgan, B., Maybery, M., & Durkin, K. (2003). Weak central coherence, poor joint attention, and low verbal ability: Independent deficits in early autism. *Developmental Psychology, 39*(4), 646–656.

Mosconi, M. W., Cody-Hazlett, H., Poe, M. D., Gerig, G., Gimpel-Smith, R., & Piven, J. (2009). Longitudinal study of amygdala volume and joint attention in 2- to 4-year-old children with autism. *Archives of General Psychiatry, 66*(5), 509–516.

Mosconi, M. W., Reznick, J., Mesibov, G., & Piven, J. (2009). The Social Orienting Continuum and Response Scale (SOC-RS): A dimensional measure for preschool-aged children. *Journal of Autism and Developmental Disorders, 39*(2), 242–250.

Munakata, Y., & McClelland, J. (2003). Connectionist models of development. *Developmental Science, 6*, 413–429.

Mundy, P. (1995). Joint attention and social-emotional approach behavior in children with autism. *Development and Psychopathology, 7*, 63–82.

Mundy, P. (2003). The neural basis of social impairments in autism: The role of the dorsal medial-frontal cortex and anterior cingulate system. *Journal of Child Psychology and Psychiatry, 44*, 793–809.

Mundy, P. (2011). The social behavior of autism: A parallel and distributed information processing perspective. In D. Amaral, G. Dawson, & D. Geschwind (Eds.), *Autism spectrum disorders* (pp. 149–171). New York: Oxford University Press.

Mundy, P., & Acra, F. (2006). Joint attention, social engagement and the development of social competence. In P. Marshall & N. Fox (Eds.), *The development of social engagement: Neurobiological perspectives* (pp. 81–117). New York: Oxford University Press.

Mundy, P., Block, J., Delgado, C., Pomares, Y., Vaughan Van Hecke, A., & Venezia Parlade, M. (2007). Individual differences and the development of infant joint attention. *Child Development, 78*, 938–954.

Mundy, P., & Burnette, C. (2005). Joint attention and neurodevelopment. In F. Volkmar, A. Klin, & R. Paul (Eds.), *Handbook of autism and pervasive developmental disorders* (3rd ed., pp. 650–681). Hoboken, NJ: Wiley.

Mundy, P., Card, J., & Fox, N. (2000). EEG correlates of the development of infant joint attention skills. *Developmental Psychobiology, 36,* 325–338.

Mundy, P., & Crowson, M. (1997). Joint attention and early social communication: Implications for research on intervention with autism. *Journal of Autism and Developmental Disorders, 27,* 653–676.

Mundy, P., Delgado, C., Block, J., Venezia-Parlade, M., Hogan, A., & Siebert, J. (2003). *The Early Social Communication Scales.* Available at *http://education. ucdavis.edu/sites/main/files/fileattachments/escs_manual_2003_2013.pdf*

Mundy, P., Fox, N., & Card, J. (2003). Joint attention, EEG coherence and early vocabulary development. *Developmental Science, 6,* 48–54.

Mundy, P., Gwaltney, M., & Henderson, H. (2010). Self-referenced processing, neurodevelopment and joint attention in autism. *Autism, 14*(5), 408–429.

Mundy, P., & Jarrold, W. (2010). Infant joint attention, neural networks and social cognition. *Neural Networks, 23*(8), 985–997.

Mundy, P., Kasari, C., & Sigman, M. (1992). Nonverbal communication, affective sharing, and intersubjectivity. *Infant Behavior and Development, 15,* 377–381.

Mundy, P., Kim, K., Swain-Lerro, L., McIntyre, N., Zajic, M., Oswald, T., & Solomon, M. (2015, May). *Joint attention and information processing in higher functioning children with ASD.* Paper presented at the International Meeting for Autism Research, Salt Lake City, UT.

Mundy, P., Mastergeorge, A., & McIntyre, N. (2012). The effects of autism on social learning and social attention. In P. Mundy & A. Mastergeorge (Eds.), *Autism for educators: Vol. 1. Translating research to schools and classrooms* (pp. 3–34). San Francisco, CA: Jossey-Bass.

Mundy, P., & Neal, A. R. (2000). Neural plasticity, joint attention, and a transactional social-orienting model of autism. *International Review of Research in Mental Retardation, 23,* 139–168.

Mundy, P., & Newell, L. (2007). Attention, joint attention and social cognition. *Current Directions in Psychological Science, 16,* 269–274.

Mundy, P., Novotny, S., Swain-Lerro, L., McIntyre, N., Zajic, M., & Oswald, T. (2015, May). *The social phenotype of ASD and parent report of joint attention in school aged children.* Paper presented at the International Meeting for Autism Research, Salt Lake City, UT.

Mundy, P., & Sigman, M. (1989a). Theoretical implications of joint attention deficits in autism. *Development and Psychopathology, 1,* 173–184.

Mundy, P., & Sigman, S. (1989b). Second thoughts on the nature of autism. *Development and Psychopathology, 1,* 213–218.

Mundy, P., & Sigman, M. (1989c). Specifying the nature of the social impairment in autism. In G. Dawson (Ed.), *Autism: Nature, diagnosis, and treatment* (pp. 3–21). New York: Guilford Press.

Mundy, P., & Sigman, M. (2006). Joint attention, social competence and developmental psychopathology. In D. Cicchetti & D. Cohen (Eds.), *Developmental psychopathology: Vol. 1. Theory and methods* (2nd ed., pp. 293–332). Hoboken, NJ: Wiley.

Mundy, P., Sigman, M., & Kasari, C. (1990). A longitudinal study of joint attention and language development in autistic children. *Journal of Autism and Developmental Disorders, 20*(1), 115–128.

Mundy, P., Sigman, M., & Kasari, C. (1993). The autistic person's theory of mind and early nonverbal joint attention deficits. In S. Baron-Cohen, H. Tager-Flusberg, D. Cohen, & F. Volkmar (Eds.), *Understanding other minds: Perspectives from autism* (pp. 181–201). Oxford, UK: Oxford University Press.

Mundy, P., Sigman, M., & Kasari, C. (1994). Joint attention, developmental level, and symptom presentation in children with autism. *Development and Psychopathology, 6*, 389–401.

Mundy, P., Sigman, M., Ungerer, J., & Sherman, T. (1986). Defining the social deficits of autism: The contribution of nonverbal communication measures. *Journal of Child Psychology and Psychiatry, 27*, 657–669.

Mundy, P., Sullivan, L., & Mastergeorge, A. M. (2009). A parallel and distributed-processing model of joint attention, social cognition and autism. *Autism Research, 2*(1), 2–21.

Mundy, P., & Vaughan Van Hecke, A. (2008). Neural systems, gaze following and the development of joint attention. In C. Nelson & M. Luciana (Eds.), *Handbook of developmental cognitive neuroscience* (pp. 819–837). New York: Oxford University Press.

Murphy, M. M., & Abbeduto, L. (2005). Indirect genetic effects and the early language development of children with genetic mental retardation syndromes: The role of joint attention. *Infants and Young Children, 18*(1), 47–59.

Naber, F., Bakermans-Kranenburg, M., van IJzendoorn, M., Dietz, C., Daalen, E., Swinkels, S. H., . . . van Engeland, H. (2008). Joint attention development in toddlers with autism. *European Child and Adolescent Psychiatry, 17*, 143–152.

Naber, F. B., Swinkels, S. H., Buitelaar, J. K., Dietz, C., van Daalen, E., Bakermans-Kranenburg, M. J., . . . van Engeland, H. (2007). Joint attention and attachment in toddlers with autism. *Journal of Abnormal Child Psychology, 35*(6), 899–911.

Nakako, T., Murai, T., Ikejiri, M., Hashimoto, T., Kotani, M., Matsumoto, K., . . . Ikeda, K. (2014). Effects of lurasidone on ketamine-induced joint visual attention dysfunction as a possible disease model of autism spectrum disorders in common marmosets. *Behavioural Brain Research, 274*, 349–354.

Naoi, N., Tsuchiya, R., Yamamoto, J. I., & Nakamura, K. (2008). Functional training for initiating joint attention in children with autism. *Research in Developmental Disabilities, 29*(6), 595–609.

Nation, K., Clarke, P., Wright, B., & Williams, C. (2006). Patterns of reading ability in children with autism spectrum disorder. *Journal of Autism and Developmental Disorders, 36*(7), 911–919.

Nation, K., & Penny, S. (2008). Sensitivity to eye gaze in autism: Is it normal? Is it automatic? Is it social? *Development and Psychopathology, 20*, 79–97.

Nelson, P. B., Adamson, L. B., & Bakeman, R. (2008). Toddlers' joint engagement experience facilitates preschoolers' acquisition of theory of mind. *Developmental Science, 11*(6), 847–852.

Neuhaus, E., Beauchaine, T. P., & Bernier, R. (2010). Neurobiological correlates of social functioning in autism. *Clinical Psychology Review, 30*(6), 733–748.

Newell, A., & Shaw, J. C. (1957). *Programming the logic theory machine.* Santa Monica, CA: RAND Corporation.

Nguyen, M., Roth, A., Kyzar, E. J., Poudel, M. K., Wong, K., Stewart, A. M., & Kalueff, A. V. (2014). Decoding the contribution of dopaminergic genes and pathways to autism spectrum disorder (ASD). *Neurochemistry International, 66*, 15–26.

Nichols, K. E., Fox, N., & Mundy, P. (2005). Joint attention, self-recognition and neurocognitive functioning. *Infancy, 7,* 35–51.

Ninio, A. (1983). Joint book reading as a multiple vocabulary acquisition device. *Developmental Psychology, 19*(3), 445–451.

Niznikiewicz, M. A., & Delgado, M. R. (2011). Two sides of the same coin: Learning via positive and negative reinforcers in the human striatum. *Developmental Cognitive Neuroscience, 1*(4), 494–505.

Norbury, C. F., Griffiths, H., & Nation, K. (2010). Sound before meaning: Word learning in autistic disorders. *Neuropsychologia, 48*(14), 4012–4019.

Norbury, C., & Nation, K. (2011). Understanding variability in reading comprehension in adolescents with autism spectrum disorders: Interactions with language status and decoding skill. *Scientific Studies of Reading, 15*(3), 191–210.

Northoff, G., Heinzel, A., de Greck, M., Bermpohl, F., Dobrowolny, H., & Panksepp, J. (2006). Self-referential processing in our brain—A meta-analysis of imaging studies on the self. *NeuroImage, 31*(1), 440–457.

Nuku, P., & Bekkering, H. (2008). Joint attention: Inferring what others perceive (and don't perceive). *Consciousness and Cognition, 17,* 339–349.

Nygren, G., Sandberg, E., Gillstedt, F., Ekeroth, G., Arvidsson, T., & Gillberg, C. (2012). A new screening programme for autism in a general population of Swedish toddlers. *Research in Developmental Disabilities, 33*(4), 1200–1210.

O'Connor, I. M., & Klein, P. D. (2004). Exploration of strategies for facilitating the reading comprehension of high-functioning students with autism spectrum disorders. *Journal of Autism and Developmental Disorders, 34,* 115–127.

O'Hearn, K., Schroer, E., Minshew, N., & Luna, B. (2010). Lack of developmental improvement on a face memory task during adolescence in autism. *Neuropsychologia, 48*(13), 3955–3960.

Ornitz, E., & Ritvo, E. (1976). Medical assessment. In E. Ritvo (Ed.), *Autism: Diagnosis, current research, and management* (pp. 7–26). New York: Spectrum.

Ortiz-Mantilla, S., Choe, M. S., Flax, J., Grant, P. E., & Benasich, A. A. (2010). Associations between the size of the amygdala in infancy and language abilities during the preschool years in normally developing children. *NeuroImage, 49*(3), 2791–2799.

Ozonoff, S., Iosif, A. M., Baguio, F., Cook, I. C., Hill, M. M., Hutman, T., . . . Young, G. S. (2010). A prospective study of the emergence of early behavioral signs of autism. *Journal of the American Academy of Child and Adolescent Psychiatry, 49*(3), 256–266.

Ozonoff, S., Young, G. S., Carter, A., Messinger, D., Yirmiya, N., Zwaigenbaum, L., . . . Stone, W. L. (2011). Recurrence risk for autism spectrum disorders: A Baby Siblings Research Consortium study. *Pediatrics, 128*(3), e488–e495.

Pack, A. A., & Herman, L. M. (2006). Dolphin social cognition and joint attention: Our current understanding. *Aquatic Mammals, 32*(4), 443–460.

Page, T. (2007, August 20). Parallel play: A lifetime of restless isolation explained. *The New Yorker.* Retrieved from *www.newyorker.com/magazine/2007/08/20/parallel-play.*

Parise, E., & Csibra, G. (2012). Electrophysiological evidence for the understanding of maternal speech by 9-month-old infants. *Psychological Science, 23,* 728–733.

Parlade, M. V., Messinger, D. S., Delgado, C. E., Kaiser, M. Y., Van Hecke, A. V., & Mundy, P. C. (2009). Anticipatory smiling: Linking early affective communication and social outcome. *Infant Behavior and Development, 32*(1), 33–43.

Paterson, S. J., Heim, S., Friedman, J. T., Choudhury, N., & Benasich, A. A. (2006). Development of structure and function in the infant brain: Implications for cognition, language and social behaviour. *Neuroscience and Biobehavioral Reviews, 30*(8), 1087–1105.

Patten, E., & Watson, L. R. (2011). Interventions targeting attention in young children with autism. *American Journal of Speech–Language Pathology, 20*(1), 60–69.

Patterson, S. Y., Elder, L., Gulsrud, A., & Kasari, C. (2014). The association between parental interaction style and children's joint engagement in families with toddlers with autism. *Autism, 18*(5), 511–518.

Paul, R., Campbell, D., Gilbert, K., & Tsiouri, I. (2013). Comparing spoken language treatments for minimally verbal preschoolers with autism spectrum disorders. *Journal of Autism and Developmental Disorders, 43*(2), 418–431.

Pellicano, E. (2010). Individual differences in executive function and central coherence predict developmental changes in theory of mind in autism. *Developmental Psychology, 46*(2), 530–544.

Pelphrey, K. A., Morris, J. P., & McCarthy, G. (2005). Neural basis of eye gaze processing deficits in autism. *Brain, 128*(5), 1038–1048.

Pelphrey, K. A., Viola, R. J., & McCarthy, G. (2004). When strangers pass processing of mutual and averted social gaze in the superior temporal sulcus. *Psychological Science, 15*(9), 598–603.

Perner, J., & Lang, B. (1999). Development of theory of mind and executive control. *Trends in Cognitive Sciences, 3*(9), 337–344.

Persson, J., Lustig, C., Nelson, J. K., & Reuter-Lorenz, P. A. (2007). Age differences in deactivation: A link to cognitive control? *Journal of Cognitive Neuroscience, 19*(6), 1021–1032.

Pessoa, L., & Adolphs, R. (2010). Emotion processing and the amygdala: From a "low road" to "many roads" of evaluating biological significance. *Nature Reviews Neuroscience, 11*(11), 773–783.

Pfeiffer, U. J., Schilbach, L., Timmermans, B., Kuzmanovic, B., Georgescu, A. L., Bente, G., & Vogeley, K. (2014). Why we interact: On the functional role of the striatum in the subjective experience of social interaction. *NeuroImage, 101,* 124–137.

Piaget, J. (1952). *The origins of intelligence in children.* New York: International Universities Press.

Pickles, A., & Angold, A. (2003). Natural categories or fundamental dimensions:

On carving nature at the joints and the rearticulation of psychopathology. *Development and Psychopathology, 15*(3), 529–551.

Pierce, K., & Redcay, E. (2008). Fusiform function in children with an autism spectrum disorder is a matter of "who." *Biological Psychiatry, 64*(7), 552–560.

Pierce, K., & Schreibman, L., (1995). Increasing complex social behaviors in children with autism: Effects of peer implemented pivotal response training. *Journal of Applied Behavior Analysis, 28*, 285–295.

Pinto, A., Greenberg, B. D., Grados, M. A., Bienvenu, O. J., Samuels, J. F., Murphy, D. L., . . . Nestadt, G. (2008). Further development of YBOCS dimensions in the OCD Collaborative Genetics study: Symptoms vs. categories. *Psychiatry Research, 160*(1), 83–93.

Pinto-Martin, J., Young, L. M., Mandell, D. S., Poghosyan, L., Giarelli, E., & Levy, S. E. (2008). Screening strategies for autism spectrum disorders in pediatric primary care. *Journal of Developmental and Behavioral Pediatrics, 29*(5), 345–350.

Piven, J., Vieland, V. J., Parlier, M., Thompson, A., O'Conner, I., Woodbury-Smith, M., . . . Szatmari, P. (2013). A molecular genetic study of autism and related phenotypes in extended pedigrees. *Journal of Neurodevelopmental Disorders, 5*(1), 30.

Poon, K. K., Watson, L. R., Baranek, G. T., & Poe, M. D. (2012). To what extent do joint attention, imitation, and object play behaviors in infancy predict later communication and intellectual functioning in ASD? *Journal of Autism and Developmental Disorders, 42*(6), 1064–1074.

Posner, M. I., & Petersen, S. E. (1990). The attention system of the human brain. *Annual Review of Neuroscience, 13*, 25–42.

Posner, M. I., & Rothbart, M. K. (2000). Developing mechanisms of self-regulation. *Development and Psychopathology, 12*(03), 427–441.

Posner, M. I., & Rothbart, M. K. (2007). Research on attention networks as a model for the integration of psychological science. *Annual Review of Psychology, 58*, 1–23.

Povinelli, D. J., & Eddy, T. J. (1996). Chimpanzees: Joint visual attention. *Psychological Science, 7*(3), 129–135.

Premack, D., & Woodruff, G. (1978). Does the chimpanzee have a theory of mind? *Behavioral and Brain Sciences, 1*(4), 515–526.

Presmanes, A. G., Walden, T. A., Stone, W. L., & Yoder, P. J. (2007). Effects of different attentional cues on responding to joint attention in younger siblings of children with autism spectrum disorders. *Journal of Autism and Developmental Disorders, 37*(1), 133–144.

Qu, S., & Chai, J. Y. (2007, April). An exploration of eye gaze in spoken language processing for multimodal conversational interfaces. In *Proceedings of the North American Chapter of the Association for Computational Linguistics–Human Language Technologies* (pp. 284–291). Rochester, NY: North American Chapter of the Association for Computational Linguistics.

Quartz, S. (1999). The constructivist brain. *Trends in Cognitive Sciences, 3*, 48–57.

Ramnani, N., Behrens, T., Penny, W., & Matthews, P. (2004). New approaches for exploring anatomical and functional connectivity in the human brain. *Biological Psychiatry, 56*, 613–619.

Randi, J., Newman, T., & Grigorenko, E. L. (2010). Teaching children with autism to read for meaning: Challenges and possibilities. *Journal of Autism and Developmental Disorders, 40*(7), 890–902.

Reaume, C. J., & Sokolowski, M. B. (2011). Conservation of gene function in behaviour. *Philosophical Transactions of the Royal Society of London: Series B. Biological Sciences, 366*(1574), 2100–2110.

Redcay, E., Dodell-Feder, D., Mavros, P. L., Kleiner, M., Pearrow, M. J., Triantafyllou, C., . . . Saxe, R. (2013). Atypical brain activation patterns during a face-to-face joint attention game in adults with autism spectrum disorder. *Human Brain Mapping, 34*(10), 2511–2523.

Redcay, E., Dodell-Feder, D., Pearrow, M. J., Mavros, P. L., Kleiner, M., Gabrieli, J. D., & Saxe, R. (2010). Live face-to-face interaction during fMRI: A new tool for social cognitive neuroscience. *NeuroImage, 50*(4), 1639–1647.

Redcay, E., Kleiner, M., & Saxe, R. (2012). Look at this: The neural correlates of initiating and responding to bids for joint attention. *Frontiers in Human Neuroscience, 6,* 169.

Redcay, E., Ludlum, R. S., Velnoskey, K. R., & Kanwal, S. (2015). Communicative signals promote object recognition memory and modulate the right posterior STS. *Journal of Cognitive Neuroscience.*

Redcay, E., Moran, J. M., Mavros, P. L., Tager-Flusberg, H., Gabrieli, J. D. E., & Whitfield-Gabrieli, S. (2013). Intrinsic functional connectivity in high-functioning adolescents with autism spectrum disorder. *Frontiers in Human Neuroscience, 7,* 573.

Reddy, V. (2003). On being the object of attention: Implications for self–other consciousness. *Trends in Cognitive Sciences, 7*(9), 397–402.

Reddy, V., Williams, E., & Vaughan, A. (2002). Sharing humour and laughter in autism and Down's syndrome. *British Journal of Psychology, 93*(2), 219–242.

Reichow, B., & Wolery, M. (2009). Comprehensive synthesis of early intensive behavioral interventions for young children with autism based on the UCLA Young Autism Project model. *Journal of Autism and Developmental Disorders, 39*(1), 23–41.

Reiersen, A. M., Constantino, J. N., Volk, H. E., & Todd, R. D. (2007). Autistic traits in a population-based ADHD twin sample. *Journal of Child Psychology and Psychiatry, 48*(5), 464–472.

Rheingold, H. L. (1966). The development of social behavior in the human infant. In H. W. Stevenson (Ed.), Concept of development. *Monographs of the Society for Research in Child Development. 31*(5, Serial No. 107), 1–17.

Rheingold, H. L., Hay, D. F., & West, M. J. (1976). Sharing in the second year of life. *Child Development, 47,* 1148–1158.

Richardson, D. C., & Dale, R. (2005). Looking to understand: The coupling between speakers' and listeners' eye movements and its relationship to discourse comprehension. *Cognitive Science, 29*(6), 1045–1060.

Richardson, D. C., Dale, R., & Kirkham, N. Z. (2007). The art of conversation is coordination: Common ground and the coupling of eye movements during dialogue. *Psychological Science, 18*(5), 407–413.

Richer, J. (1978). The partial noncommunication of culture to autistic children—An application of human ethology. In M. Rutter & E. Schopler (Eds.), *Autism* (pp. 47–61). New York: Springer.

Ricketts, J. (2011). Research review: Reading comprehension in developmental disorders of language and communication. *Journal of Child Psychology and Psychiatry, 52*(11), 1111–1123.

Ricketts, J., Jones, C. R., Happé, F., & Charman, T. (2013). Reading comprehension in autism spectrum disorders: The role of oral language and social functioning. *Journal of Autism and Developmental Disorders, 43*(4), 807–816.

Rimland, B. (1964). *Infantile autism: The syndrome and its implications for a neural theory of behavior.* New York: Appleton-Century-Crofts.

Rizzolatti, G., & Arbib, M. A. (1998). Language within our grasp. *Trends in Neurosciences, 21*(5), 188–194.

Robins, D. L., Fein, D., Barton, M. L., & Green, J. A. (2001). The Modified Checklist for Autism in Toddlers: An initial study investigating the early detection of autism and pervasive developmental disorders. *Journal of Autism and Developmental Disorders, 31*(2), 131–144.

Robson, K. (1967). The role of eye-to-eye contact in maternal infant attachment. *Journal of Child Psychology and Psychiatry, 8*, 13–25.

Rocha, M., Schriebman, L., & Stahmer, A. (2007). Effectiveness of training parents to teach joint attention with children with autism. *Journal of Early Intervention, 29*, 154–172.

Roeyers, H., Van Oost, P., & Bothuyne, S. (1998). Immediate imitation and joint attention in young children with autism. *Development and Psychopathology, 10*, 441–450.

Rogers, S. J. (2009). What are infant siblings teaching us about autism in infancy? *Autism Research, 2*(3), 125–137.

Rogers, S. J., & Dawson, G. (2010). *Early Start Denver Model for young children with autism: Promoting language, learning, and engagement.* New York: Guilford Press.

Rogers, S. J., Hayden, D., Hepburn, S., Charlifue-Smith, R., Hall, T., & Hayes, A. (2006). Teaching young nonverbal children with autism useful speech: A pilot study of the Denver model and PROMPT interventions. *Journal of Autism and Developmental Disorders, 36*(8), 1007–1024.

Rogers, S. J., Hepburn, S. L., Stackhouse, T., & Wehner, E. (2003). Imitation performance in toddlers with autism and those with other developmental disorders. *Journal of Child Psychology and Psychiatry, 44*(5), 763–781.

Rogers, S. J., & Pennington, B. F. (1991). A theoretical approach to the deficits in infantile autism. *Development and Psychopathology, 3*(2), 137–162.

Rogers, S. J., Vismara, L., Wagner, A. L., McCormick, C., Young, G., & Ozonoff, S. (2014). Autism treatment in the first year of life: A pilot study of Infant Start, a parent-implemented intervention for symptomatic infants. *Journal of Autism and Developmental Disorders, 44*(12), 2981–2995.

Rogoff, B., Mistry, J., Goncu, A., & Mosier, C. (1993). Guided participation in cultural activity by toddlers and caregivers. *Monographs of the Society for Research in Child Development, 58*(8, Serial No. 236), 1–179.

Romero-Fernandez, W., Borroto-Escuela, D. O., Agnati, L. F., & Fuxe, K. (2013).

Evidence for the existence of dopamine D2–oxytocin receptor heteromers in the ventral and dorsal striatum with facilitatory receptor–receptor interactions. *Molecular Psychiatry, 18*, 849–855.

Ronald, A., Happé, F., & Plomin, R. (2005). The genetic relationship between individual differences in social and nonsocial behaviours characteristic of autism. *Developmental Science, 8*(5), 444–458.

Rose, S. A., Feldman, J. F., Wallace, I. F., & Cohen, P. (1991). Language: A partial link between infant attention and later intelligence. *Developmental Psychology, 27*(5), 798–806.

Rosenberg, S. A., Zhang, D., & Robinson, C. C. (2008). Prevalence of developmental delays and participation in early intervention services for young children. *Pediatrics, 121*(6), e1503–e1509.

Rossano, F., Carpenter, M., & Tomasello, M. (2012). One-year-old infants follow others' voice direction. *Psychological Science, 23*(11), 1298–1302.

Rothbart, M. K., & Bates, J. E. (1998). Temperament. In W. Damon (Series Ed.) & N. Eisenberg (Vol. Ed.), *Handbook of child psychology: Vol. 3. Social, emotional, and personality development* (5th ed., pp. 105–176). New York: Wiley.

Roux, A. M., Herrera, P., Wold, C. M., Dunkle, M. C., Glascoe, F. P., & Shattuck, P. T. (2012). Developmental and autism screening through 2-1-1: Reaching underserved families. *American Journal of Preventive Medicine, 43*(6), S457–S463.

Rozga, A., Hutman, T., Young, G. S., Rogers, S. J., Ozonoff, S., Dapretto, M., & Sigman, M. (2011). Behavioral profiles of affected and unaffected siblings of children with autism: Contribution of measures of mother–infant interaction and nonverbal communication. *Journal of Autism and Developmental Disorders, 41*(3), 287–301.

Rutgers, A. H., Bakermans-Kranenburg, M. J., van IJzendoorn, M. H., & van Berckelaer-Onnes, I. A. (2004). Autism and attachment: A meta-analytic review. *Journal of Child Psychology and Psychiatry, 45*, 1123–1134.

Rutherford, M., Young, G., Hepburn, S., & Rogers, S. (2007). A longitudinal study of pretend play in autism. *Journal of Autism and Developmental Disorders, 37*, 1024–1039.

Rutter, M. (1968). Concepts of autism: A review of research. *Journal of Child Psychology and Psychiatry, 9*(1), 1–25.

Rutter, M. (1978). Diagnosis and definition of childhood autism. *Journal of Autism and Childhood Schizophrenia, 8*(2), 139–161.

Rutter, M. (1986). Child psychiatry: Looking 30 years ahead. *Journal of Child Psychology and Psychiatry, 27*(6), 803–840.

Rutter, M., Bailey, A., & Lord, C. (2003). *The Social Communication Questionnaire: Manual.* Los Angeles, CA: Western Psychological Services.

Ryan, C. J., Roguev, A., Patrick, K., Xu, J., Jahari, H., Tong, Z., . . . Krogan, N. J. (2012). Hierarchical modularity and the evolution of genetic interactomes across species. *Molecular Cell, 46*(5), 691–704.

Saby, J. N., Marshall, P. J., & Meltzoff, A. N. (2012). Neural correlates of being imitated: An EEG study in preverbal infants. *Social Neuroscience, 7*(6), 650–661.

Sacrey, L. A. R., Armstrong, V. L., Bryson, S. E., & Zwaigenbaum, L. (2014).

Impairments to visual disengagement in autism spectrum disorder: A review of experimental studies from infancy to adulthood. *Neuroscience and Biobehavioral Reviews, 47*, 559–577.

Safiulina, D., & Kaasik, A. (2013). Energetic and dynamic: How mitochondria meet neuronal energy demands. *PLoS Biology, 11*(12), e1001755.

Sahley, T. L., & Panksepp, J. (1987). Brain opioids and autism: An updated analysis of possible linkages. *Journal of Autism and Developmental Disorders, 17*(2), 201–216.

Saito, D. N., Tanabe, H. C., Izuma, K., Hayashi, M. J., Morito, Y., Komeda, H., . . . Sadato, N. (2010). "Stay tuned": Inter-individual neural synchronization during mutual gaze and joint attention. *Frontiers in Integrative Neuroscience, 4*, 127.

Sajonz, B., Kahnt, T., Margulies, D. S., Park, S. Q., Wittmann, A., Stoy, M., . . . Bermpohl, F. (2010). Delineating self-referential processing from episodic memory retrieval: Common and dissociable networks. *NeuroImage, 50*(4), 1606–1617.

Salt, J., Shemilt, J., Sellars, V., Boyd, S., Coulson, T., & McCool, S. (2002). The Scottish Centre for Autism Preschool Treatment Programme II: The results of a controlled treatment outcome study. *Autism, 6*(1), 33–46.

Sato, W., Uono, S., Okada, T., & Toichi, M. (2010). Impairment of unconscious, but not conscious, gaze-triggered attention orienting in Asperger's disorder. *Research in Autism Spectrum Disorders, 4*(4), 782–786.

Saxon, T. F., & Reilly, J. T. (1999). Joint attention and toddler characteristics: Race, sex and socioeconomic status. *Early Child Development and Care, 149*(1), 59–69.

Scaife, M., & Bruner, J. (1975). The capacity for joint visual attention in the infant. *Nature, 253*, 265–266.

Scarpa, A., Reyes, N. M., Patriquin, M. A., Lorenzi, J., Hassenfeldt, T. A., Desai, V. J., & Kerkering, K. W. (2013). The Modified Checklist for Autism in Toddlers: Reliability in a diverse rural American sample. *Journal of Autism and Developmental Disorders, 43*(10), 2269–2279.

Scassellati, B. (1999). Imitation and mechanisms of joint attention: A developmental structure for building social skills on a humanoid robot. In C. L. Nehaniv (Ed.), *Computation for metaphors, analogy, and agents* (pp. 176–195). Berlin: Springer-Verlag.

Schertz, H. H., & Odom, S. L. (2007). Promoting joint attention in toddlers with autism: A parent-mediated developmental model. *Journal of Autism and Developmental Disorders, 37*(8), 1562–1575.

Schertz, H. H., Odom, S. L., Baggett, K. M., & Sideris, J. H. (2013). Effects of Joint Attention Mediated Learning for toddlers with autism spectrum disorders: An initial randomized controlled study. *Early Childhood Research Quarterly, 28*(2), 249–258.

Schietecatte, I., Roeyers, H., & Warreyn, P. (2012). Can infants' orientation to social stimuli predict later joint attention skills? *British Journal of Developmental Psychology, 30*(2), 267–282.

Schilbach, L., Bzdok, D., Timmermans, B., Fox, P. T., Laird, A. R., Vogeley, K.,

& Eickhoff, S. B. (2012). Introspective minds: Using ALE meta-analyses to study commonalities in the neural correlates of emotional processing, social and unconstrained cognition. *PloS One, 7*(2), e30920.

Schilbach, L., Eickhoff, S. B., Cieslik, E. C., Kuzmanovic, B., & Vogeley, K. (2012). Shall we do this together?: Social gaze influences action control in a comparison group, but not in individuals with high-functioning autism. *Autism, 16*, 151–162.

Schilbach, L., Wilms, M., Eickhoff, S. B., Romanzetti, S., Tepest, R., Bente, G., . . . Vogeley, K. (2010). Minds made for sharing: Initiating joint attention recruits reward-related neurocircuitry. *Journal of Cognitive Neuroscience, 22*(12), 2702–2715.

Schilbach, L., Wohlschlaeger, A. M., Kraemer, N. C., Newen, A., Shah, N. J., Fink, G. R., & Vogeley, K. (2006). Being with virtual others: Neural correlates of social interaction. *Neuropsychologia, 44*(5), 718–730.

Schriber, R. A., Robins, R. W., & Solomon, M. (2014). Personality and self-insight in individuals with autism spectrum disorder. *Journal of Personality and Social Psychology, 106*(1), 112–122.

Schultz, R. T. (2005). Developmental deficits in social perception in autism: The role of the amygdala and fusiform face area. *International Journal of Developmental Neuroscience, 23*(2), 125–141.

Schultz, R. T., Gauthier, I., Klin, A., Fulbright, R. K., Anderson, A. W., Volkmar, F., . . . Gore, J. C. (2000). Abnormal ventral temporal cortical activity during face discrimination among individuals with autism and Asperger syndrome. *Archives of General Psychiatry, 57*(4), 331–340.

Schultz, R. T., Grelotti, D. J., Klin, A., Kleinman, J., Van der Gaag, C., Marois, R., & Skudlarski, P. (2003). The role of the fusiform face area in social cognition: Implications for the pathobiology of autism. *Philosophical Transactions of the Royal Society of London: Series B. Biological Sciences, 358*(1430), 415–427.

Schulze, C., Grassmann, S., & Tomasello, M. (2013). 3-year-old children make relevance inferences in indirect verbal communication. *Child Development, 84*(6), 2079–2093.

Schwartz, C. B., Henderson, H. A., Inge, A. P., Zahka, N. E., Coman, D. C., Kojkowski, N. M., . . . Mundy, P. C. (2009). Temperament as a predictor of symptomotology and adaptive functioning in adolescents with high-functioning autism. *Journal of Autism and Developmental Disorders, 39*(6), 842–855.

Sebanz, N., Bekkering, H., & Knoblich, G. (2006). Joint action: Bodies and minds moving together. *Trends in Cognitive Sciences, 10*(2), 70–76.

Seibert, J. M., Hogan, A. E., & Mundy, P. C. (1982). Assessing interactional competencies: The Early Social-Communication Scales. *Infant Mental Health Journal, 3*, 244–258.

Senju, A. (2013). Atypical development of spontaneous social cognition in autism spectrum disorders. *Brain and Development, 35*(2), 96–101.

Senju, A., & Johnson, M. H. (2009). The eye contact effect: Mechanisms and development. *Trends in Cognitive Sciences, 13*(3), 127–134.

Senju, A., Johnson, M. H., & Csibra, G. (2006). The development and neural basis of referential gaze perception. *Social Neuroscience, 1*(3–4), 220–234.

Senju, A., Southgate, V., Snape, C., Leonard, M., & Csibra, G. (2011). Do 18-month-olds really attribute mental states to others?: A critical test. *Psychological Science, 22*(7), 878–880.

Shad, M. U., Brent, B. K., & Keshavan, M. S. (2011). Neurobiology of self-awareness deficits in schizophrenia: A hypothetical model. *Asian Journal of Psychiatry, 4*(4), 248–254.

Shattuck, P. T., Seltzer, M. M., Greenberg, J. S., Orsmond, G. I., Bolt, D., Kring, S., . . . Lord, C. (2007). Change in autism symptoms and maladaptive behaviors in adolescents and adults with an autism spectrum disorder. *Journal of Autism and Developmental Disorders, 37*(9), 1735–1747.

Sheinkopf, S., Mundy, P., Claussen, A., & Willoughby, J. (2004). Infant joint attention skill and preschool behavioral outcomes in at-risk children. *Development and Psychopathology, 16*, 273–293.

Sherer, M. R., & Schreibman, L. (2005). Individual behavioral profiles and predictors of treatment effectiveness for children with autism. *Journal of Consulting and Clinical Psychology, 73*(3), 525–538.

Shih, P., Shen, M., Öttl, B., Keehn, B., Gaffrey, M. S., & Müller, R. A. (2010). Atypical network connectivity for imitation in autism spectrum disorder. *Neuropsychologia, 48*(10), 2931–2939.

Shockley, K., Richardson, D. C., & Dale, R. (2009). Conversation and coordinative structures. *Topics in Cognitive Science, 1*(2), 305–319.

Shook, B. L., Schlag-Rey, M., & Schlag, J. (1991). Primate supplementary eye field: II. Comparative aspects of connections with the thalamus, corpus striatum, and related forebrain nuclei. *Journal of Comparative Neurology, 307*(4), 562–583.

Siever, L. J., & Davis, K. L. (2004). The pathophysiology of schizophrenia disorders: Perspectives from the spectrum. *American Journal of Psychiatry, 161*, 398–413.

Sigman, M., Cohen, S. E., & Beckwith, L. (1997). Why does infant attention predict adolescent intelligence? *Infant Behavior and Development, 20*(2), 133–140.

Sigman, M., & Kasari, C. (1995). Joint attention across contexts in normal and autistic children. In C. Moore & P. J. Dunham (Eds.), *Joint attention: Its origins and role in development* (pp. 189–203). Hillsdale, NJ: Erlbaum.

Sigman, M. D., Kasari, C., Kwon, J. H., & Yirmiya, N. (1992). Responses to the negative emotions of others by autistic, mentally retarded, and normal children. *Child Development, 63*(4), 796–807.

Sigman, M., & McGovern, C. (2005). Improvement in cognitive and language skills from preschool to adolescence in autism. *Journal of Autism and Developmental Disorders, 35*(1), 15–23.

Sigman, M., & Mundy, P. (1989). Social attachments in autistic children. *Journal of the American Academy of Child and Adolescent Psychiatry, 28*(1), 74–81.

Sigman, M., Mundy, P., Sherman, T., & Ungerer, J. (1986). Social interactions of autistic, mentally retarded, and normal children and their caregivers. *Journal of Child Psychology and Psychiatry, 27*, 647–656.

Sigman, M., Ruskin, E., Arbelle, S., Corona, R., Dissanayake, C., Espinosa, M., . . . Zierhut, C. (1999). Continuity and change in the social competence of children with autism, Down syndrome, and developmental delays. *Monographs of the Society for Research in Child Development, 64*(1, Serial No. 256), 1–114.

Sigman, M., & Ungerer, J. (1984). Attachment behaviors in autistic children. *Journal of Autism and Related Disabilities, 14*, 231–244.

Siller, M., & Sigman, M. (2002). The behaviors of parents of children with autism predict the subsequent development of their children's communication. *Journal of Autism and Developmental Disorders, 32*(2), 77–89.

Siller, M., & Sigman, M. (2008). Modeling longitudinal change in the language abilities of children with autism: Parent behaviors and child characteristics as predictors of change. *Developmental Psychology, 44*(6), 1691.

Simms, M. L., Kemper, T. L., Timbie, C. M., Bauman, M. L., & Blatt, G. J. (2009). The anterior cingulate cortex in autism: Heterogeneity of qualitative and quantitative cytoarchitectonic features suggests possible subgroups. *Acta Neuropathologica, 118*(5), 673–684.

Sinzig, J., Morsch, D., Bruning, N., Schmidt, M. H., & Lehmkuhl, G. (2008). Inhibition, flexibility, working memory and planning in autism spectrum disorders with and without comorbid ADHD-symptoms. *Child and Adolescent Psychiatry and Mental Health, 2*(1), 4.

Skarratt, P. A., Cole, G. G., & Kuhn, G. (2012). Visual cognition during real social interaction. *Frontiers in Human Neuroscience, 6*, 196.

Skinner, B. F. (1957). *Verbal behavior.* New York: Appleton-Century-Crofts.

Skuse, D. H., & Gallagher, L. (2009). Dopaminergic–neuropeptide interactions in the social brain. *Trends in Cognitive Sciences, 13*(1), 27–35.

Slessor, G., Phillips, L. H., & Bull, R. (2008). Age-related declines in basic social perception: Evidence from tasks assessing eye-gaze processing. *Psychology and Aging, 23*(4), 812–819.

Smith, L., & Thelen, E. (2003). Development as a dynamic system. *Trends in Cognitive Sciences, 7*, 343–348.

Smith, T., Eikeseth, S., Klevstrand, M., & Lovaas, O. I. (1997). Intensive behavioral treatment for preschoolers with severe mental retardation and pervasive developmental disorder. *American Journal on Mental Retardation, 102*(3), 238–249.

Smith, T., Groen, A. D., & Wynn, J. W. (2000). Randomized trial of intensive early intervention for children with pervasive developmental disorder. *American Journal on Mental Retardation, 105*(4), 269–285.

Smith, V., Mirenda, P., & Zaidman-Zait, A. (2007). Predictors of expressive vocabulary growth in children with autism. *Journal of Speech, Language, and Hearing Research, 50*, 149–160.

Soproni, K., Miklósi, Á., Topál, J., & Csányi, V. (2001). Comprehension of human communicative signs in pet dogs (*Canis familiaris*). *Journal of Comparative Psychology, 115*(2), 122–126.

Spencer, J. P., Clearfield, M., Corbetta, D., Ulrich, B., Buchanan, P., & Schöner, G. (2006). Moving toward a grand theory of development: In memory of Esther Thelen. *Child Development, 77*(6), 1521–1538.

Sperling, G., & Weichselgartner, E. (1995). Episodic theory of the dynamics of spatial attention. *Psychological Review, 102*, 503–532.

Spreng, R. N., & Grady, C. L. (2010). Patterns of brain activity supporting auto-biographical memory, prospection, and theory of mind, and their relationship to the default mode network. *Journal of Cognitive Neuroscience, 22*(6), 1112–1123.

Spreng, R. N., Sepulcre, J., Turner, G. R., Stevens, W. D., & Schacter, D. L. (2013). Intrinsic architecture underlying the relations among the default, dorsal attention, and frontoparietal control networks of the human brain. *Journal of Cognitive Neuroscience, 25*(1), 74–86.

Stagg, S. D., Davis, R., & Heaton, P. (2013). Associations between language development and skin conductance responses to faces and eye gaze in children with autism spectrum disorder. *Journal of Autism and Developmental Disorders, 43*(10), 2303–2311.

Staudte, M., Koller, A., Garoufi, K., & Crocker, M. W. (2012). Using listener gaze to augment speech generation in a virtual 3D environment. In N. Miyake, D. Peebles, & R. P. Cooper (Eds.), *Proceedings of the 34th Annual Meeting of the Cognitive Science Society* (pp. 1007–1012). Austin, TX: Cognitive Science Society. Retrieved from *http://mindmodeling.org/cogsci2012*

Stavropoulos, K. K., & Carver, L. J. (2013). Research review: Social motivation and oxytocin in autism–implications for joint attention development and intervention. *Journal of Child Psychology and Psychiatry, 54*(6), 603–618.

Steels, L. (2003). Evolving grounded communication for robots. *Trends in Cognitive Sciences, 7*(7), 308–312.

Stojanovick, V., Perkins, M., & Howard, S. (2006). Linguistic heterogeneity in Williams syndrome. *Clinical Linguistics and Phonetics, 20*(7–8), 547–552.

Stone, W., Coonrod, E., & Ousley, C., (1997). Brief report: Screening Tool for Autism in Two Year Olds (STAT): Development and preliminary data. *Journal of Autism and Developmental Disorders, 30*, 607–612.

Stone, W. L., Coonrod, E. E., Turner, L. M., & Pozdol, S. L. (2004). Psychometric properties of the STAT for early autism screening. *Journal of Autism and Developmental Disorders, 34*(6), 691–701.

Stone, W. L., McMahon, C. R., & Henderson, L. M. (2008). Use of the Screening Tool for Autism in Two-Year-Olds (STAT) for children under 24 months: An exploratory study. *Autism, 12*(5), 557–573.

Störmer, V. S., Passow, S., Biesenack, J., & Li, S. C. (2012). Dopaminergic and cholinergic modulations of visual–spatial attention and working memory: Insights from molecular genetic research and implications for adult cognitive development. *Developmental Psychology, 48*(3), 875–879.

Strain, P. S., Kerr, M. M., & Ragland, E. U. (1979). Effects of peer-mediated social initiations and prompting/reinforcement procedures on the social behavior of autistic children. *Journal of Autism and Developmental Disorders, 9*(1), 41–54.

Striano, T., Chen, X., Cleveland, A., & Bradshaw, S. (2006). Joint attention social cues influence infant learning. *European Journal of Developmental Psychology, 3*, 289–299.

Striano, T., Reid, V., & Hoel, S. (2006). Neural mechanisms of joint attention in infancy. *European Journal of Neuroscience, 23*, 2819–2823.

Striano, T., & Stahl, D. (2005). Sensitivity to triadic attention in early infancy. *Developmental Science, 8*(4), 333–343.

Striano, T., Stahl, D., Cleveland, A., & Hoehl, S. (2007). Sensitivity to triadic attention between 6 weeks and 3 months of age. *Infant Behavior and Development, 30*(3), 529–534.

Suda, S., Iwata, K., Shimmura, C., Kameno, Y., Anitha, A., Thanseem, I., . . . Mori, N. (2011). Decreased expression of axon-guidance receptors in the anterior cingulate cortex in autism. *Molecular Autism, 2*(1), 14.

Sullivan, M., Finelli, J., Marvin, A., Garrett-Mayer, E., Bauman, M., & Landa, R. (2007). Response to joint attention in toddlers at risk for autism spectrum disorder: A prospective study. *Journal of Autism and Developmental Disorders, 37*(1), 37–48.

Supekar, K., Uddin, L. Q., Khouzam, A., Phillips, J., Gaillard, W. D., Kenworthy, L. E., . . . Menon, V. (2013). Brain hyperconnectivity in children with autism and its links to social deficits. *Cell Reports, 5*(3), 738–747.

Sutton, S. K., Burnette, C. P., Mundy, P. C., Meyer, J., Vaughan, A., Sanders, C., & Yale, M. (2005). Resting cortical brain activity and social behavior in higher functioning children with autism. *Journal of Child Psychology and Psychiatry, 46*(2), 211–222.

Syal, S., & Finlay, B. L. (2011). Thinking outside the cortex: Social motivation in the evolution and development of language. *Developmental Science, 14*(2), 417–430.

Tager-Flusberg, H. (2014). Editorial: Promoting communicative speech in minimally verbal children with autism spectrum disorder. *Journal of the American Academy of Child and Adolescent Psychiatry, 53,* 612–613.

Tamietto, M., & de Gelder, B. (2010). Neural bases of the non-conscious perception of emotional signals. *Nature Reviews Neuroscience, 11*(10), 697–709.

Taylor, B. A., & Hoch, H. (2008). Teaching children with autism to respond to and initiate bids for joint attention. *Journal of Applied Behavior Analysis, 41*(3), 377–391.

Taylor, J. L., & Seltzer, M. M. (2010). Changes in the autism behavioral phenotype during the transition to adulthood. *Journal of Autism and Developmental Disorders, 40*(12), 1431–1446.

Thelen, E. (1989). The (re)discovery of motor development: Learning new things from an old field. *Developmental Psychology, 25*(6), 946–962.

Thomas, C., Avidan, G., Humphreys, K., Jung, K. J., Gao, F., & Behrmann, M. (2009). Reduced structural connectivity in ventral visual cortex in congenital prosopagnosia. *Nature Neuroscience, 12*(1), 29–31.

Thompson-Schill, S. L., Ramscar, M., & Chrysikou, E. G. (2009). Cognition without control: When a little frontal lobe goes a long way. *Current Directions in Psychological Science, 18*(5), 259–263.

Thurm, A., Lord, C., Lee, L., & Newschaffer, C. (2007). Predictors of language acquisition in preschool children with autism spectrum disorders. *Journal of Autism and Developmental Disorders, 37,* 1721–1734.

Tiegerman, E., & Primavera, L. H. (1984). Imitating the autistic child: Facilitating communicative gaze behavior. *Journal of Autism and Developmental Disorders, 14*(1), 27–38.

Tinbergen, E. A., & Tinbergen, N. (1972). *Early childhood autism: An ethological approach.* Berlin: Parey.

Tinbergen, N., & Tinbergen, E. A. (1983). *Autistic children: New hope for a cure.* London: Allen & Unwin.

Tomasello, M. (1988). The role of joint attentional processes in early language development. *Language Sciences, 10*(1), 69–88.

Tomasello, M. (2008). Why don't apes point? *Trends in Linguistics: Studies and Monographs, 197,* 375–394.

Tomasello, M., & Call, J. (1997). *Primate cognition.* Oxford, UK: Oxford University Press.

Tomasello, M., & Carpenter, M. (2007). Shared intentionality. *Developmental Science, 10*(1), 121–125.

Tomasello, M., Carpenter, M., Call, J., Behne, T., & Moll, H. (2005). Understanding sharing intentions: The origins of cultural cognition. *Behavioral and Brain Sciences, 28,* 675–691.

Tomasello, M., Carpenter, M., & Hobson, R. P. (2005). The emergence of social cognition in three young chimpanzees. *Monographs of the Society for Research in Child Development, 70*(1, Serial No. 179), 1–152.

Tomasello, M., & Farrar, M. J. (1986). Joint attention and early language. *Child Development, 57,* 1454–1463.

Tomasello, M., Hare, B., & Fogleman, T. (2001). The ontogeny of gaze following in chimpanzees, *Pan troglodytes,* and rhesus macaques, *Macaca mulatta. Animal Behaviour, 61*(2), 335–343.

Tomasello, M., Hare, B., Lehman, H., & Call, J. (2006). Reliance on head versus eyes in the gaze following of great apes and humans: The cooperative eyes hypothesis. *Journal of Human Evolution, 52,* 314–320.

Tomasello, M., & Todd, J. (1983). Joint attention and lexical acquisition style. *First Language, 4*(12), 197–211.

Tompa, P., & Fuxreiter, M. (2008). Fuzzy complexes: Polymorphism and structural disorder in protein–protein interactions. *Trends in Biochemical Sciences, 33*(1), 2–8.

Tost, H., Kolachana, B., Hakimi, S., Lemaitre, H., Verchinski, B. A., Mattay, V. S., . . . Meyer–Lindenberg, A. (2010). A common allele in the oxytocin receptor gene (OXTR) impacts prosocial temperament and human hypothalamic-limbic structure and function. *Proceedings of the National Academy of Sciences USA, 107*(31), 13936–13941.

Toth, K., Munson, J., Meltzoff, A., & Dawson, G. (2006). Early predictors of communication development in young children with autism spectrum disorders: Joint attention, imitation and toy play. *Journal of Autism and Developmental Disorders, 36,* 993–1005.

Townsend, J., Courchesne, E., Covington, J., Westerfield, M., Harris, N. S., Lyden P., . . . Press, G. (1999). Spatial attention deficits in patients with acquired or developmental cerebellar abnormality. *Journal of Neuroscience, 19,* 5632–5643.

Tremblay, H., & Rovira, K. (2007). Joint visual attention and social triangular engagement at 3 and 6 months. *Infant Behavior and Development, 30*(2), 366–379.

Trevarthen, C. (1979). Communication and cooperation in early infancy: A description of primary intersubjectivity. In M. Bullowa (Ed.), *Before speech:*

The beginning of interpersonal communication (pp. 321–347). New York: Cambridge University Press.

Trevarthen, C., & Hubley, P. (1978). Secondary intersubjectivity: Confidence, confiding and acts of meaning in the first year. In A. Lock (Ed.), *Action, gesture and symbol: The emergence of language* (pp. 183–229). New York: Academic Press.

Trezza, V., Damsteegt, R., Achterberg, E. M., & Vanderschuren, L. J. (2011). Nucleus accumbens μ-opioid receptors mediate social reward. *Journal of Neuroscience, 31*(17), 6362–6370.

Tribushinina, E. (2014). Comprehension of degree modifiers by preschool children: What does it mean to be 'a bit cold'? *Folia Linguistica, 48*, 255–276.

Tronick, E. (2005). Why is connection with others so critical?: The formation of dyadic states of consciousness and the expansion of individuals' states of consciousness: Coherence governed selection and the co-creation of meaning out of messy meaning making. In J. Nadel & D. Muir (Eds.), *Emotional development: Recent research advances* (pp. 293–315). New York: Oxford University Press.

Tsao, L. L., & Odom, S. L. (2006). Sibling-mediated social interaction intervention for young children with autism. *Topics in Early Childhood Special Education, 26*(2), 106–123.

Uddin, L. Q., & Menon, V. (2009). The anterior insula in autism: Under-connected and under-examined. *Neuroscience and Biobehavioral Reviews, 33*(8), 1198–1203.

Uekermann, J., Kraemer, M., Abdel-Hamid, M., Schimmelmann, B. G., Hebebrand, J., Daum, I., & Kis, B. (2010). Social cognition in attention-deficit hyperactivity disorder (ADHD). *Neuroscience and Biobehavioral Reviews, 34*(5), 734–743.

Ungerer, J., & Sigman, M. (1981). Symbolic play and language comprehension in autistic children. *Journal of the American Academy of Child Psychiatry, 20*(2), 318–337.

Uppal, N., Wicinski, B., Buxbaum, J. D., Heinsen, H., Schmitz, C., & Hof, P. R. (2014). Neuropathology of the anterior midcingulate cortex in young children with autism. *Journal of Neuropathology and Experimental Neurology, 73*(9), 891–902.

Vaidya, C. J., Foss-Feig, J., Shook, D., Kaplan, L., Kenworthy, L., & Gaillard, W. D. (2011). Controlling attention to gaze and arrows in childhood: An fMRI study of typical development and autism spectrum disorders. *Developmental Science, 14*(4), 911–924.

Vallender, E. J., Mekel-Bobrov, N., & Lahn, B. T. (2008). Genetic basis of human brain evolution. *Trends in Neurosciences, 31*(12), 637–644.

Van der Paelt, S., Warreyn, P., & Roeyers, H. (2014). Effect of community interventions on social-communicative abilities of preschoolers with autism spectrum disorder. *Research in Autism Spectrum Disorder, 8*, 518–528.

Vanderwert, R., & Nelson, C. (2014). The use of near-infrared spectroscopy in the study of typical and atypical development. *NeuroImage, 85*, 264–271.

Van Honk, J., & Schutter, D. (2006). From affective valence to motivational direction: The frontal asymmetry of emotion revised. *Psychological Science, 17*, 963–965.

Vaughan, A., Mundy, P., Block, J., Burnette, C., Delgado, C., Gomez, Y., . . . Pomares, Y. (2003). Child, caregiver, and temperament contributions to infant joint attention. *Infancy, 4*(4), 603–616.

Vaughan Van Hecke, A., Stevens, S., Carson, A. M., Karst, J. S., Dolan, B., Schohl, K., . . . Brockman, S. (2013). Measuring the plasticity of social approach: A randomized controlled trial of the effects of the PEERS intervention on EEG asymmetry in adolescents with autism spectrum disorders. *Journal of Autism and Developmental Disorders, 45*(2), 316–335.

Vaughan Van Hecke, A., Mundy, P. C., Acra, C. F., Block, J. J., Delgado, C. E., Parlade, M. V., . . . Pomares, Y. B. (2007). Infant joint attention, temperament, and social competence in preschool children. *Child Development, 78*(1), 53–69.

Vaughan Van Hecke, A., Mundy, P., Block, J. , Delgado, C., Parlade, M., Pomares, Y., & Hobson, J. (2012). Infant responding to joint attention, executive processes, and self-regulation in preschool children. *Infant Behavior and Development, 35*(2), 303–311.

Vaughan Van Hecke, A., Oswald, T., & Mundy, P. (2015). Joint attention and the social phenotype of autism spectrum disorder: A perspective from developmental psychopathology. In D. Cicchetti (Ed.), *Developmental psychopathology* (3rd ed., pp. 116–151). Hoboken, NJ: Wiley.

Venezia, M., Messinger, D., Thorp, D., & Mundy, P. (2004). Timing changes: The development of anticipatory smiling. *Infancy, 6*, 397–406.

Ventola, P., Kleinman, J., Pandey, J., Wilson, L., Esser, E., Boorstein, H., . . . Fein, D. (2007). Differentiating between autism spectrum disorders and other developmental disabilities in children who failed a screening instrument for ASD. *Journal of Autism and Developmental Disorders, 37*(3), 425–436.

Vismara, L. A., Colombi, C., & Rogers, S. J. (2009). Can one hour per week of therapy lead to lasting changes in young children with autism? *Autism, 13*(1), 93–115.

Vismara, L. A., & Lyons, G. L. (2007). Using perseverative interests to elicit joint attention behaviors in young children with autism: Theoretical and clinical implications for understanding motivation. *Journal of Positive Behavior Interventions, 9*(4), 214–228.

Vismara, L. A., & Rogers, S. J. (2008). The Early Start Denver Model: A case study of an innovative practice. *Journal of Early Intervention, 31*(1), 91–108.

Vivanti, G., & Dissanayake, C. (2014). Propensity to imitate in autism is not modulated by the model's gaze direction: An eye-tracking study. *Autism Research, 7*(3), 392–399.

Volkmar, F. R., Cohen, D. J., Bregman, J. D., Hooks, M. Y., & Stevenson, J. M. (1989). An examination of social typologies in autism. *Journal of the American Academy of Child and Adolescent Psychiatry, 28*, 82–86.

Von Der Heide, R. J., Skipper, L. M., Klobusicky, E., & Olson, I. R. (2013). Dissecting the uncinate fasciculus: Disorders, controversies and a hypothesis. *Brain, 136*(Pt. 6), 1692–1707.

Voos, A. C., Pelphrey, K. A., Tirrell, J., Bolling, D. Z., Vander Wyk, B., Kaiser, M. D., . . . Ventola, P. (2013). Neural mechanisms of improvements in social motivation after pivotal response treatment: Two case studies. *Journal of Autism and Developmental Disorders, 43*(1), 1–10.

Vygotsky, L. (1962). *Thought and language.* Cambridge, MA: MIT Press.

Wachs, T. D. (2000). *Necessary but not sufficient: The respective roles of single and multiple influences on individual development.* Washington, DC: American Psychological Association.

Wade, M., Hoffmann, T. J., Wigg, K., & Jenkins, J. M. (2014). Association between the oxytocin receptor (OXTR) gene and children's social cognition at 18 months. *Genes, Brain and Behavior, 13*(7), 603–610.

Wade, M., Moore, C., Astington, J. W., Frampton, K., & Jenkins, J. M. (2015). Cumulative contextual risk, maternal responsivity and social cognition at 18 months. *Developmental Psychopathology, 27*(1), 189–203.

Warneken, F., Chen, F., & Tomasello, M. (2006). Cooperative activities in young children and chimpanzees. *Child Development, 77*(3), 640–663.

Wass, S. (2011). Distortions and disconnections: disrupted brain connectivity in autism. *Brain and Cognition, 75*(1), 18–28.

Weng, S. J., Wiggins, J. L., Peltier, S. J., Carrasco, M., Risi, S., Lord, C., & Monk, C. S. (2010). Alterations of resting state functional connectivity in the default network in adolescents with autism spectrum disorders. *Brain Research, 1313*, 202–214.

Werner, H., & Kaplan, B. (1963). *Symbol formation.* New York: Wiley.

Wetherby, A., Allen, L., Cleary, J., Kublin, K., & Goldstein, H. (2002). Validity and reliability of the Communication and Symbolic Behavior Scales Developmental Profile with very young children. *Journal of Speech, Language, and Hearing Research, 45*(6), 1202–1218.

Wetherby, A., & Prizant, B. (2002). *Communication and Symbolic Behavior Scales: Developmental Profile.* Baltimore, MD: Brookes.

Wetherby, A., & Prutting, C. (1984). Profiles of communicative and cognitive-social abilities in autistic children. *Journal of Speech and Hearing Research, 27*, 367–377.

Whalen, C., & Schreibman, L. (2003). Joint attention training for children with autism using behavior modification procedures. *Journal of Child Psychology and Psychiatry, 44*(3), 456–468.

Whalen, C., Schreibman, L., & Ingersoll, B. (2006). The collateral effects of joint attention training on social initiations, positive affect, imitation, and spontaneous speech for young children with autism. *Journal of Autism and Developmental Disorders, 36*, 655–664.

White, P. J., O'Reilly, M., Streusand, W., Levine, A., Sigafoos, J., Lancioni, G., . . . Aguilar, J. (2011). Best practices for teaching joint attention: A systematic review of the intervention literature. *Research in Autism Spectrum Disorders, 5*(4), 1283–1295.

Wicker, B., Fonlupt, P., Hubert, B., Tardif, C., Gepner, B., & Deruelle, C. (2008). Abnormal cerebral effective connectivity during explicit emotional processing in adults with autism spectrum disorder. *Social Cognitive and Affective Neuroscience, 3*(2), 135–143.

Wicker, B., Ruby, P., Royet, J. P., & Fonlupt, P. (2003). A relation between rest and the self in the brain? *Brain Research Reviews, 43*(2), 224–230.

Wilkowski, B. M., Robinson, M. D., & Friesen, C. K. (2009). Gaze-triggered orienting as a tool of the belongingness self-regulation system. *Psychological Science, 20*(4), 495–501.

Williams, J. (2008). Self–other relations in social development and autism: Multiple roles for mirror neurons and other brain bases. *Autism Research, 1,* 73–90.

Williams, J. H., Waiter, G. D., Perra, O., Perrett, D. I., & Whiten, A. (2005). An fMRI study of joint attention experience. *NeuroImage, 25*(1), 133–140.

Wilson, E. O. (1975). *Sociobiology: The new synthesis.* Cambridge, MA: Belknap Press of Harvard University Press.

Wimmer, H., & Perner, J. (1983). Beliefs about beliefs: Representation and constraining function of wrong beliefs in young children's understanding of deception. *Cognition, 13*(1), 103–128.

Wing, L., & Gould, J. (1979). Severe impairments of social interaction and associated abnormalities in children: Epidemiology and classification. *Journal of Autism and Developmental Disorders, 9,* 11–29.

Wing, L., Gould, J., & Gillberg, C. (2011). Autism spectrum disorders in the DSM-V: Better or worse than the DSM-IV? *Research in Developmental Disabilities, 32*(2), 768–773.

Wing, L., Gould, J., Yeates, S. R., & Brierly, L. M. (1977). Symbolic play in severely mentally retarded and in autistic children. *Journal of Child Psychology and Psychiatry, 18*(2), 167–178.

Wing, L., & Potter, D. (2002). The epidemiology of autistic spectrum disorders: Is the prevalence rising? *Mental Retardation and Developmental Disabilities Research, 8,* 151–161.

Wing, L., & Ricks, D. (1977). The aetiology of childhood autism: A criticism of the Tinbergens' ethological theory. *Psychological Medicine, 6,* 533–543.

Witkin, H. A., Moore, C. A., Goodenough, D. R., & Cox, P. W. (1977) Field-dependent and field-independent cognitive styles and their educational implications. *Review of Educational Research, 69,* 1–64.

Wolf, I., Dziobek, I., & Heekeren, H. R. (2010). Neural correlates of social cognition in naturalistic settings: A model-free analysis approach. *NeuroImage, 49*(1), 894–904.

Wolff, J. J., Bodfish, J. W., Hazlett, H. C., Lightbody, A. A., Reiss, A. L., & Piven, J. (2012). Evidence of a distinct behavioral phenotype in young boys with fragile X syndrome and autism. *Journal of the American Academy of Child and Adolescent Psychiatry, 51*(12), 1324–1332.

Wong, C., & Kasari, C. (2012). Play and joint attention of children with autism in the preschool special education classroom. *Journal of Autism and Developmental Disorders, 42*(10), 2152–2161.

Wong, C. S., Kasari, C., Freeman, S., & Paparella, T. (2007). The acquisition and generalization of joint attention and symbolic play skills in young children with autism. *Research and Practice for Persons with Severe Disabilities, 32*(2), 101–109.

Wong, P. C., Morgan-Short, K., Ettlinger, M., & Zheng, J. (2012). Linking neurogenetics and individual differences in language learning: The dopamine hypothesis. *Cortex, 48*(9), 1091–1102.

Woodward, A. L. (2003). Infants' developing understanding of the link between looker and object. *Developmental Science, 6*(3), 297–311.

World Health Organization. (1977). *Manual of the international statistical classification of diseases, injuries and causes of death* (9th rev.). Geneva, Switzerland: Author.

Wu, N., & Su, Y. (2015). Oxytocin receptor gene relates to theory of mind and prosocial behavior in children. *Journal of Cognition and Development, 16*(2), 302–313.

Wu, R., Gopnik, A., Richardson, D. C., & Kirkham, N. Z. (2010). Social cues support learning about objects from statistics in infancy. In S. Ohlsson & R. Catrambone (Eds.), *Proceedings of the 32nd Annual Meeting of the Cognitive Science Society* (pp. 1228–1233). Austin, TX: Cognitive Science Society. Retrieved from *http://mindmodeling.org/cogsci2010*.

Wu, R., & Kirkham, N. Z. (2010). No two cues are alike: Depth of learning during infancy is dependent on what orients attention. *Journal of Experimental Child Psychology, 107*(2), 118–136.

Wu, Z., Pan, J., Su, Y., & Gros-Louis, J. (2013). How joint attention relates to cooperation in 1- and 2-year-olds. *International Journal of Behavioral Development, 37*(6), 542–548.

Xiao, Z., Qiu, T., Ke, X., Xiao, X., Xiao, T., Liang, F., . . . Liu, Y. (2014). Autism spectrum disorder as early neurodevelopmental disorder: Evidence from the brain imaging abnormalities in 2–3 years old toddlers. *Journal of Autism and Developmental Disorders, 44*(7), 1633–1640.

Yates, D. (2011). Neuroanatomy: Mapping neural function alongside connectivity. *Nature Reviews Neuroscience, 12*(5), 245–245.

Yawata, S., Yamaguchi, T., Danjo, T., Hikida, T., & Nakanishi, S. (2012). Pathway-specific control of reward learning and its flexibility via selective dopamine receptors in the nucleus accumbens. *Proceedings of the National Academy of Sciences USA, 109*(31), 12764–12769.

Yoder, P., & Stone, W. (2006). Randomized comparison of two communication interventions for preschoolers with autism spectrum disorders. *Journal of Consulting and Clinical Psychology, 74*, 426–435.

Yoder, P., Stone, W. L., Walden, T., & Malesa, E. (2009). Predicting social impairment and ASD diagnosis in younger siblings of children with autism spectrum disorder. *Journal of Autism and Developmental Disorders, 39*(10), 1381–1391.

Young, G. S., Merin, N., Rogers, S. J., & Ozonoff, S. (2009). Gaze behavior and affect at 6 months: Predicting clinical outcomes and language development in typically developing infants and infants at risk for autism. *Developmental Science, 12*(5), 798–814.

Young, M., Neggers, B., Zandbelt, B., & Schall, J. (2014). Comparative connectivity of frontal eye field and striatum between humans and macaques. *Journal of Vision, 14*(10), 1217–1217.

Yuen, R., Thiruvahindrapuram, B., Merico, D., Walker, S. Tammimies, K. . . .

Scherer, S. (2015). Whole-genome sequencing of quartet families with autism spectrum disorder. *Nature Medicine, 21*(2), 185–191.

Zelazo, P. D., Qu, L., Müller, U., & Schneider, W. (2005). Hot and cool aspects of executive function: Relations in early development. In W. Schneider, R. Schumann-Lengsteler, & B. Sodian (Eds.), *Young children's cognitive development: Interrelationships among executive functioning, working memory, verbal ability, and theory of mind* (pp. 71–93). Hove, UK: Psychology Press.

Zercher, C., Hunt, P., Schuler, A., & Webster, J. (2001). Increasing joint attention, play and language through peer supported play. *Autism, 5*(4), 374–398.

Zwaigenbaum, L., Bryson, S., Rogers, T., Roberts, W., Brian, J., & Szatmari, P. (2005). Behavioral manifestations of autism in the first year of life. *International Journal of Neuroscience, 23*, 143–152.

Index

Note: f following a page number indicates a figure; *t* indicates a table.

336